ACCLAIM FOR
meals that heal – ᴏ

MW00576514

"It's one thing to understand chronic inflammation and how your eating habits can prevent, reduce, or eliminate it, but putting that knowledge into action in the kitchen is another. Thankfully, with *Meals That Heal – One Pot*, Carolyn has you covered. In clear, easy-to-understand language, she breaks down the topic of inflammation to help you discover your best path forward. And, perhaps most importantly, she eliminates the stumbling block of how to make healthy eating actually happen in your kitchen—with your busy schedule. As a busy mom herself, Carolyn has made sure to fill this book with recipes that your whole family will love and that you'll be proud to serve."

—**ANN TAYLOR PITTMAN,** James Beard Award–winning food writer, former executive editor at *Cooking Light*, and author of *The New Way to Cook Light* and *Everyday Whole Grains*

"*Meals That Heal – One Pot* is an excellent guide to understanding the whats, whys, and hows of chronic inflammation, but it doesn't stop there. Importantly, it also gives you the tools to help you keep inflammation in check and prevent disease by eating better, with lots of quick, tasty, and customizable recipes. I highly recommend this excellent book."

—**ELLIE KRIEGER, RDN,** Food Network and PBS cooking show host, *Washington Post* contributor, and best-selling cookbook author

"Carolyn's recipes and expertise, as illustrated throughout this book, demonstrate perfectly how food should not only taste great, but should also make you feel just as great inside."

—**NICOLE MCLAUGHLIN,** chef, culinary video producer, and host of Allrecipes's *You Can Cook That*

"Preparing meals at home is one of the most reliable ways to benefit from food as medicine, but the inconvenience of cooking, and cleaning up after, gets in the way. In this terrific book, Carolyn Williams empowers us all with a bounty of convenient, no-muss, no-fuss options for great food and great nutrition."

—**DR. DAVID L. KATZ,** founder and CEO of DietID, Inc., and the True Health Initiative, former president of the American College of Lifestyle Medicine, and coauthor of *What to Eat* with Mark Bittman

"Any cookbook that includes vibrant, appealing recipes that are also healthy *and* made in one pot is like a unicorn: exceedingly rare and worth celebrating! I'm already inspired by Carolyn's actionable suggestions on how to jump start healthier eating, and my meal plan for the week has practically made itself thanks to recipes like the Southwestern Caesar Salad, Beef Bulgogi Skillet, and Sheet Pan Jambalaya. Yum!"

—**JENNA HELWIG,** food director at *Real Simple* and author of *Bare Minimum Dinners*

"It's not every day that the food you eat can help you be healthier with each bite — but that's exactly what the meals in *Meals That Heal – One Pot* do. Carolyn turns science and research into delicious meals that you want to eat again and again. She also breaks down the daunting task of understanding why inflammation happens and what you can do to stop it. That's a win-win!"

—**KIMBERLY HOLLAND,** senior digital food editor at *Southern Living* and author of *Collagen Handbook*

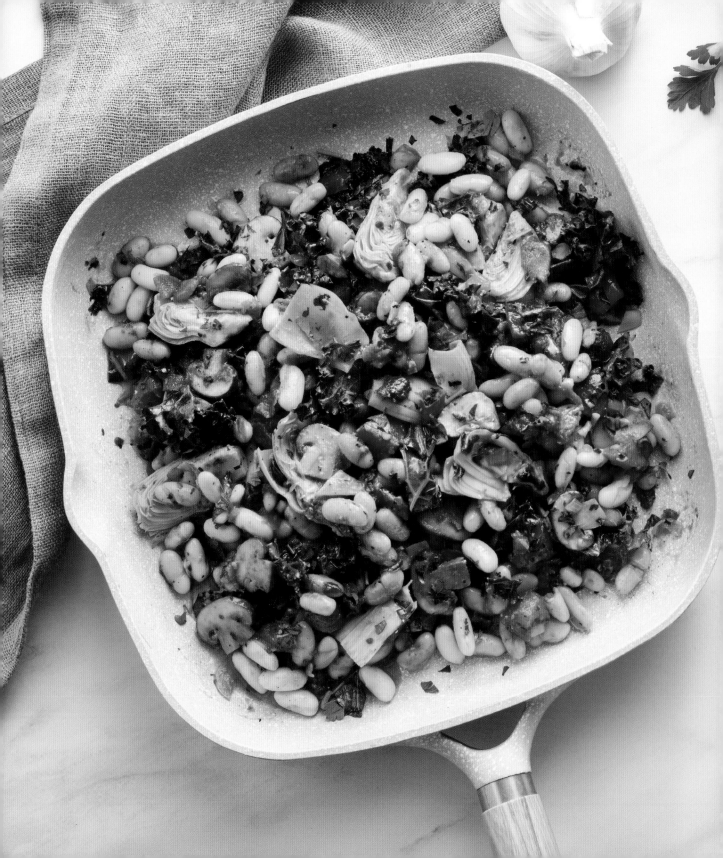

meals
that
heal
one p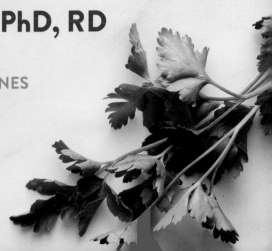t

100+ Recipes for Your Stovetop, Sheet Pan, Instant Pot, and Air Fryer

REDUCE INFLAMMATION FOR WHOLE-BODY HEALTH

CAROLYN WILLIAMS, PhD, RD

PHOTOGRAPHY BY ANNA JONES
Food styling by Melissa Mileto

THE EXPERIMENT
NEW YORK

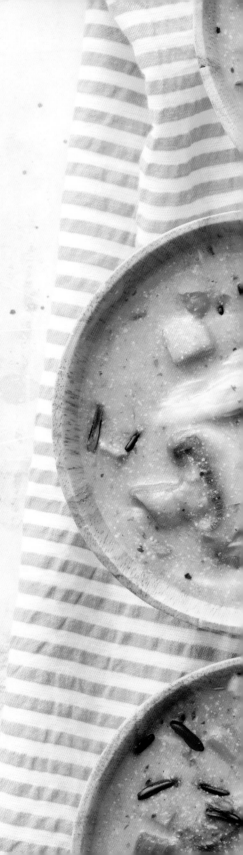

MEALS THAT HEAL – ONE POT: *100+ Recipes for Your Stovetop, Sheet Pan, Instant Pot, and Air Fryer—Reduce Inflammation for Whole-Body Health*
Text copyright © 2022 by Carolyn Williams
Photographs copyright © 2022 by Anna Jones
Photographs on pages 16, 20, 22, 27, 32, 33, 43, 45, 48, 52, 60, 75, 78, 79, 84, and 184 copyright © Adobe Stock

The Experiment, LLC
220 East 23rd Street, Suite 600
New York, NY 10010-4658
theexperimentpublishing.com

This book contains the opinions and ideas of its author. It is intended to provide helpful and informative material on the subjects addressed in the book. It is sold with the understanding that the author and publisher are not engaged in rendering medical, health, or any other kind of personal professional services in the book. The author and publisher specifically disclaim all responsibility for any liability, loss, or risk—personal or otherwise—that is incurred as a consequence, directly or indirectly, of the use and application of any of the contents of this book.

THE EXPERIMENT and its colophon are registered trademarks of The Experiment, LLC. Many of the designations used by manufacturers and sellers to distinguish their products are claimed as trademarks. Where those designations appear in this book and The Experiment was aware of a trademark claim, the designations have been capitalized.

The Experiment's books are available at special discounts when purchased in bulk for premiums and sales promotions as well as for fundraising or educational use. For details, contact us at info@theexperimentpublishing.com.

Library of Congress Cataloging-in-Publication Data available upon request

ISBN 978-1-61519-822-1
Ebook ISBN 978-1-61519-823-8

Cover and text design by Beth Bugler
Additional text design by Stacy Wakefield Forte
Author photograph by Jeana Rutledge

Manufactured in China

First printing September 2022
10 9 8 7 6 5 4 3 2 1

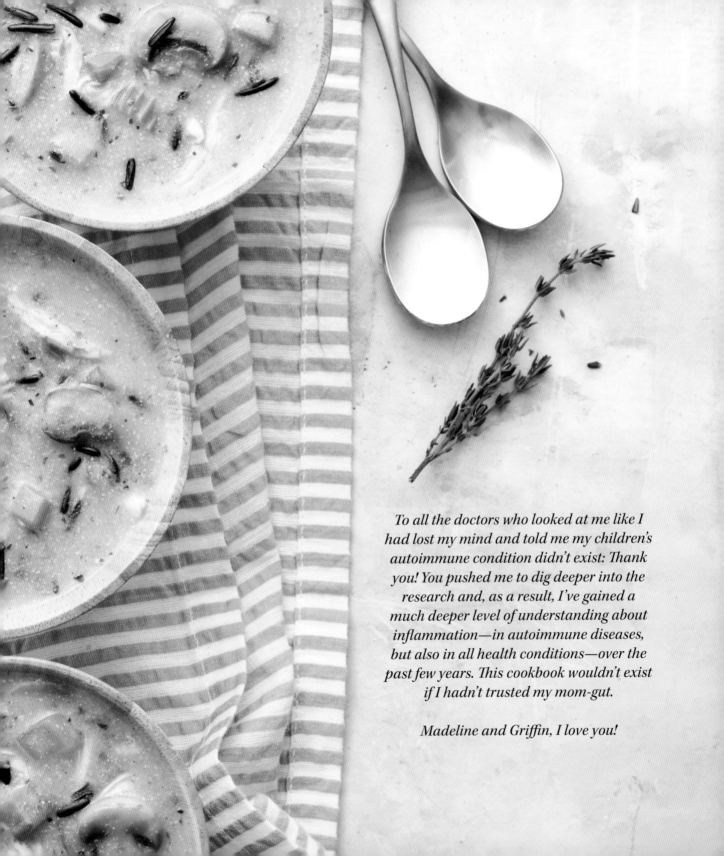

To all the doctors who looked at me like I had lost my mind and told me my children's autoimmune condition didn't exist: Thank you! You pushed me to dig deeper into the research and, as a result, I've gained a much deeper level of understanding about inflammation—in autoimmune diseases, but also in all health conditions—over the past few years. This cookbook wouldn't exist if I hadn't trusted my mom-gut.

Madeline and Griffin, I love you!

contents

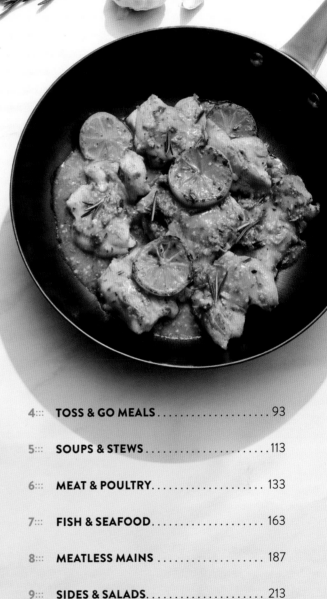

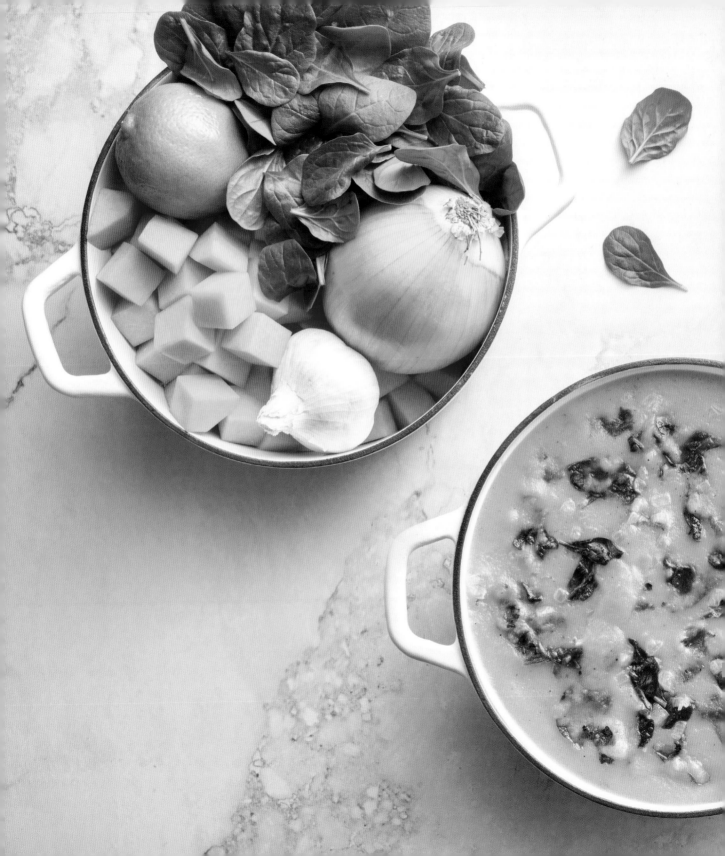

preface

WHY DIDN'T I DISCOVER ONE-POT MEALS SOONER?

ONE-POT, ONE-DISH, and one–sheet pan meals really are the epitome of quick and easy cooking. In fact, I'm not sure why I didn't write a cookbook about them sooner!

With "one-pot" meals, you've essentially got all you need in one pot, dish, or pan. The entrée recipes in this book all offer adequate to substantial protein, vegetables, healthy fats, and sometimes complex carbs to keep you nourished and satisfied. Anything additional that's needed or recommended for serving is super simple, like a frozen veggie or ready-to-heat grain. If you want to add a little more to your plate, turn to the Sides & Salads (page 213) and Snacks, Treats & Drinks (page 245) chapters.

the benefits of one-pot meals

- **SIMPLICITY IN PREP:** These recipes simplify meals by combining your protein, veggies, healthy fats, and sometimes complex carbs in one dish or pot. After a long day, this kind of cooking seems more doable and less overwhelming than preparing a protein and sides separately.

- **LESS TIME AND CLEANUP:** Fewer things to prep and cook shaves down kitchen time and leaves you with fewer pots in the sink. Hands-on prep time is 15 minutes or less. While you may still need to be nearby for a quick stir or to listen for a timer during cooking, the short prep times mean you can multitask while cooking.

- **ENHANCED FLAVOR:** When creating these recipes, I discovered that many had a ton of flavor naturally, due to the ingredients cooking all in one pot. This didn't stop me from pumping up the flavor with additional spices, herbs, salt, and pepper, but I did find that many didn't need quite as much seasoning as an entrée and sides that didn't cook together.

Can you tell how excited I am about all the helpful information and recipes jam-packed into this cookbook? I can't wait to share it with you!

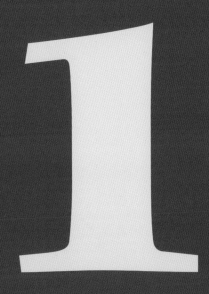

1

:·:·:·:·:·:·:·:·:·:·:·:

INFLAMMATION:
*the good, the bad
& how it affects you*

Did you know that you likely have some level of inflammation right now, regardless of health status or age?

Things like allergies, high blood pressure, wrinkles, or finding yourself slowly gaining weight are all early signs of inflammation, and ongoing inflammation can lead to conditions like diabetes, heart disease, autoimmune diseases, or cancer. Have no fear, though, because this book is here to help!

what is inflammation?

Most people are surprised to learn these two things about inflammation:

1 Inflammation isn't a diagnosed disease or condition. Rather, it's more like a fire in the body, one that starts small and contained but can easily be provoked and spread, increasing your susceptibility to chronic conditions.

2 Not all inflammation is bad. There are two types, one of which keeps you healthy!

Here's an overview of inflammation and how it impacts your health.

"good" or acute inflammation

Inflammation is a natural immune system response designed to keep the body healthy. In fact, we need short-term or **acute inflammation** for survival to fight off foreign bodies and heal the body. Foreign invaders include pathogens (harmful microbes), such as bacteria and viruses; physical objects, like splinters; and compounds, like chemicals and toxins. Collectively, these foreign invaders are referred to as antigens.

When the immune system detects an antigen, it triggers an inflammatory response, sending white blood cells to the area under attack and secreting inflammatory compounds known as cytokines. What follows is a mounted attack by the white blood cells and cytokines to get rid of the antigen or, in the case of an injury, stop additional tissue damage and assist in blood clotting. Like a real battle, there's some collateral damage, but macrophages, a type of white blood cell, tend to the damage and remove debris once the situation is under control. Noticeable signs of this include swelling, pain, redness, fever, or pus, which flare up quickly but go away as the attack and inflammatory response subsides.

This acute response is known as innate immunity, and it is the body's broad, first line of defense. When the innate response needs additional help, the body's

KEY TERMS

PATHOGEN
a harmful microbe like a bacteria, virus, parasite, or fungus

CYTOKINES
inflammatory compounds secreted by white blood cells

ADAPTIVE IMMUNITY
the body's more specific, second line of defense

ANTIGEN
pathogen or substance that the body perceives as a foreign invader or threat

INNATE IMMUNITY
the body's first line of defense that is general and nonspecific

ANTIBODIES
proteins designed to identify and attack a specific antigen

adaptive immune response (a much more targeted defense against the specific antigen attacking the body) steps up and rallies white blood cells known as B cells and T cells. B cells produce antibodies (proteins designed to identify and attack a specific antigen), and T cells attack antigens directly and release additional cytokines. Another inflammatory battle ensues, like the innate defense but more complex, to rid the body of the antigen. Sometimes antibiotics or other treatments may be needed to help the healing process along, but the overall response is acute and slowly dissipates.

The key to "good" inflammation is that it's acute; the inflammatory response goes away once the antigen is destroyed. This is crucial for overall health for two primary reasons:

1. After the acute inflammation goes away, the immune system can take a quick "breather" and rest, which is necessary to maintain immune system health. This brief downtime is what allows the immune system to function effectively and at full capacity in the future.

2. During these battles, friendly fire from the immune system's artillery (white blood cells or higher levels of circulating cytokines) harms a few healthy bystander cells. Since the acute inflammatory response is brief or acute though, the injuries are minor, especially in terms of overall health. However, the damage to healthy cells accumulates if the response continues, which is why long-term inflammation is so harmful.

"bad" or chronic inflammation

Chronic inflammation occurs when an inflammatory response is triggered, and it doesn't resolve or go away. Instead, it sticks around. The problem with chronic inflammation is the ongoing inflammatory response slowly wears down the immune system, causing it to be less effective in fighting off antigens that we encounter daily (such as the pathogens that cause the common cold or flu).

It also becomes dysregulated and hyperreactive to environmental and lifestyle factors. These are things like toxins in our food and water supply, inflammatory foods, a lack of adequate sleep, a sedentary lifestyle, and unmanaged or ongoing stress, all of which are addressed later in this chapter.

Sometimes chronic inflammation happens when an antigen is resistant to attacks by antibodies and antibiotics. This is the case with some bacteria and viruses. However, most chronic inflammation today is due to a combination of environmental exposures and lifestyle factors (See **Environmental and Lifestyle Causes of Chronic Inflammation**). A dysregulated, hypersensitive immune system can perceive these factors as antigens or irritants that elicit, aggravate, and escalate the existing inflammatory response. And because they are such constants, they establish a low level of chronic inflammation that sticks around until lifestyle changes are made.

Regular intake of inflammatory foods

A lack of anti-inflammatory foods

Toxins in our food, water supply, and environment

Allergies and sensitivities

Routinely high intakes of calories, carbohydrates, sodium, or alcohol

ENVIRONMENTAL AND LIFESTYLE CAUSES OF CHRONIC INFLAMMATION

Being overweight, obese, or having excess belly fat

A lack of regular physical activity

Sitting most of the day

Ongoing or frequent stress in any form

Lack of adequate, good-quality sleep

While none of this is good, the bigger issue is that the immune system isn't separate or siloed from the rest of the body. Both the nervous and endocrine systems are intricately connected to the immune system, as each system relies on interactions with the other two to maintain homeostasis. Chronic inflammation is a type of immune dysregulation, so as it develops, it leads to altered responses from the nervous and endocrine systems, which then begins to create a snowball of inflammatory effects that cause cell and tissue damage. Immune dysregulation, coupled with environmental toxins and lifestyle irritants, promotes gene expression. This refers to the activation of certain genetic variants that can also cause cell damage and "turn on" genes that you may have a predisposition for, such as autoimmune conditions (see page 26 for more information on gene expression).

Ongoing inflammation causes the immune system to become dysregulated and hyperreactive, which in turn disrupts nervous system activation and signaling and hormone regulation.

An inflammatory cascade of effects is set in motion due to dysregulation occurring in and among all three systems (immune, nervous, and endocrine) and gene expression.

Tissue damage results, compounding dysregulation and inflammation. Signs are often evident (excess body fat and/or high blood pressure, triglycerides, and blood glucose) but others (like mutated precancerous cells and autoimmunity) may not be.

All combined, these inflammatory effects pave the way for disease onset. In fact, inflammation plays a role in the development, progression, or underlying etiology for top health conditions affecting Americans today, such as hypertension, high cholesterol, obesity, insulin resistance, and depression. It also plays a role in most of the leading causes of death in the world, including heart disease, stroke, type 2 diabetes, cancer, Alzheimer's, and chronic lung and kidney diseases.

Signs worsen to meet diagnostic criteria for conditions such as diabetes, heart disease, thyroid and adrenal dysfunction, reproductive issues, joint deterioration, cancer, and autoimmune disorders.

Inflammation is hard to avoid, but the good news is that small changes to daily habits reduce ongoing inflammation, and it's never too late to start. What's even better is that upgrading and changing the foods you eat is one of the quickest, most impactful ways to do this!

reducing chronic inflammation

☑ Improves and maintains physical and mental health

☑ Decreases susceptibility to everyday illnesses like colds and infections

☑ Slows the aging process

☑ Stops the progression of many chronic diseases and eases symptoms

☑ Reduces risk and prevents the onset of chronic diseases

☑ Aids in management of autoimmune conditions and flare-ups

☑ Prevents additional cell and tissue damage

☑ Allows for hormonal balance

how do you know if you have chronic inflammation?

Most American adults have some level of ongoing inflammation in their bodies, which fluctuates based on health habits and life events. The inflammation may be tiny and contained, with signs that only pop up during stressful periods, or it may be bigger, with signs and symptoms that are easier to identify. If nothing is done, these small inflammatory fires can start new fires in other parts of the body. As this happens, symptoms and signs become more overt and measurable. These small fires begin to feed off each other, slowly progressing to systemic inflammation and finally resulting in diabetes, heart disease, dementia, and other inflammatory conditions.

Now, here's the good news: Low levels of chronic inflammation can usually be resolved with small lifestyle changes, and the earlier you act, the easier this can be. Identifying and addressing the cause of these warning signs and indicators is what prevents inflammation from progressing, so use the **Early Warning Signs and Early Indicators of Chronic Inflammation** to help you identify inflammation. Then, use the recommendations in chapter 2 to help you reduce and prevent it.

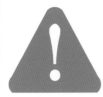

EARLY WARNING SIGNS

Think of these signs and symptoms as "check engine" lights for your body. They don't necessarily mean that you have chronic inflammation. However, they are associated with an inflammatory response that could be associated with existing chronic or acute inflammation, which could progress to being chronic.

MENTAL HEALTH SIGNS	PHYSICAL SIGNS	MEASURABLE SIGNS
☐ Decreased motivation, ability to concentrate, or forgetfulness ☐ Depression, anxiety, or decreased enjoyment in life ☐ Irritability and mood swings	☐ Acid reflux ☐ Being overweight or carrying excessive body fat, particularly in the abdominal area ☐ Constipation, bloating, gas, or other changes to digestive and bathroom habits ☐ Eye puffiness or constant dark circles ☐ Feeling "tired and wired" at the same time ☐ Feeling tired when you wake up in the morning ☐ Frequent hangry episodes and blood sugar imbalances ☐ Insomnia ☐ Increased "need" or cravings for carbs, sugar, salt, or caffeine ☐ Increased susceptibility to things like colds, UTIs, and sinus and yeast infections ☐ Low sex drive ☐ Regular headaches ☐ Sleepiness, hives, or itching after eating ☐ Stiffness, aches, or joint pain ☐ Weight gain or inability to lose weight	☐ Elevated blood pressure: ≥130 mm Hg on the top (systolic) and/or ≥85 mm Hg on the bottom (diastolic) ☐ Elevated fasting blood glucose (≥100 mg/dL) or elevated hemoglobin A1c (>5.7%) ☐ Elevated LDL cholesterol: ≥100 mg/dL ☐ Elevated triglycerides: ≥150 mg/dL ☐ Needing to take medication for the management of any of the above

why hasn't my doctor mentioned chronic inflammation?

Inflammation's connection to health disparities and disease onset is clear and well-established in medical research, yet many health care professionals never bring up inflammation or the impact that reducing it could have on a patient's health. Why is this? The problem seems to lie in the translation of this research to conventional medical training and treatment.

Conventional or Western medicine is focused on treating symptoms and diseases using evidence-based findings. This allows it to be targeted, focused, and have defined protocols and treatments, and it's ideal when treating one specific issue or body part. The downside is that health care providers aren't trained to look at symptoms from a whole-body perspective to identify underlying causes. They're also rarely trained to think outside established diagnostic criteria and protocols and are sometimes even discouraged to do so. Furthermore, health factors that don't have a defined treatment protocol and whose treatments need to be individualized (like mental wellbeing and past trauma) are rarely even addressed.

Instead, the focus is on symptom management, using a black-and-white approach (caused by typical medical training as well as insurance companies). This is fine when you're talking about a health issue like a broken bone or pregnancy, and there are very clear options for diagnosis: broken or not broken; pregnant or not pregnant. But this isn't an appropriate approach for most health issues and doesn't allow providers to consider the whole body in the diagnosis and treatment. Currently, the tendency is to say "you're fine" if a test result doesn't meet the clinically defined threshold, even if the results are high or concerning.

Your doctor also may not have mentioned chronic inflammation because there isn't a clear-cut diagnostic test for it. A few lab tests aid in identifying it, and there are health care providers that combine conventional medicine with a whole-body approach. This isn't limited to a certain type of provider, so it's best to explore options among practitioners who take a whole-body approach but also incorporate evidence-based practice.

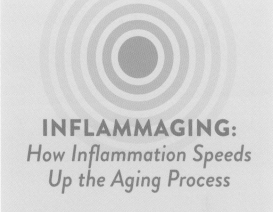

INFLAMMAGING:
How Inflammation Speeds Up the Aging Process

Acute inflammation is a natural part of our skin's aging process, but low-grade inflammation can amplify the rate at which our appearance ages. In fact, chronic inflammation and stress are associated with reduced skin elasticity, an increase in wrinkles, and a perceived older age based on physical appearance. UV rays and past skin damage are major contributors to skin's aging, but factors that contribute to low-grade inflammation, like diet, stress, and gut health, are now considered key contributors to the rate at which visible signs of aging occur. This means that adopting an anti-inflammatory diet is good for the body both inside and out!

my 4-step anti-inflammatory eating approach

No one food or nutrient can solve all of your inflammation issues. Inflammation looks different for every person—the location and causes, as well as genetics and lifestyle factors. However, research clearly points to four components of diet and lifestyle that are essential for reducing inflammation and preventing future inflammation:

STEP #1
Increase Anti-Inflammatory Foods

STEP #2
Decrease Dietary Inflamers

STEP #3
Nourish Your Gut

STEP #4
Reduce Stressors and Lifestyle Irritants

step #1
increase anti-inflammatory foods

This first step is key, but it's not always where people expect me to tell them to start. Diet culture has trained many of us to feel that eliminating foods is the first step. This approach tends to encourage an all-or-nothing mindset, which isn't helpful for long-term changes. And when it comes to inflammation, cutting food out—at least initially—shouldn't be your first priority. Instead, focus on incorporating more anti-inflammatory foods on a daily basis.

There's so much potential healing power in certain foods and nutrients, and most people are consuming them way below the recommended amounts. Anti-inflammatory eating isn't about restriction or following a diet. Rather, it's an eating approach where you emphasize anti-inflammatory foods and decrease dietary inflamers. Eating a diet of predominantly anti-inflammatory foods gives you the freedom to then enjoy an occasional less healthy one.

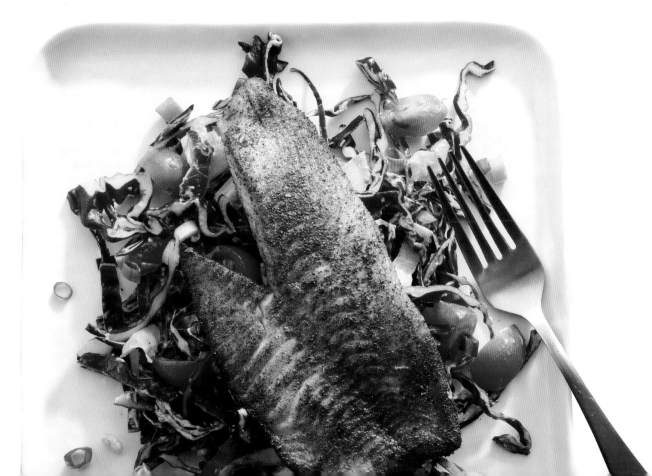

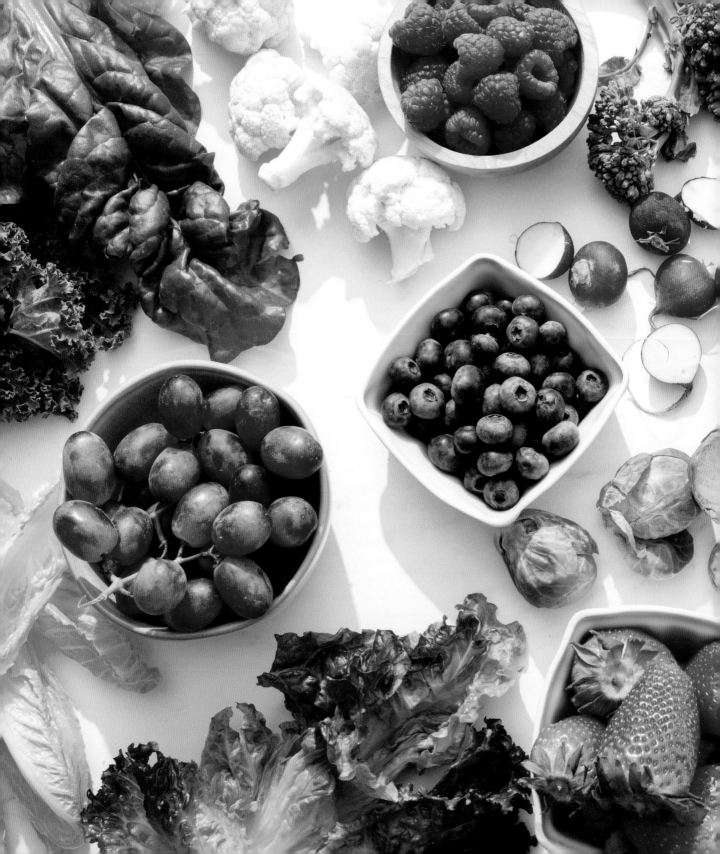

my top 3 anti-inflammatory food groups

The data and findings are overwhelmingly strong when it comes to the power of these food groups to tamp down and stop inflammation. Incorporating more of these three foods is the first place to start when adopting an anti-inflammatory eating approach.

	LEAFY GREENS	CRUCIFEROUS VEGETABLES	RED-PURPLE FRUITS
Examples	Cruciferous greens Dandelion greens Lettuces (such as green leaf, red leaf, radicchio, and romaine) Spinach Swiss chard	Arugula Broccoli Brussels sprouts Cabbage* (all types, including bok choy) Cauliflower Collard and mustard greens* Horseradish Kale* Kohlrabi Radish Rutabaga Turnips Wasabi Watercress*	Blackberries Blueberries Boysenberries Cherries Cranberries Grapes Strawberries Raspberries
Anti-Inflammatory Component(s)	Carotenoids (beta-carotene, lutein, and zeaxanthin) Lipoic acid Vitamin C	Glucosinolates (indoles and isothiocyanates) Lignans Lipoic acid Vitamin C	Anthocyanins Lignans Resveratrol Vitamin C
Frequency	At least 6 cups per week or 1 cup per day	At least 5 servings per week	At least 2 cups per week

*Indicates those in the cruciferous vegetable list

KEY SUPPORTING PLAYERS

	OTHER VIBRANT PRODUCE	HEALTHY FATS AND OILS	NUTS AND SEEDS
Examples	Citrus fruits, green beans, peppers, sweet potatoes, summer squash, tomatoes, winter squash, zucchini	Avocados Cold-water fish, such as mackerel, salmon, sardines, trout, and tuna Extra virgin olive oil	Almonds, Brazil nuts, cashews, flaxseeds, hazelnuts, macadamia nuts, peanuts, pecans, pistachios, pumpkin seeds, sesame seeds, walnuts
Anti-Inflammatory Component(s)	Carotenoids (such as beta-carotene, lycopene, lutein, and zeaxanthin), flavonols (such as quercetin and kaempferol), flavanones, fiber	Oleocanthal, omega-3 fatty acids EPA and DHA, vitamin E	Coenzyme Q10, phytosterols, lignans, omega-3 fatty acid ALA, vitamin E
Frequency	Daily	Daily	1-ounce (28 g) 5 times per week

	TEA	SPICES, HERBS, ALLIUMS, AND ROOTS	GUT PROMOTERS
Examples	Black, green, oolong, and white teas	Black pepper, cayenne pepper, cinnamon, cumin, garlic, ginger, leeks, mint, onion, oregano, parsley, rosemary, scallions, shallots, turmeric	Probiotics: found in fermented and cultured foods Prebiotics: found in high-fiber produce
Anti-Inflammatory Component(s)	Catechins	Capsaicin, curcumin, flavones, flavonols, organosulfur compounds	An ample and diverse supply of good bacteria (see page 30)
Frequency	Daily	Daily	Daily

jump start:

EASY WAYS TO EAT MORE TOP ANTI-INFLAMMATORY FOODS NOW

1. Make a smoothie with berries, leafy greens, and yogurt.

2. Snack on fruits and nuts.

3. Swap pasta and refined starches for veggie spirals and riced cauliflower.

4. Make a cup of green tea, iced or hot.

5. Order fish when you eat out if you don't cook it regularly at home.

6. Eat at least one salad a day.

7. Roast vegetables for dinner or a pre-dinner snack.

8. Cook with a new spice or herb each week.

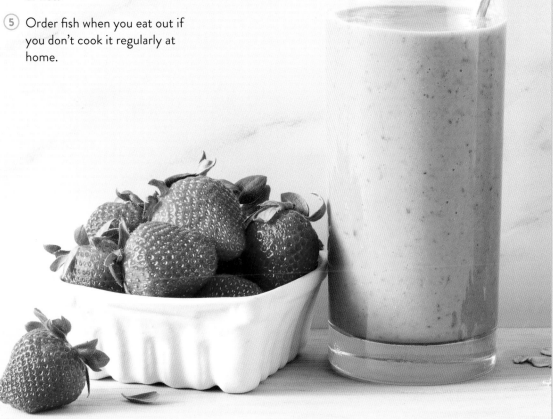

step #2
decrease dietary inflamers

While certain foods have powerful anti-inflammatory properties, others have the opposite effect. Dietary inflamers don't typically initiate low-grade inflammation. Instead, they fuel the intensity of existing inflammation, slowly pushing the body toward more serious health issues. Dietary inflamers originate in different places within our food system, and they don't affect everyone in the same ways. For simplicity, I've found it helpful to group dietary inflamers into three categories.

3 types of dietary inflamers

1 dietary inflamers for everyone

2 potential inflammatory foods and food components for some

3 inflammatory toxins, chemicals, and compounds in our food and water supply

1. dietary inflamers for everyone

Many of these dietary inflamers are fine in small to moderate amounts as part of a healthy diet. The problem, though, is that our intake has drastically increased over the past seaveral decades. At the same time, intake of foods with anti-inflammatory properties has decreased. These shifts are largely due to the advances in food processing and increased availability of food at any time of day. These charts list commonly consumed inflammatory components in foods and how to avoid them. Chapter 2 provides more information on healthier food choices to eat instead.

TOP DIETARY INFLAMERS FOR EVERYONE

INFLAMERS	HOW TO AVOID
Added sugars	• Avoid sugary drinks, like lemonades, punches, soft drinks, and sweet tea; candy; and processed foods with added sugars. • Aim to keep daily added sugar ≤ 25 g (6 teaspoons) for women and ≤ 36 g (9 teaspoons) for men. Less is ideal when possible. • Use added sugar values to monitor intake and choose products lower in added sugars.
Higher-glycemic, refined carbohydrate sources	• Avoid baked goods, breads, pastas, pastries, and snack foods made with refined flours and refined starchy foods like french fries and potato chips. • Watch out for breads and pastas labeled "wheat" or "multigrain" as these do not indicate the product is 100 percent whole-grain or even made predominantly from whole grains.
Trans fats	• Avoid or minimize fast food, fried foods, and packaged foods. • Avoid products that use "hydrogenated" or "partially hydrogenated" oils, such as margarines, microwave popcorn, prepacked pastries, and shortening-based foods, like frostings.
Saturated fats	• Choose lean meats and poultry; remove the skin and/or trim visible fat. • Minimize butter and animal fats. • Avoid tropical oils like palm, palm kernel, and refined and hydrogenated coconut oils.
High omega-6 to omega-3 ratio	• Minimize usage of products containing corn, peanut, safflower, soybean, sunflower, and vegetable oils. • When using oils with a higher proportion of omega-6 fatty acids, choose higher quality sources such as extra virgin olive oil and canola oil. • Increase fats and oil with a higher proportion of omega-3 fatty acids, such as fatty fish, flaxseeds and flaxseed oil, and walnuts and walnut oil. See page 16 for more guidance on choosing healthy fats and oils.
Processed meats	• Avoid processed meats like hot dogs, smoked and cured processed meats, and meat products like sausage and bacon. See page 51 for more information on processed meats.
Artificial sweeteners	• Minimize use of artificial sweeteners, particularly those in the pink, blue, or yellow packets. • Opt for a plant-based sweetener like stevia (green packets) or monk fruit, if using one.
Excessive intake of calories, alcohol, or sodium	• Avoid going excessively above energy needs on a regular basis. • Limit alcohol to no more than 1 drink per day for women and no more than 2 drinks per day for men. • Keep daily sodium to <2300 mg.

2. potential inflammatory foods and food components for some

Unlike the dietary inflamers on the previous page, the inflammatory potential of these foods and dietary components vary by individual, and there are two main categories: food allergies and food reactions (also known as sensitivities or intolerances).

- **FOOD ALLERGIES:** Allergens are proteins in food that elicit a specific immune response by the body, triggering the release of histamine. Symptoms are immediate and range from mild to severe, even life-threatening, and require an antihistamine or epinephrine to stop them. Approximately 90 percent of food allergies are caused by allergens in eight foods: milk, eggs, peanuts, tree nuts, fish, shellfish, wheat, and soy.

- **FOOD REACTIONS (SENSITIVITIES AND INTOLERANCES):** Adverse physiological reactions to food that aren't quick or apparent in their occurrence when compared to allergies. They may be caused by a less pronounced and nonthreatening immune response or an inability to digest certain components like lactose. These components act as irritants to the body, causing inflammation. When low-grade inflammation is already present, the body may be particularly sensitive and more susceptible to their irritation. Food reactions are subtler and harder to identify but determining and avoiding the foods that are irritants to your body is an essential part of keeping inflammation at bay and managing inflammatory conditions.

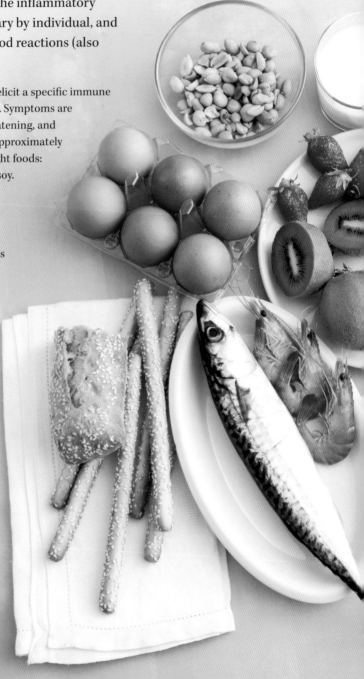

FOOD REACTIONS

	IMMUNE-MEDIATED *(Commonly referred to as a food sensitivity)*	NONIMMUNE-MEDIATED *(Commonly referred to as a food intolerance)*
Differences	• Triggered by an immune response • Don't always occur when irritant is eaten; reaction may be related to other compounds and irritants in the food, level of inflammation in the body, and stress	• Not triggered by an immune response • Due to an inability to digest certain foods or components or an abnormal response to them • May be dose-dependent
Similarities	• Delayed onset with less clear or apparent symptoms in comparison to a food allergy • Not life-threatening but can impact quality of life and aggravate existing inflammation and inflammatory conditions • Some foods may cause both immune and nonimmune-mediated reactions • Symptoms are very similar regardless of immune system involvement	
Symptoms	Abdominal pain, bloating, brain fog, cramping, diarrhea, fatigue, gas, headaches (including migraines), joint pain, nausea, sore throat, or congestion due to increased mucus production	
Common Triggers	• Artificial food coloring and dyes (such as Yellow 5, Yellow 6, Red 40, Blue 1, Blue 3) • Aspartame • Citrus • Corn • Dairy or lactose • Eggs • Fish and seafood • FODMAPs (Fermentable Oligosaccharides, Disaccharides, Monosaccharides, and Polyols; certain sugars and starches naturally found in some grains, fruit, and dairy foods)	• Food additives (such as sulfites, sodium benzoate, nitrates, MSG) • Gluten (found in products made with wheat, barley, and rye) • Histamines (common in aged cheeses, wine, cured and processed meats) • Legumes • Nightshades (eggplant, tomatoes, peppers, white potatoes) • Nuts • Soy • Yeast

Note: This is not meant to be an exhaustive list. Consult a dietitian or other knowledgeable health care provider for guidance in identifying others and managing more complex sensitivities, such as FODMAPs.

celiac and non-celiac gluten sensitivity

For individuals with a gluten sensitivity, avoiding foods with gluten (any foods containing wheat, barley, or rye) minimizes symptoms and can be a key part of reducing overall inflammation in the body. Consuming gluten will bring back symptoms and inflammation, but gluten itself does not cause damage to the body. This is different from celiac disease, in which gluten triggers an autoimmune attack on the small intestine. Those with celiac must avoid gluten completely, since even very small amounts can cause intestinal damage and lead to severe GI discomfort and an increased risk of nutrition deficiencies.

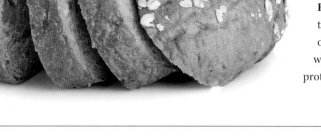

how to identify a food sensitivity or intolerance

Testing is an effective way to pinpoint food allergies, but the process for identifying sensitivities and intolerances is much more difficult and rarely comes with clear-cut answers. This is due to symptoms being subtle and delayed in onset, but it's also because there are few medical lab tests with the specificity and sensitivity to identify problematic foods. At-home sensitivity tests are popular, but there's skepticism about their accuracy, and they may provide false negatives and false positives.

The best way to identify problematic foods is through an elimination diet where you remove potential foods and food irritants for several days. Then you add individual foods back into your diet to see if your body reacts. A true elimination diet is 8 to 10 weeks and very restrictive because you remove all foods with potential irritants at the same time. A food-specific elimination approach is much less restrictive and often very effective in identifying key problematic foods (see **A Modified Elimination Protocol**. I encourage you to try this approach if you suspect a sensitivity or intolerance, and then to find a dietitian who can guide you in a stricter elimination protocol if needed.

WHO MIGHT BENEFIT FROM DOING AN ELIMINATION DIET?

- You've had several symptoms listed above with no clear reason or diagnosis.
- You think you've noticed an increase in symptom(s) when certain foods are consumed.
- You have a chronic inflammatory-related condition.
- You have an autoimmune disorder or condition or have a family history.
- You have a condition that is commonly associated with food sensitivities or intolerances (see list).

a modified elimination protocol

This approach is useful if you think there may be one or two primary food culprits causing your symptoms. This protocol is only for sensitivities and intolerances and should never be used to identify food allergens or celiac disease.

here's how to do it:

1 Choose one food or dietary component to eliminate (such as artificial sweeteners, dairy, dyes, or gluten).

2 Avoid eating that food and food products containing it for at least two weeks.

3 "Challenge" the body by slowly adding that food back to your diet and watch for symptoms. Remember that sensitivities and intolerance reactions may take 48 to 72 hours to become apparent.

QUESTIONS AND CONSIDERATIONS DURING THIS ELIMINATION PROCESS

- Did symptoms improve when eliminated in step 2?

- Did symptoms return or new ones present when you added back in step 3?

- If you didn't have noticeable symptoms prior, did you notice any changes in how your body felt (such as energy levels, sleep quality, sensitivity to other environmental factors, thought clarity, or anxiety levels) during the elimination period?

WHAT TO DO WITH YOUR FINDINGS

If you answered "yes" to any of these questions, you likely have some level of sensitivity or intolerance. Many people find benefits in avoiding that food as much as possible going forward. For others, the long-term benefits may not seem worthwhile right now, and this is fine. If that's the case, consider eliminating this food temporarily if you notice signs and symptoms of low-grade inflammation or during stressful periods when the immune system and body are hypersensitive and reactive. Doing this can be key in helping to calm early chronic inflammation.

3. inflammatory toxins, chemicals, and compounds in our food and water supply

Toxins are harmful chemicals or compounds that can accumulate in the body, causing irritation and disrupting homeostasis. The most common ones today are human-made chemicals and compounds used in farming, food production and processing, plastics, household products, and beauty products; environmental pollutants, such as smoke and exhaust; and heavy metals, such as mercury, lead, arsenic, and cadmium that have seeped into soil and water supplies.

Toxins are harmful because they cause disturbances that can potentially lead to cell damage and gene expression that cause imbalances or altered biological mechanisms—all of which trigger inflammation. In the past, attention has primarily focused on the carcinogenic effects. However, there are two lesser-known categories or effects—endocrine-disrupting and neurotoxic effects—that appear almost as damaging to health and much more pervasive.

- **CARCINOGENS**: increase risk for cancer

- **ENDOCRINE DISRUPTORS**: interfere or alter hormones and hormone balance

- **NEUROTOXINS**: alter nervous system or structure, which can affect development, behavior, and degenerative brain diseases like Alzheimer's and Parkinson's diseases

Exposure to and ingestion of toxins is unavoidable, and while toxins with obvious health implications are banned, there are many others that aren't considered safe but are allowed and regularly used. This will be the case until there's substantial additional data to support banning their usage, and this is a slow process. Even once they're banned, many will still be present in soil and water. Becoming an educated consumer when it comes to toxins is the best way to reduce exposure.

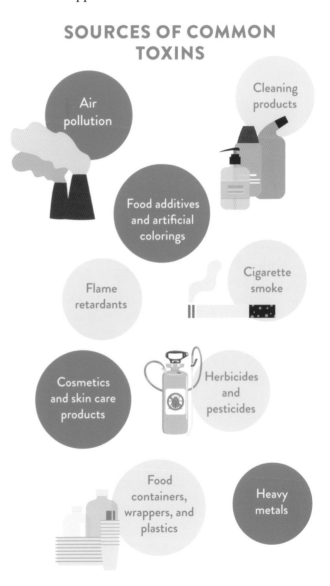

SOURCES OF COMMON TOXINS

Air pollution

Cleaning products

Food additives and artificial colorings

Flame retardants

Cigarette smoke

Cosmetics and skin care products

Herbicides and pesticides

Food containers, wrappers, and plastics

Heavy metals

TOP THREATS IN FOOD, FOOD-CONTACT MATERIALS, AND WATER

Looking into environmental toxins can quickly become overwhelming and all-consuming—trust me! This chart lists the most common toxins associated with food, food products, and water, where they're found, and their potential effects. Use this chart, along with **Jump Start: 12 Easy Ways to Reduce Toxins & Chemicals in Food (page 27)**, to start making small changes to reduce toxin exposure and ingestion.

TOXIN	WHERE IT'S FOUND	POTENTIAL EFFECTS
Arsenic	Drinking water, fruit juices, rice	Carcinogenic and endocrine-disrupting
Bisphenols such as bisphenol-A (BPA)	Disposable utensils, linings of canned goods, plastic food storage, receipts, water bottles	Endocrine-disrupting
Mercury	Fish	Possibly carcinogenic and neurotoxic
Persistent Organic Pollutants (Includes dioxins, PCBs, furans, flame retardants known as PBDEs, and PFAS)	Breast milk; herbicides; fat in meat, poultry, and dairy; skin on poultry and fish	Carcinogenic, endocrine-disrupting, and neurotoxic
Pesticides (Includes organophosphates, carbamates, chlorophenoxy herbicides, and pyrethroids)	Residue in and on food and in water sources, treated sports fields	Carcinogenic, endocrine-disrupting, and neurotoxic
Phthalates	Beauty products, food packaging, food storage containers, fragrances, plastic bottles, toys	Endocrine-disrupting and potentially neurotoxic
Polyfluoroalkyl substances (PFAS)	Stain-resistant clothing and carpets, Teflon and other nonstick coatings on pans	Possibly carcinogenic, endocrine-disrupting, and potentially neurotoxic

what is gene expression?

Genetics "load the gun," and the environment pulls the trigger.

   This is my favorite description of gene-environment interaction because of the clear picture it paints for what can be a complex and overwhelming topic. It's important to have a basic understanding of the role that genetics play in inflammatory disease development and your health.

- The **genome** refers to all the genetic material in the body. It consists of DNA found in chromosomes; sections of DNA are referred to as **genes**.

- DNA sequencing in genes can vary among individuals, and these differences are known as **gene variants.** Gene variations are what make DNA unique to each person.

- **Gene expression** is a regulated process in which cells use the instructions in DNA to make certain proteins or compounds. It's highly regulated to make sure cells produce only what is needed and is turned "on" and "off" using feedback mechanisms.

Gene expression can also be triggered by environmental exposures, leading to altered regulation or production of the cell's proteins or compounds that vary in impact. Certain gene variants increase a person's risk for disease if they come into contact with an environmental exposure that triggers their expression (see page 7 for more on environmental factors).

   But there's another way gene-environment interaction can lead to harmful gene expression: **epigenetics.** Over time, environmental toxins and irritants create "marks" on DNA. These marks, **epigenetic modifications,** don't change DNA, but rather they alter healthy gene expression and regulation. Epigenetic changes can occur at any time and are transgenerational, meaning they get passed down to offspring. Exposure to environmental toxins and trauma early in life are considered key causes of epigenetic modifications.

MORE ON ENDOCRINE DISRUPTORS

The endocrine system is a network of glands (such as the pancreas, thyroid, and adrenal glands) that secrete hormones to control functions in the body related to growth, reproduction, metabolism, neurotransmitters, nervous system activation, bone health, mood, fluid balance, and sleep. Endocrine-disrupting compounds (EDCs) interfere with normal hormone balance and function. They have been associated with increased risk for the following:

- Altered kidney function and increased blood pressure

- Breast and prostate cancers

- Endometriosis, uterine fibroids, and polycystic ovarian syndrome

- Impaired thyroid function

- Increased anxiety and depression

- Infertility and reproductive issues

- Issues related to behavior, memory

- Obesity

- Premature sexual development

- Type 2 diabetes

- Weakened immune system

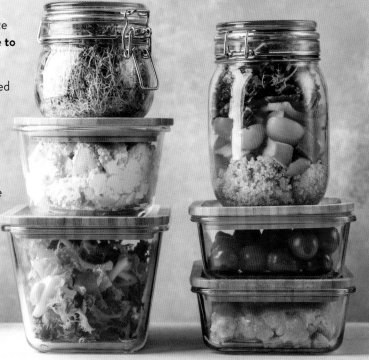

jump start: 12 EASY WAYS TO REDUCE TOXINS & CHEMICALS IN FOOD

1. Rinse rice before cooking and purchase rice grown in California, India, or Pakistan, which are lowest in arsenic.

2. Transfer food to glass or nonplastic microwave-safe containers before reheating.

3. Let food cool before storing in plastic containers or covering with plastic wrap.

4. Choose lower-mercury fish and seafood choices (see page 185).

5. Choose organic and/or local produce when possible; prioritize organic purchases (see **Produce to Prioritize, page 28**).

6. Use cast-iron or ceramic-coated skillets in place of Teflon or nonstick coated pans.

7. Use a water filter.

8. Choose plastics with the numbers 2, 4, or 5. Avoid those with the numbers 3, 6, and 7.

9. Use stainless steel, glass, or porcelain water bottles and containers.

10. Handwash plastic containers instead of using the dishwasher.

11. Choose fresh, frozen, or dried produce over canned.

12. Wash fruits and vegetables well before eating, cutting, or cooking.

conventional versus organic produce

All produce has chemical remnants from pesticides, herbicides, insecticides, and soil and water contaminants—including organic produce. Organic fruits and vegetables are lower in residue amounts and types, but regular produce can still be a healthy option. Here's what you need to know about both:

Organic produce still has chemical and compound residues, but in lower levels.

Both organic and conventional produce should be washed prior to eating and preparing, especially those with edible exposures. Residue is located primarily on the produce peel and outside skin, and washing appears to be the best way to minimize it.

Certain produce may have higher levels due to the plant's texture or growing process. Prioritize purchasing organic versions of those that may have higher levels (such as the **Produce to Prioritize**) and that don't have an outer husk, peel, or covering that will get discarded before eating (such as grapes, berries, and tomatoes).

Don't take an all-or-nothing approach by not eating produce unless it's organic. The benefits of produce consumption are so profound that overall intake is what's most important to health. My weekly groceries include a mix of both organic and conventional produce.

PRODUCE TO PRIORITIZE

The Environmental Working Group publishes an annual list of the top twelve "dirty" produce using data gathered by the USDA's Pesticide Data Program. It's important to mention that these lists are criticized by federal agencies and some health professionals for causing undue alarm and doing more harm than good, and I'll admit that I used to fall into that category.

However, my concern about our food supply has increased significantly over the course of my research the past few years. While I don't recommend using the EWG's Dirty Dozen or Clean Fifteen (a list of fruits and vegetables with the lowest pesticide residue) as definitive lists (and definitely not as a list of foods to avoid), I do think it's important to be aware, and these lists may be helpful in deciding which produce to try to purchase organic.

DIRTY DOZEN LIST

Strawberries

Spinach

Kale and dark leafy greens

Nectarines

Apples

Grapes

Peppers

Cherries

Peaches

Pears

Celery

Tomatoes

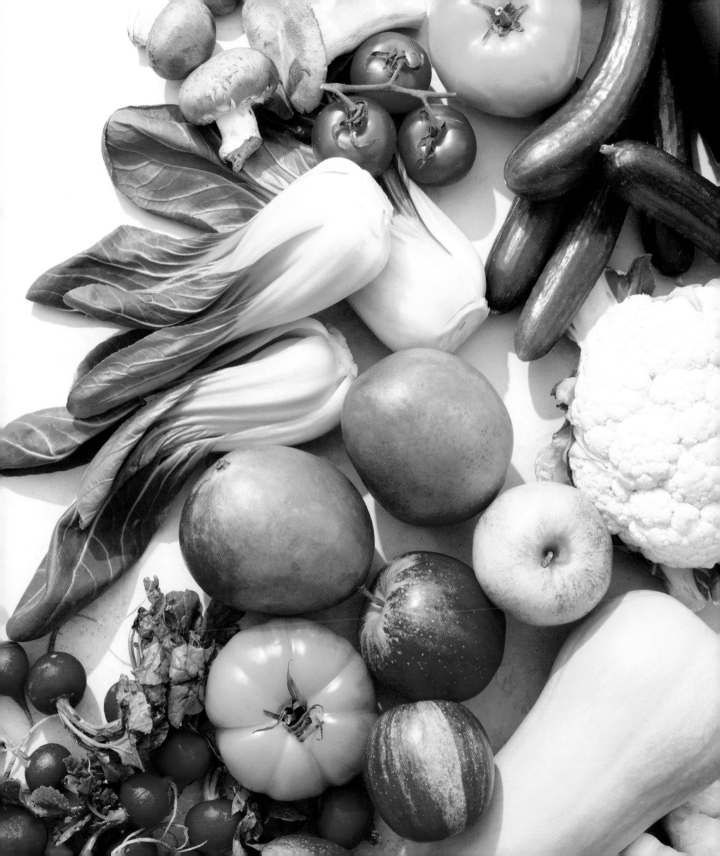

step #3
nourish your gut

While huge advances have been made in the four years since I wrote the first *Meals That Heal* cookbook, there is still so much we don't know about gut health. However, two things are clear:

1 The gut plays a much larger, more powerful role in our physical and mental health than we ever imagined.

2 The gut's influence on our health is largely determined by the makeup of our microbiome (the diversity, supply, variety, and balance of bacteria and other beneficial organisms in the gut).

Approximately 70 to 80 percent of the immune system is housed in the gut, so our immune cells interact regularly with gut bacteria. This means that diet, through changes in the microbiome, has a direct influence on overall health, including immune health and inflammation. In fact, changes and imbalances in the microbiome have been linked to most major health issues affecting Americans today: obesity, high blood pressure, depression, diabetes, cancer, autoimmune conditions, Alzheimer's, dementia, thyroid issues, and hormonal imbalances, which are all conditions also connected to chronic inflammation.

A healthy gut (one that has an ample, diverse, and balanced population of bacteria) supports healthy immune function by serving as a protective lining over the intestinal walls, preventing many irritants and inflamers in food from being absorbed and entering the body. The bacteria in a healthy microbiome also produce compounds needed for the rest of the body to function properly, such as neurotransmitters, enzymes, hormones, vitamins, amino acids, and short-chain fatty acids.

When the microbiome is disrupted, the makeup of gut bacteria is altered and unbalanced (this is known as gut dysbiosis). This creates holes or "leaks" in the protective lining, meaning some irritants and inflamers in the foods we consume are now able to pass through the intestinal walls into the body. These include things like toxins, antigens, and microbes, all of which can trigger or exacerbate inflammation once in the bloodstream. Disruptions to the microbiome can be caused by medications like antibiotics, lifestyle factors like stress and lack of sleep, and environmental exposures.

Restoring and nourishing your gut is key to help the microbiome bounce back from disruptions, and diet appears to have the best, most impactful way to do this. While over-the-counter probiotics can be an easy place to turn, your primary focus should be on increasing those foods and beverages that protect, feed, and repopulate your gut microbes. A probiotic supplement may be used in conjunction with diet to potentially offer additional support, but it shouldn't be used as your primary method of gut support.

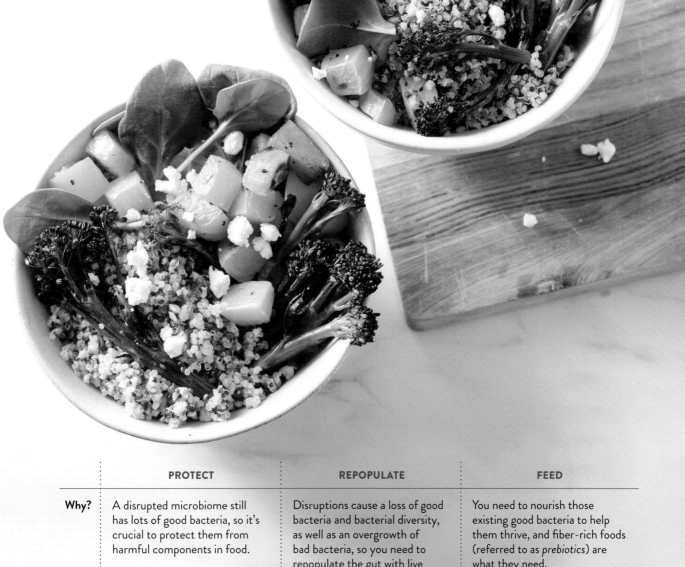

	PROTECT	**REPOPULATE**	**FEED**
Why?	A disrupted microbiome still has lots of good bacteria, so it's crucial to protect them from harmful components in food.	Disruptions cause a loss of good bacteria and bacterial diversity, as well as an overgrowth of bad bacteria, so you need to repopulate the gut with live strains of good bacteria.	You need to nourish those existing good bacteria to help them thrive, and fiber-rich foods (referred to as *prebiotics*) are what they need.
How?	1. Minimize added sugars, saturated fats, excessive protein intake, excessive alcohol, and highly processed foods. 2. Wash produce to reduce pesticide residue. 3. Manage stress. 4. Brush your teeth.	1. Regularly incorporate fermented foods, such as kimchi, kombucha, miso, sauerkraut, and tempeh, and cultured dairy products with live, active strains such as cottage cheese, kefir, and yogurt. 2. Consider taking a multi-strain probiotic.	1. Increase daily fiber intake by adding fruits, vegetables, nuts and seeds, legumes, and some whole grains. 2. Incorporate foods that are good sources of prebiotic fibers: apples, artichokes, asparagus, bananas, chickpeas, flaxseed, garlic, leeks, oats, onions, and soybeans.

INCORPORATE MORE FERMENTED FOODS NOW!

(1) **Kimchi** is a Korean dish made with vegetables like cabbage, radishes, and cucumbers, which are brined and then fermented. It has a tangy, spicy, slightly sweet flavor.

(2) **Kombucha** is a fermented tea drink, often flavored with fruit, made by adding good bacteria and yeast to lightly sweetened green or black tea.

(3) **Miso** is a traditional Japanese seasoning paste made from fermented soybeans that has a salty, umami flavor.

(4) **Sauerkraut** is salted cabbage that's fermented by lactobacillus bacteria naturally found on the vegetable. It has a salty, slightly sour taste. Made with just salt and water, other vegetables can be fermented this same way.

(5) **Tempeh** is made by fermenting cooked soybeans into a dense block. It has a nutty flavor and is a good source of probiotics, as well as protein and fiber.

(6) **Other fermented foods:** yogurt, kefir, some cheeses like cottage cheese with live active cultures

here are some ideas for incorporating more fermented foods.

Since they contain live organisms, it's best to add them at the end of the cooking process when possible.

Add sauerkraut to coleslaw or chopped salads.

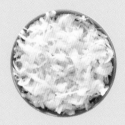

Add kefir to smoothies.

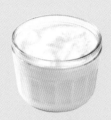

Blend or process kimchi with plain yogurt to create a dip for raw vegetables.

Add sauerkraut or kimchi as a condiment or topping to sandwiches or wraps.

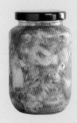

Sip on kombucha instead of a cocktail.

Add miso paste to flavor broth for soups and stews.

Whisk small amounts of miso paste into salad dressings and marinades to add a salty, savory flavor (similar to soy sauce).

Add miso paste to stir-fry sauce ingredients like rice vinegar, mirin, sesame oil, and soy sauce or tamari, starting small to avoid excessive saltiness.

Use kimchi liquid as a base to make salad dressings or add a tablespoon or two to mayonnaise for a flavorful spread.

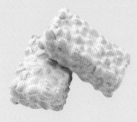

Substitute crumbled tempeh for ground meat and poultry in stir-fries and skillet dishes.

Top cooked rice or grain bowls with a spoonful or two of kimchi.

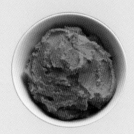

step #4
reduce stressors and lifestyle irritants

Stress is a normal and unavoidable part of life, but the body's stress response enables us to handle it—at least to a certain degree and for a period of time. When stress is continuous or frequent, this healthy stress response turns inflammatory and begins to negatively impact physical and mental health. While we tend to focus on stress' psychological causes and effects, the reality is this:

- Anything that threatens the body's homeostasis (psychological, mental, physical, lifestyle-induced, or environmental) is a stressor or cause of stress.

- Stressors trigger a physiological stress response that involves the nervous, endocrine, and immune systems.

Looking at it from another perspective, anything that makes you question your ability to cope or manage a situation (or makes our body question its ability) initiates the body's stress response. Here are some of the most common stressors today.

PHYSICAL & PHYSIOLOGICAL
Stressors on the Body

- Inadequate and/ or poor-quality sleep

- A lack of regular physical activity

- Sitting for long periods each day

- Excessive exercise

- Regular heavy labor or bouts of excessive exercise or activity without adequate rest

- Exposure to environmental toxins and chemicals

- Infections from pathogens like bacteria and viruses

- Excess body fat

- Dehydration

- Malnutrition

- Poor metabolic detoxification

- Temperature extremes

- Acute and chronic pain

- Food and environmental allergies

- Food sensitivities and intolerances

- Trauma and injuries

- Excessive alcohol or caffeine

- Substance abuse

- Radiation

- Harmful UV exposure

- Vaccinations

- Acute and chronic inflammation

COGNITIVE & PSYCHOLOGICAL
Stressors on the Body

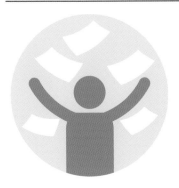

- Information and sensory overload

- Environmental "noise" (such as alarms, notifications, crowds, and bright lights)

- Deadlines and time constraints

- Uncertainty and unpredictability

- Financial constraints and concerns

- Chronic pain

- A lack of engagement or participation in life

- Being overscheduled or overcommitted

- An inability to say "no"

- Unhealthy relationships and commitments

- Caretaking of a family member or friend

- Worry and concerns about children

- Isolation or human contact limited to a very small group of the same individuals (intentional or unintentional)

- Grief, resentment, anger, frustration, or guilt

- Conflict or an inability to resolve conflict

- Moral and ethical worry and concerns (such as inequality, climate change, politics, etc.)

- Fears and anxiety-producing thoughts

- Conflict with family members or friends

- Conflict at work or within an organization

- Making difficult decisions

- Feeling like you have no control

- Recognition of memory loss or cognitive decline

- Feelings or memories associated with past trauma or stressful events

- Any major life change (divorce, moving, job change, death, birth)

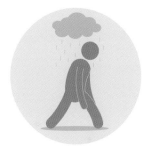

the danger of ongoing stressors

Like the inflammatory response, the stress response is designed to be short-term and temporary. So, when the stressor sticks around, the response keeps the body in fight-or-flight overdrive, with cortisol levels elevated. The result is an overstimulated nervous system and a dysregulated endocrine system, which begins to impact the immune system since these three systems are intricately connected. Consequently, there's a cascade of inflammatory effects, first from the stress and initial stress response and then from the changes that occur from the ongoing stress response. Additional stressors act as irritants, aggravating and intensifying chronic inflammation and perpetuating existing inflammatory feedback cycles. This is why ongoing stress is even more harmful when low-grade inflammation already exists.

daily habits to improve stress management

Stress is a constant throughout life, so learning how to manage and minimize the effects is important to reduce inflammation and improve overall health. While incorporating stress management tips and tools to reduce stress are helpful, you've first got to establish a foundation that will allow you to manage and overcome stress. There are three lifestyle habits for this that are often overlooked:

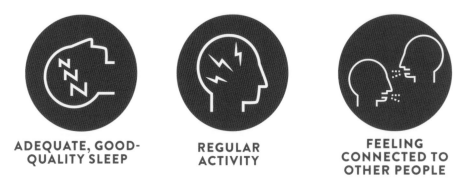

ADEQUATE, GOOD-QUALITY SLEEP

REGULAR ACTIVITY

FEELING CONNECTED TO OTHER PEOPLE

These often seem so basic that they can be easy to overlook. Yet, they're fundamental to our coping skills and health when it comes to stress. Prioritizing each on a weekly basis is associated with reduced inflammation and lower inflammatory blood markers. Conversely, skipping out on any of the three is associated with low-grade inflammation.

Inflammation-Related Effects of
ONGOING OR FREQUENT STRESSORS

Dysregulation among the immune, nervous, and endocrine systems due to ongoing stress leads to:

- Increased susceptibility to illness and infection
- Slow wound healing
- Sleep disruptions or insomnia
- Exacerbation of existing inflammation
- Changes to gut bacteria
- Activation of latent viruses in the body (such as Epstein-Barr)
- Autoimmunity and a break in autoimmunity tolerance
- Increased sensitivity to irritants in foods and in the environment
- Development of several chronic inflammation signs (see page 10)
- Weight gain and insulin resistance
- Changes to appetite
- Cravings for foods high in carbohydrates or added sugars or for beverages with caffeine
- Menstrual irregularities
- A need to use caffeine to "wake up" and alcohol to "chill out"

Risks of long-term stress include:

- Cell damage and mutations due to gene expression
- Onset of an autoimmune disorder or condition
- Onset of a chronic disease
- Onset or worsening of depression, anxiety, or other mental health issues

jump start: EASY WAYS TO REDUCE STRESS NOW

1. Get a brief change of scenery. Run an errand or walk around the office—anything that temporarily prevents your mind from being solely focused on the stressor or situation.

2. Find an app that guides you in a quick breathing exercise or desk yoga.

3. Turn on music or listen to a podcast.

4. Go outside for 10 minutes. It doesn't matter if you sit and relax, eat lunch, or move; you'll still get the benefits of fresh air and greenspace.

5. Read a book or magazine for 10 minutes.

6. Sip on a cup of green tea.

7. Connect with a friend and vent, if needed!

8. Journal or make lists to help you feel organized and to reduce anxiety or worry.

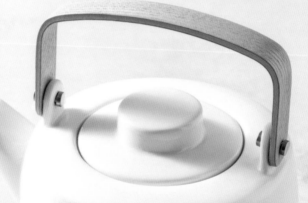

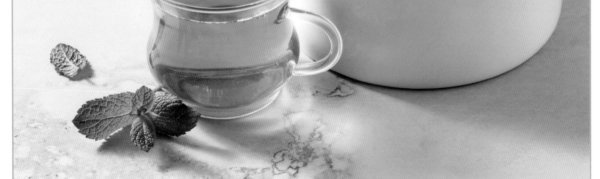

where do you start?

Chronic inflammation affects everyone in some capacity, regardless of age or health status, so addressing and preventing it is essential for health and long-term quality of life for everyone, too. Inflammation looks very different for each person, which means there's no exact blueprint or right-or-wrong way to follow an anti-inflammatory eating and lifestyle approach. But I know this may also lead you to become overwhelmed and unsure where to start, so here are recommendations for how to use this cookbook.

focus on the big picture for YOU

What are your big takeaways or concepts from this chapter, specifically the ones that hit home when it comes to your health? What are your biggest health concerns? What's your top one?

start small and build

Reducing inflammation is a gradual, ongoing process, and that's also how you should approach incorporating anti-inflammatory diet and lifestyle changes. Once you've determined your top health concern, identify the inflamer (diet, sleep, stress, lack of activity, etc.) with the largest influence. Then, set small goals to lessen this inflamer that you approach one at time. Chapter 2 provides focuses on anti-inflammatory foods choices, a blueprint for an anti-inflammatory diet and lifestyle, and the best ways to set goals and get started.

make it easy

Eating healthy should be easy, simple, and delicious if you're going to stick with it long-term. Chapter 3 shares all of my tricks, hacks, and shortcuts for simplifying planning, prep, and getting dinner on the table, and chapters 4 to 10 give you over 100 recipes that you and your family will love!

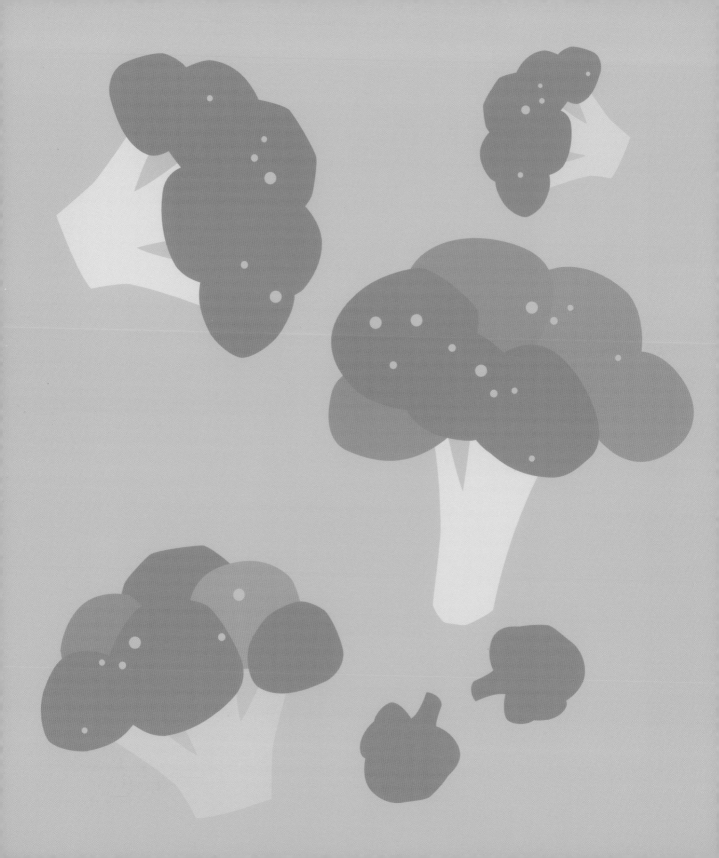

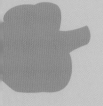

2

·············

your everyday guide to
NO-FUSS,
ANTI-INFLAMMATORY
EATING

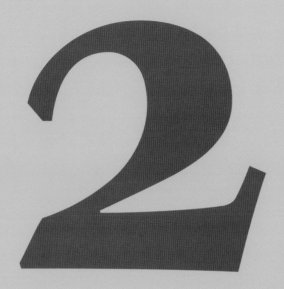

Now it's time for more fun stuff—and likely the reason you bought this cookbook: food and what to eat!

I think it's crucial for you to have a basic understanding of inflammation and its influence on health, but I also totally get that chapter 1 may have left you unsure of what to eat or even where to start.

But don't worry, because this chapter is going to tell you what foods to eat and which to avoid, as well as everything you need to know for shopping, meal planning, and cooking. All recommendations incorporate and build upon the 4-step process I shared in chapter 1 (see page 12)—increase anti-inflammatory foods, decrease dietary inflamers, nourish your gut, reduce stressors and lifestyle irritants—to guide you in adopting an anti-inflammatory diet and lifestyle.

In this chapter, you'll find daily and weekly eating recommendations by food group, including food lists, servings, and details to know when shopping. I'll also share information on how meal timing and the role that time-restricted eating or fasting can play in an anti-inflammatory eating approach.

daily and weekly eating goals to reduce inflammation

These goals and recommendations are key components of anti-inflammatory eating, so use them as your guide when choosing foods each day and over the course of a week. You'll find more details on each of these food groups on the following pages.

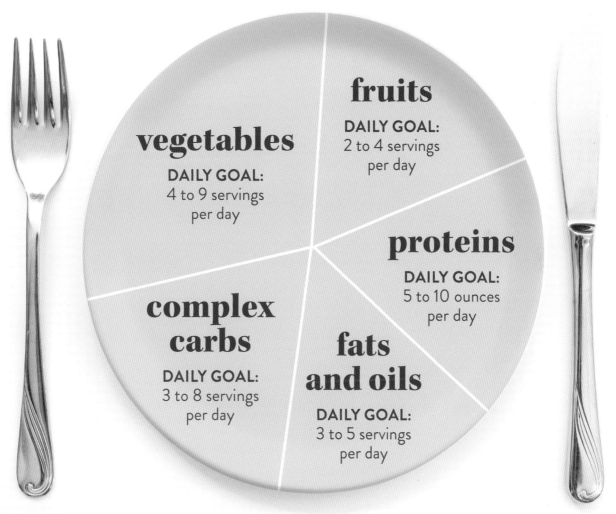

vegetables
DAILY GOAL:
4 to 9 servings
per day

fruits
DAILY GOAL:
2 to 4 servings
per day

proteins
DAILY GOAL:
5 to 10 ounces
per day

complex carbs
DAILY GOAL:
3 to 8 servings
per day

fats and oils
DAILY GOAL:
3 to 5 servings
per day

Note: The ranges in the food group servings are designed to provide flexibility for accommodating a variety of macronutrient and energy needs ranging from 1400 to 2200 calories. Athletes and very active individuals who have higher energy and nutrient needs should increase servings as needed.

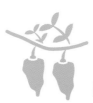

—vegetables—

DAILY GOAL: 4 to 9 servings per day

- Include at least 1 cup of leafy greens each day.
- Include cruciferous vegetables 4 or more times per week.
- Aim for variety in type and color (but don't let this limit overall intake).

leafy greens	cruciferous vegetables	other vegetables	
Cruciferous greens (kale, mustard greens, turnip greens, watercress, arugula)	Bok choy and napa cabbages	Artichokes	Iceberg lettuce
Leaf lettuces (romaine, red leaf, green leaf)	Broccoli (including broccoli rabe and broccolini)	Asparagus	Mushrooms
Mesclun, spring mix, and other mixed greens	Brussels sprouts	Beets	Okra
Radicchio	Cauliflower	Carrots	Onions
Spinach	Green and red cabbages	Celery	Peppers
Swiss chard	Kohlrabi	Cucumber	Summer squash and zucchini
	Radishes	Eggplant	Sweet potatoes
	Rutabaga	Green beans and snap peas	Winter squash (acorn, butternut, delicata, spaghetti)
	Turnips	Leeks	Tomatoes
	Cruciferous greens (listed above)		

ONE SERVING IS EQUIVALENT TO

1 cup raw cut vegetables

½ cup cooked vegetables (including leafy greens)

1 cup raw leafy greens

DO "OTHER VEGETABLES" OFFER ANY BENEFITS?

Yes! Each one provides a unique assortment of anti-inflammatory nutrients and compounds and contains different forms of fiber to support gut health. Eating a variety of these "others" to meet daily vegetable goals is just as important as eating your cruciferous and leafy green vegetables.

Leafy Greens & Cruciferous Veggies:
WHAT'S THE BIG DEAL?

These two vegetable families offer some of the strongest anti-inflammatory benefits. Prioritize meeting recommendations for both and then use a variety of other vegetables to meet daily intake recommendations. Here's why:

LEAFY GREENS contain a powerful combination of the antioxidant vitamin C and three phytochemicals in the carotenoid family: beta-carotene, lutein, and zeaxanthin. Collectively, all four stop free radicals to prevent new inflammation and exacerbation of existing inflammation, but carotenoids also interfere with inflammatory signaling pathways that create altered proteins and enzymes through faulty gene expression. Regular consumption of leafy greens is associated with a lower risk of heart disease, type 2 diabetes, Alzheimer's disease, Parkinson's disease, cancer, and mental health issues, such as depression and anxiety.

CRUCIFEROUS VEGETABLES are unique in that that they contain glucosinolates, a phytochemical family of sulfur-containing compounds. Cooking breaks down glucosinolates into biologically active forms that the body can use (such as isothiocyanates and indoles), but it's also why many of these vegetables have a slight sulfur odor when cooking. Glucosinolates offer anti-inflammatory, antibacterial, and antiviral protection, but it's their impact on cancer that may be the greatest. Research suggests they may have the potential to prevent the mutation of healthy cells into cancer cells; inhibit enzymes needed for the growth and metastasis of cancer cells; kill both benign and malignant cancer cells; and alter hormone metabolism to decrease the risk of hormone-sensitive cancers, such as breast cancer.

jump start:

12 WAYS TO SNEAK MORE LEAFY GREENS AND CRUCIFEROUS VEGGIES IN TODAY!

1. Make a salad for breakfast with a hard-boiled or fried egg for protein.

2. Wilt baby spinach into soups, stews, and saucy skillet dishes just before serving.

3. Puree vegetables like spinach and cauliflower florets in sauces and soups.

4. Toss a handful of greens in the blender when making a smoothie.

5. Skip the heavy pizza toppings; top with 2 to 3 cups of spring mix or tender greens tossed in a light vinaigrette.

6. Add spinach (and other veggies like tomatoes, peppers, and onions) to an omelet or egg scramble.

7. Substitute mashed or riced cauliflower for rice, pasta, or potatoes.

8. Add sliced or shredded bok choy or napa cabbage to stir-fries.

9. Use large, sturdy lettuce leaves in place of a wrap or tortilla.

10. Toss a handful of spinach or kale inside a quesadilla or grilled cheese before cooking.

11. Use broccoli florets and radish slices for hummus and dips.

12. Snack on kale chips instead of potato chips or other snack foods.

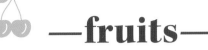

—fruits—

DAILY GOAL: 2 to 4 servings per day

Include a serving of berries most days or a minimum of 4 times per week.

Choose fruit that is bright or deep in color (think purples, blues, reds, deep yellows, oranges).

Consume servings at different times of the day (rather than 2 to 3 servings at one sitting).

If you're relatively healthy and not prone to hypoglycemia, choose fruits with a low to moderate glycemic index value; enjoy high glycemic ones on occasion.

Choose whole fruit over juice.

If you're prone to hypoglycemia, blood sugar fluctuations, or have metabolic syndrome or diabetes, focus primarily on fruits with a low glycemic index value.

Apples	Citrus (oranges, grapefruit, tangerines)	Papaya	Pomegranates
Apricots		Peaches	Prunes
Avocados*	Dates	Pears	Watermelon
Bananas	Figs	Pineapple	Unsweetened dried fruits
Berries (blueberries, blackberries, raspberries, strawberries)	Grapes	Plums	
Cantaloupe	Honeydew		
Cherries	Lychee		
Cranberries	Mango		

ONE SERVING IS EQUIVALENT TO

½ cup fresh or frozen fruit

½ large piece of fruit such as apple, grapefruit, orange, peach, or pear

1 small banana, peach, apple, or orange, or 1 to 2 clementine or kiwis

¼ cup dried fruit or ½ cup (120 ml) 100 percent juice

*Avocados are in the fruit family but are considered with the fats and oils for meal planning purposes.

fruit and glycemic response

Sugars naturally found in fruits (which differ from inflammatory sugars added to foods) are what give them their sweetness. This makes them a great quick energy source that also offers anti-inflammatory perks, thanks to their fiber, antioxidant, and phytochemical content. Blood glucose increases after eating fruit (as it will following consumption of any carbohydrate-containing food), and this response varies among fruits. A food's glycemic index (GI) value indicates the rate and intensity of this increase, which can be used as a tool to guide you in fruit choices.

Fruits with a lower glycemic index (GI) are your best choices in terms of avoiding blood sugar surges, which are associated with inflammation. Fruits with a high GI trigger the greatest glycemic response, and while you don't necessarily have to avoid them, you should be aware of their potential impact and consume them in moderation. Glycemic response to carbohydrates, including fruits, varies by individual, so pay attention to those that trigger a greater response. Signs of this can be hyperglycemia or hypoglycemia one to three hours after eating. Grapes and certain tropical fruits, like pineapple, may react more like high GI fruits in some people.

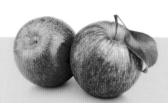

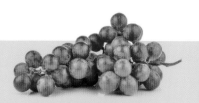

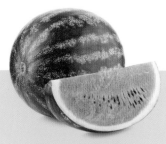

LOW GI FRUITS

Apples

Apricots (fresh or dried)

Avocados

Berries (blueberries, blackberries, raspberries, strawberries)

Cantaloupe

Cherries (fresh)

Cranberries (fresh)

Citrus (oranges, grapefruit, tangerines)

Honeydew

Peaches

Pears

Plums

Pomegranates

Prunes

MODERATE GI FRUITS

Banana (yellow, ripe)

Cranberries (dried)

Figs (fresh or dried)

Grapes

Kiwi

Lychee

Mango

Papaya

Pineapple

Raisins

HIGH GI FRUITS

Bananas (overripe)

Dates (fresh or dried)

Watermelon

Most dried, sweetened fruits

jump start: LOAD UP ON FROZEN BERRIES TODAY!

The common assumption is that fresh produce is superior to frozen, but this isn't necessarily the case—especially for berries. The powerful nutrients in berries are often at their peak right when harvested, after which the levels of many, like vitamin C and some phytochemicals, slowly decline. Depending on harvest location, this means fresh berries can lose some of their anti-inflammatory power if they don't reach grocery shelves for 3 to 7 days. Buying in-season produce from local and regional sources helps alleviate this, but so does freezing. Many farmers flash-freeze berries within hours of being picked, which halts this loss and means some frozen fruits have slightly more nutrients and phytochemicals than fresh.

One frozen berry that I encourage people to look for is wild blueberries. These aren't "wild" in the sense that they might be picked from a bush in your backyard or in the woods. Rather, wild blueberries are a specific type of berry harvested in the northeastern United States.

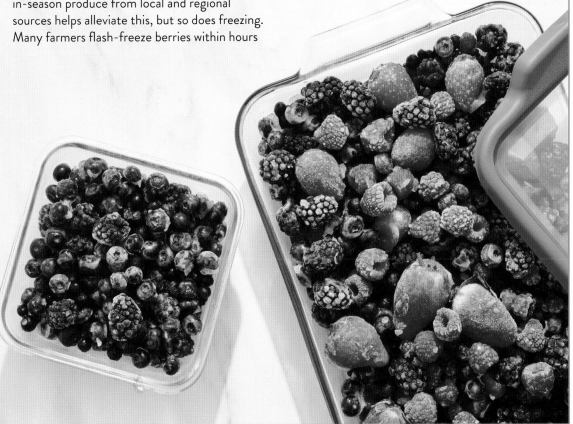

—proteins—

DAILY GOAL: 5 to 10 ounces per day

Protein intake should be from a variety of sources, which may include both plant-based and lean animal proteins.

Prioritize incorporating a variety of plant proteins in meals and snacks.

For those who eat both plant and animal-based proteins, include lower-mercury fish and seafood sources 2 to 3 times per week. Skinless poultry or lean white meat can be eaten up to 3 times per week and lean cuts of red meat up to 2 times per week.

Avoid processed, smoked, and cured meat and poultry products.

plant-derived sources

Soy foods (such as edamame, tofu, tempeh, and soy-derived products)

Legumes (bean, lentils, and peas)*

Nuts and seeds

Peanut butter

Almond butter and other nut butters

fish and seafood sources**

Anchovies	Monkfish
Bass	Perch
Butterfish	Pollock
Catfish	Sablefish
Cod	Salmon
Flounder	Sardines
Grouper	Sole
Haddock	Tilapia
Mackerel	Trout
Mahi-mahi	Tuna

Shellfish (such as clams, crabs, lobster, shrimp, scallops, and oysters)

poultry and meat

Eggs

Skinless chicken, turkey, and other lean poultry

Lean white meats such as pork

Lean red meat such as beef, lamb, and wild game

ONE OUNCE OF PROTEIN IS EQUIVALENT TO

1 ounce (28 g) of cooked fish, seafood, poultry, or meat

1 egg

¼ to ⅓ cup cooked beans, lentils, peas, or soybeans

1 ½ to 2 ounces (42 to 56 g) cooked tempeh or tofu

1 tablespoon peanut butter, almond butter, or other nut butter

½ ounce (14 g) nuts or seeds

*Foods within the legume family are also listed on page 52 since they are also a primary source of complex carbohydrates.

**See a breakdown of best and better choices based on mercury levels on page 185.

minimizing a top inflamer— processed meats

Processed meats, including bacon, sausage, cured meats, smoked meats, hot dogs, cold cuts, and jerky, are a top inflamer in the American diet. The term "processed meat" refers to any animal protein that has been altered through a process like salting, curing, preserving, canning, or other method to improve flavor or extend shelf-life. But it's the addition of compounds or chemicals during this that increases the inflammatory effects and health risks.

Frequent consumption of processed meats is associated with inflammation that can lead to diabetes and heart disease, but the connection to cancer is strongest. In fact, the World Health Organization has classified processed meats as a Group 1 carcinogen, the same rating as asbestos and tobacco smoke. Researchers haven't pinpointed one specific ingredient or processing additive as the main culprit. Many speculate that nitrates added during processing play a role in this, and there's substantial evidence that other harmful compounds are created when these meats are cooked: AGEs (advanced glycation end products), HCAs (heterocyclic amines), and PAHs (polycyclic aromatic hydrocarbons).

If you're a bacon lover, here are ways to minimize intake and reduce risks from processed meats:

- Avoid using high temperatures when cooking; don't consume any charred meats.

- Skip products that contain the words *nitrate*, *nitrite*, *cured*, or *salted* in the ingredient list.

- Cook turkey or chicken breasts to thinly slice for sandwiches instead of purchasing deli meats.

- Order a sandwich with grilled chicken or grilled fish instead of deli meats.

- Consider skipping the meat altogether by opting for a veggie sandwich with hummus or cheese.

- Reduce portion size and eat less frequently when or if you consume processed meats.

- *Nitrate-free* or *uncured* labels often signify that a vegetable-based preservative like celery powder is used for curing or preserving the meat. These may be lower in nitrates, but they're not nitrate-free.

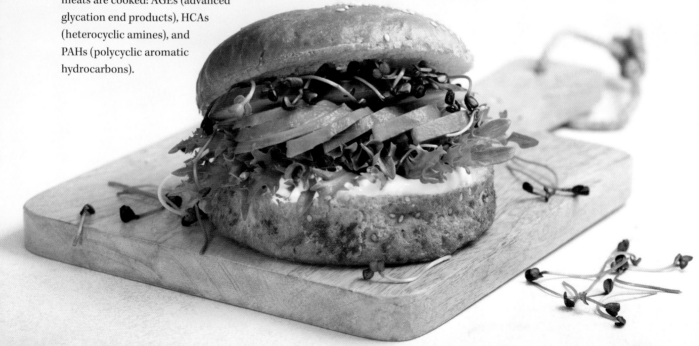

—complex carbs—

DAILY GOAL: 3 to 8 servings per day

Choose whole food sources followed by minimally processed grain products.

Prioritize getting daily carbs from vegetables (including starchy ones), fruits, and legumes; then fill in the gaps with whole grains and, if desired, dairy products.

Keep tabs on daily carbohydrate intake.

Avoid refined grains and highly processed foods with added sugars.

Because there are so many sources of complex carbs, the foods listed below, which have a low to moderate glycemic index in most people, should be prioritized over other sources.

legumes and other starchy vegetables	whole grains	minimally processed carbohydrate sources
Beans (like adzuki, black, cannellini, chickpeas, edamame, fava, great northern, kidney, and pinto)	Amaranth	100 percent whole-grain breads, crackers, and cereals
Lentils (all colors)	Barley*	Pastas made from whole-grain flours
Peas (like black-eyed, green, and split peas)	Brown rice	Pastas made from legume or nut-based flours (such as chickpea or almond flours)
Potatoes (small red and sweet)	Buckwheat	Corn tortillas
Butternut squash	Bulgur	Cauliflower and/or whole-grain pizza crusts
Parsnips	Corn	Cereal made with whole grains and minimal added sugar
Yams	Millet	
	Oats	
	Quinoa	
	Wheat* (including forms like einkorn, farro, freekeh, and spelt), wild rice	

SERVING SIZE EQUIVALENTS

½ cup cooked whole-grain or pasta

1 slice bread (approximately 1 oz/28 g)

3 cups (24 g) popcorn

1 cup whole-grain cereal

5 to 7 crackers

*Indicates grains that contain gluten

carbs and inflammation

Carbohydrates exert a powerful influence on inflammation in the body, which can be positive when they're a source of fiber, antioxidants, and phytochemicals by promoting gut health and preventing free radical damage. But they can also have a negative impact, and there are two primary determinants for this potential: glycemic impact and total carb load or amount consumed.

- **GLYCEMIC IMPACT:** The impact that a carbohydrate-rich food has on blood glucose levels (referred to as *glycemic impact*) is a key factor when choosing carb-rich foods. Foods with a low to moderate GI index value should be prioritized. The foods listed in the table above have low to moderate GI values. Thanks to their fiber, antioxidant, and phytochemical content, these foods usually have a positive impact on inflammation.

- **TOTAL CARBOHYDRATE:** The other determinant is the total amount consumed at a meal and within a day. Most people consume more carbohydrates than they need or realize, and excessive carbohydrate intake at meals or over a period of days can lead to weight gain and insulin resistance, both of which create additional inflammation. Research suggests that moderate to low carbohydrate consumption is beneficial in reducing inflammatory blood markers for many, but this varies by individual.

low and lower-carb eating approaches

Many find that eating a low- or lower-carb diet is an effective way to lose weight and reduce inflammation. But it's important to know that there's no precise or fixed definition for "low-carb"—meaning there are lots of ways to approach it. Two of the most well-known low-carb diets are the Atkins diet and the ketogenic diet, but eating approaches like paleo and Whole30 also tend to be low or lower in carb intake. Most popular diets usually fall into one of these three categories below, depending on level of carbohydrate restrictions. Regardless of total carbohydrate grams, what's key for them all is focusing on vegetables, healthy fats and oils, and high-fiber plant and/or lean animal proteins, and then sprinkling in a few higher-fiber complex carbs and low GI fruits.

- **CONSUME 100 TO 175 GRAMS OF CARBOHYDRATES:** This may seem like a lot, but it's a half to two-thirds lower than what is recommended based on guidelines for a 1600 to 2000 calorie diet. If you're active, engaged in sports, or want to ease into cutting back carbs, this is a good place to start. This is the approximate range for weight maintenance for those following a plan like the Atkins diet.

- **CONSUME 50 TO 100 GRAMS OF CARBOHYDRATES:** Eating at this level takes a little more planning to make sure you consume adequate calories through the addition of vegetables, healthy fats and oils, and some lean protein. It also still allows for the incorporation of some fruits and legumes.

- **CONSUME LESS THAN 50 GRAMS OF CARBOHYDRATES:** Eating at this level takes a lot more planning, and it can be much harder to consume adequate calories and key anti-inflammatory foods like fruits and vegetables. The ketogenic diet falls into the lower half of this category as consumption is often limited to 20 grams net carbohydrates or less. The tendency is to compensate by adding extra animal proteins since plant proteins have some carbohydrates, but calories really need to come from additional healthy fats and oils like nuts, high-fiber plant protein foods, and some lean poultry and meat.

EASY ANTI-INFLAMMATORY CARB SWAPS

Check out the quick swaps that are higher in fiber and lower in glycemic index. A few even sneak in some vegetables, fruits, or healthy foods.

INSTEAD OF ...	TRY
Flour tortillas or wraps	Corn tortillas Lettuce leaves
Traditional spaghetti and other pastas	Pastas made with whole-grain flours Pastas made with legume or lentil-based flours Veggie spirals like zucchini or butternut squash "noodles" Spaghetti squash **Caprese Zoodles** (page 229) **Semi-Homemade Bolognese with Zoodles** (page 146) **Pork Piccata over Zoodles** (page 159)
Instant flavored oatmeal	Steel-cut oats or groats
Potato chips, crackers, pretzels, and other processed or refined snack foods	Whole-grain or veggie-based crackers, pretzels Toasted chickpeas, nuts, yogurt, trail mix, fruit **Crispy Ranch Chickpeas** (page 250) **Marinated Feta-Veggie Skewers** (page 252) **Rosemary-Parmesan Cauliflower Crisps** (page 255)
White or wheat bread	100 percent whole-grain bread or breads that use nut-based flours (like almond flour) and/or legume-based flours (like chickpea flour)
Sodas, lemonade, or other sweetened beverages	Seltzer or water with lemon

INSTEAD OF . . .	TRY
Croutons	Toasted nuts
Rice (all types)	Cauliflower or broccoli "rice"

Cheesy Chicken, Broccoli, and "Rice" Casserole
(page 134)

Tzatziki "Rice" Bowls with Gyro Meatballs
(page 154)

Wild Mushroom "Risotto"
(page 234)

INSTEAD OF . . .	TRY
Traditional pizza crust	100 percent whole-grain or cauliflower pizza crust
French fries	Roasted sweet potato wedges or fries Zucchini chips or wedges Oven "fried" vegetables like eggplant or parsnips

Roasted Parmesan Zucchini
(page 230)

INSTEAD OF . . .	TRY
Chips or crackers for dips and sauce	Baby carrots, broccoli florets, celery, cherry tomatoes, or cucumber slices
Mashed potatoes	Mashed cauliflower or a combination of mashed cauliflower and potatoes Mashed celeriac or parsnips

Lower-Carb Mashed Potatoes
(page 238)

Twice-Baked Cauliflower Casserole
(page 241)

INSTEAD OF . . .	TRY
Flavored yogurt	Plain yogurt that you add fruit or nuts to and, if needed, a touch of honey or maple syrup

—fats and oils—

DAILY GOAL: 3 to 5 servings per day

> Prioritize eating and cooking with the "best oils" and "best food sources" below.

> Choose a cooking oil based on its smoke point.

> Avoid hydrogenated and trans fats.

> Minimize saturated fats by opting for lean animal proteins and avoiding excessive or frequent consumption of high-fat dairy products and coconut and palm oils.

> Avoid vegetable oil and highly refined plant and seed oils (see Fats and Oils to Minimize)

best oils for low to medium heat cooking and uncooked dishes
(Smoke point ranges from 225 to 350°F/110 to 175°C)

Extra virgin olive oil (avoid "pure olive oil" or "light olive oil")

Walnut oil

Flaxseed oil

best oils for medium-high to high heat
(Smoke point ranges from 390 to 525°F/200 to 275°C)

Avocado oil

Expeller pressed canola oil

Expeller pressed grapeseed oil

Sesame oil

best food sources

Fish higher in fat

Nuts and seeds

Avocados

Mayonnaise and salad dressings that use one or more of the identified best oils

FATS AND OILS TO MINIMIZE

Coconut oil

Corn oil

Cottonseed oil

Safflower oil

Sunflower oil

Soybean oil

Skin on poultry and excessive fat or marbling in meats

FATS AND OILS TO AVOID

Palm or palm kernel oil

Vegetable oil

Lard

Vegetable shortening

Any type of oil with the words *hydrogenated* or *partially hydrogenated*

SERVING SIZE EQUIVALENTS

1 tablespoon of any oil or measurable fat

1 ounce (28 g) of nuts or seeds

½ of an avocado

3 to 4 ounces (85 to 113 g) of higher-fat fish

coconut oil: healthy or harmful?

Coconut oil is primarily composed of saturated fatty acids, the "bad" fats that are also associated with fat in animal food. For years, the recommendation has been to minimize saturated fat since higher intakes are associated with higher LDL cholesterol, which increases risk for heart disease. So, coconut oil, which is comprised of 82 percent saturated fatty acids, was considered totally off limits. But the harmful effects (and potential benefits) of consuming coconut oil are now being questioned as many rethink the emphasis that has been placed on saturated fat. This is due to more recent knowledge that:

1 Total cholesterol by itself is not a good indicator of heart disease risk, and looking at indicators like levels of triglycerides, HDL level, and CRP in the blood is best.

2 Fats aren't the only thing that impact heart disease risk; added sugars and refined carbohydrates play a huge role that we're still trying to fully understand.

Minimizing saturated fat intake is still important, but these shifts in knowledge have opened the door to exploring coconut oil's potential health value, primarily because its saturated fatty acids are made up of medium-chain triglycerides (MCTs). This sets coconut oil apart from animal fats (which are primarily long-chain triglycerides). Research findings are conflicting, but they suggest that MCTs may be used more readily as an energy source (so the body is more apt to burn them rather than store them) and may potentially offer protection or improve brain health. Several of these MCTs in coconut oil (such as lauric acid) also have antibacterial, antiviral, and antifungal effects in the body.

key takeaways for cooking with coconut oil

- Use it on occasion or in place of other saturated fats like butter, but not as your primary fat source.

- Choose one with minimal refining (look for "virgin coconut oil" or "pure coconut oil" on the label).

- Keep cooking temps low to moderate (unrefined coconut oil has a smoke point of 350°F/175°C).

jump start: **SNACK ON NUTS DAILY**

Choosing a handful of nuts for a snack is one of the best anti-inflammatory choices you can make because they contain so many healthy nutrients and compounds. These include the omega-3 fatty acid known as ALA, fiber, vitamin E, and a group of phytochemicals known as phytosterols. Research suggests eating nuts (in portion sizes of 1 to 1 ½ ounces/28 to 42 g) supports weight loss and is associated with lower body weights. Aim to incorporate 1 ounce (28 g) of nuts like walnuts, almonds, and pistachios into your diet three to five times a week.

understanding what determines an oil's healthfulness

With the low-fat and fat-free days behind us, people are recognizing the value that fat provides when it comes to not just flavor and texture when cooking but also to satiety and overall health. Healthy eating recommendations prioritize oils over solid fats (such as butter or lard), but this doesn't mean that all oils are necessarily healthy or good for you. Here are three factors that determine an oil's healthfulness.

① **FATTY ACID COMPOSITION:** All oils contain a mix of polyunsaturated, monounsaturated, and saturated fatty acids, and an oil is often classified based on which one is predominant. Unsaturated fats include monosaturated fats (which have more omega-6 fatty acids) and polyunsaturated fats (which have more omega-3), and these are often referred to as "good fats." While this is still the case, US consumption of omega-6 fatty acids is excessive in comparison to omega-3s (largely due to the use of vegetable oils like corn, soybean, and sunflower in processed foods), and this imbalance is a source of inflammation.

How to minimize inflammation: Consume more polyunsaturated fats by eating higher-fat fish, walnuts, flaxseeds, and sunflower seeds. Choose less refined sources of monounsaturated oils (such as extra virgin olive oil, expeller pressed canola oil, and avocado oil).

② **COOKING HEAT AND SMOKE POINT:** Every oil has a unique smoke point, the temperature at which its structure becomes unstable and starts to break down. When this happens, the fatty acids are oxidized, generating free radicals and acrolein, an inflammatory compound also found in tobacco smoke. This is why you should be cautious about cooking with extra virgin olive oil over medium to high heats.

How to minimize inflammation: Choose oils that have a smoke point appropriate for each heat level using the table above.

③ **LEVEL OF REFINING:** The process by which oils are extracted from their source is also a factor to consider. Extraction can be done using chemical solvents or through pressing, and methods that use a cold pressing technique and little to no chemicals are considered healthier. Most oils on the market use chemical and heat pressing for extraction, which slightly changes the structure of the oil and leaves chemical remnants.

How to minimize inflammation: Choose "cold-pressed" extra virgin or virgin olive oils and "expeller pressed" canola or grapeseed oils. Or choose oils that don't need much refinement, like avocado oil.

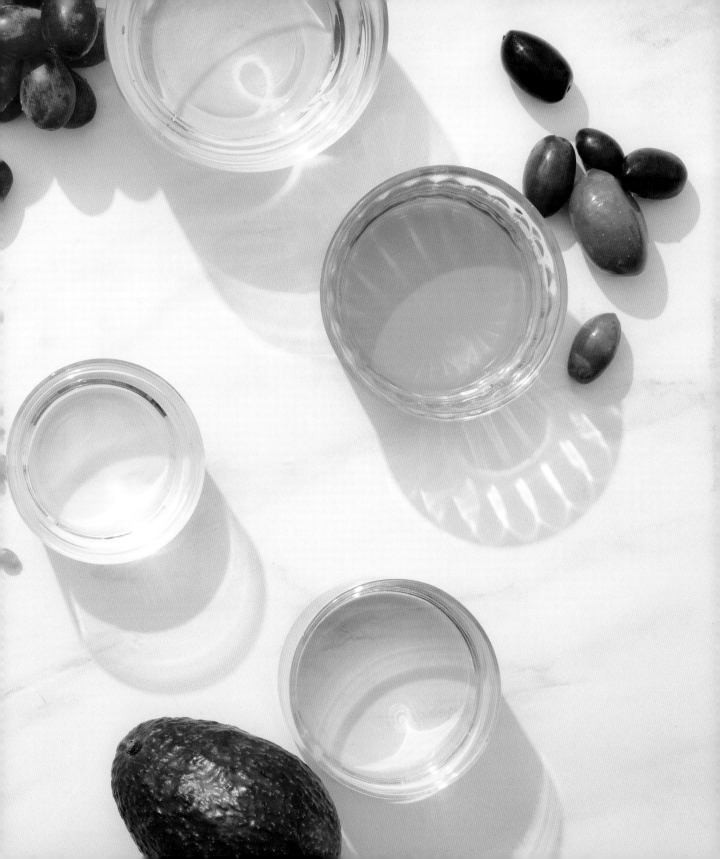

what about milk and dairy products?

Consuming dairy isn't a key or required component for anti-inflammatory eating—but this doesn't mean it's off limits, either. In fact, you may be able to incorporate a few servings of yogurt, cheese, and milk each week if you choose. A 2017 study that reviewed the findings from fifty-two clinical human trials that examined inflammatory blood markers in relation to dairy consumption found the opposite. Consumption of dairy had a weak yet statistically significant anti-inflammatory effect in the body. However, dairy can be inflammatory in anyone with an identified milk allergy, sensitivity, or intolerance, like lactose intolerance.

WHO MIGHT BENEFIT FROM AVOIDING DAIRY?

People with an identified allergy, sensitivity, or intolerance should avoid dairy altogether or, in some cases of lactose intolerance, only consume products that the body is able to digest without producing symptoms. If you suspect a sensitivity, briefly eliminating dairy or following a brief elimination diet (see pages 22–23) may be a good idea. Existing low-grade inflammation in the body tends to make the body hyperactive and sensitive to foods like dairy, and eliminating it can play a key role in reducing that inflammation. This doesn't necessarily mean you'll have to eliminate dairy forever. Once the inflammation in the body has calmed down, slowly add it back and watch for reactions. You may find that your body can tolerate dairy or that it's best to continue avoiding. Note that this is only recommended for a sensitivity and never an allergy.

RECOMMENDATIONS IF YOU NEED TO AVOID DAIRY

- Plant-based milk beverages and yogurts can be great sources of calcium and vitamin D when consumed several times a week. Make sure you have an alternative source of nutrients

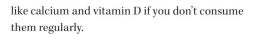

like calcium and vitamin D if you don't consume them regularly.

- A good alternative to butter for many with a dairy intolerance or sensitivity is ghee. Ghee is clarified butter, from which most of the lactose and casein (a milk protein that is often a cause of inflammation) is removed. Ghee isn't dairy-free, though, so it should not be used by those with a dairy allergy.

RECOMMENDATIONS IF YOU DON'T HAVE A KNOWN DAIRY ALLERGY, SENSITIVITY, OR INTOLERANCE

- Yogurt and dairy products with active, live cultures appear to strengthen "leaky" holes in the gut that allow inflammatory irritants into the body, so you might consider incorporating them several times a week as a probiotic source.

- Higher-fat dairy provides satiety but also is a source of saturated fat, which, in excess, causes inflammation. This doesn't mean you have to choose fat-free or low-fat sources but do keep tabs on overall intake if consuming full-fat varieties.

- Choose cheeses with moderate to strong flavors like feta, Parmesan, and blue cheese, where a little goes a long way.

- Plant-based milk beverages and yogurts can be a great source of calcium and vitamin D, even for those who don't have to avoid dairy.

YOUR ANTI-INFLAMMATORY BLUEPRINT FOR OVERALL HEALTH AND WELLNESS

Don't you love a good plan? I do, so that's exactly what I've included below. Here, you'll find a blueprint for an anti-inflammatory diet and lifestyle for overall health and wellness. This plan is focused on reducing inflammation, supporting immune system function, and slowing the aging process. It's appropriate for most all people and ages. This is where I encourage you to start, and it's a solid, effective plan to use long-term.

Overall Diet Emphasis	• Eat to meet personal daily energy and nutrient needs by using the food group recommendations on page 43. • Choose whole or minimally processed food sources (see page 76). • Incorporate gut-promoting foods regularly (see pages 30–33). • Avoid going excessively above personal daily energy needs on a regular basis. • Keep daily sodium to <2300 mg. • Keep daily added sugar intake to ≤25 g for women and ≤36 g for men. • Avoid top inflamers such as processed meats, fried foods, fast food, and highly processed foods. • Avoid foods that trigger a reaction due to an allergy, sensitivity, or intolerance (see page 21).
Key Lifestyle Habits	• Aim for 7 to 9 hours of adequate, restful sleep. • Be active each day. Engage in planned exercise or activity that increases your heart rate several times per week, as well as strength work. • Identify stressors in your life that are ongoing or routinely pop up during the year. Make a plan for how to cope and manage that stress more effectively. • Limit alcoholic drinks (≤1 drink per day for women, ≤2 drinks per day for men).
Other Things to Consider	• Adopt habits to decrease toxins, antibiotics, and hormones in food (see page 24). • Consume food within a daily window of 12 hours or less. • Prioritize organic produce and organic or grass-fed animal proteins when possible. • Incorporate green tea and fermented foods daily (see pages 32–33).

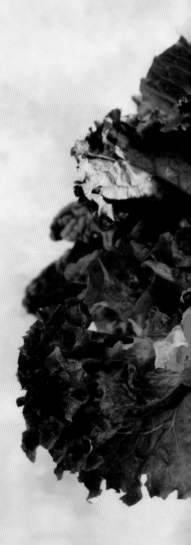

jump start:

WHERE TO START AND WHAT'S MOST IMPORTANT?

So, how do you start your anti-inflammatory journey? The biggest mistake you can make is trying to completely overhaul your diet overnight. Instead, focus on one to three changes. Once you get the hang of those, then tackle a few more. If you need help determining what your initial focus should be, I've got two simple approaches.

Option 1: Keep track of everything you consume for 3 to 4 days. Then compare each day to the daily and weekly eating recommendations above. What are you not getting enough of? What are you getting too much of? What do you think is having the greatest impact on your health? Your biggest issues or priorities are usually apparent. Write them down, and then pick your top two (or two that feel doable) as an initial focus.

Option 2: Another approach (and the one I like best) is to increase your daily consumption of leafy greens, cruciferous vegetables, and berries. Try to hit your daily and weekly goals for each of these, and begin to incorporate healthier oils and fat sources like nuts. While this approach may sound overly simplistic, it usually creates a mindset and eating approach where many of the other recommendations naturally fall into place. Or, it will get you to a place where you are more ready to take a closer look at your diet and health.

Keeping your goals simple and attainable is key. Now, use my tips and tricks in chapter 3 to make achieving those goals easy and stress-free.

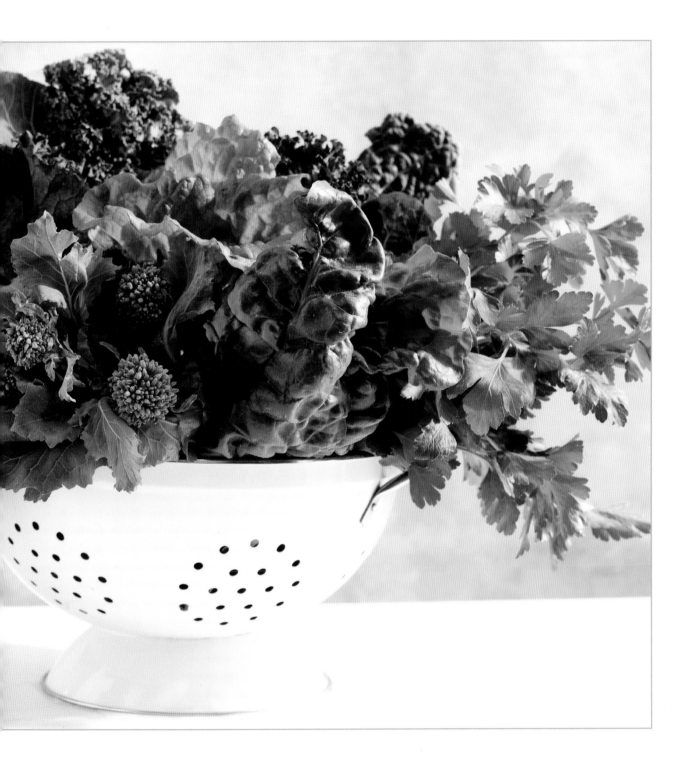

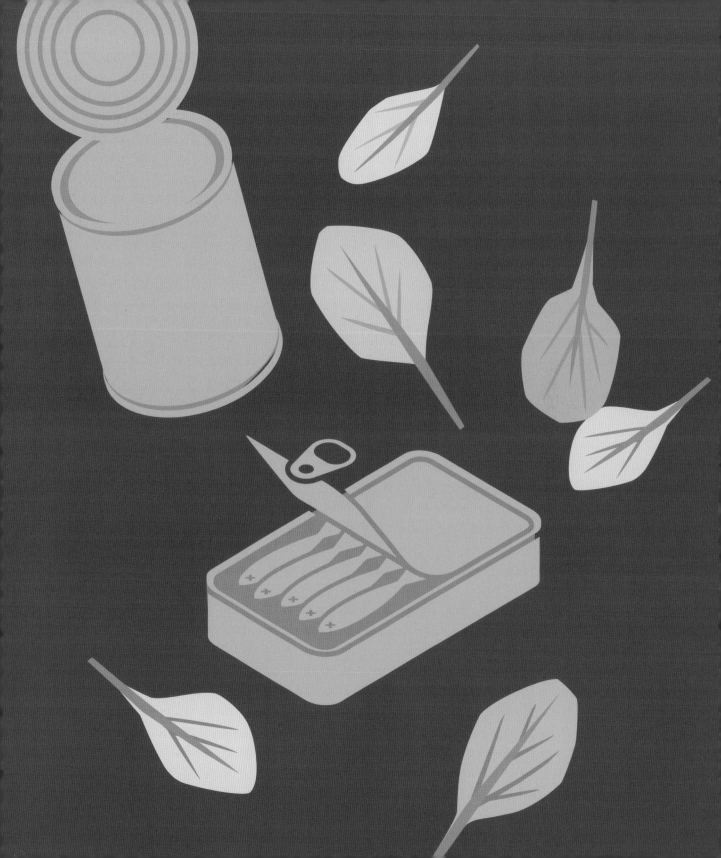

3

SIMPLIFYING MEALS:
*ingredients & tricks
to minimize planning
and prep*

Who's ready to eat? Chapters 1 and 2 threw a lot of information at you, but chapter 3 is all about preparing and eating delicious anti-inflammatory meals—and, even more importantly, making it quick and simple! In this chapter, I'll share my tips, tricks, and shortcuts for how you can make anti-inflammatory eating a realistic, long-term way of life.

my 4-step process for simple, fuss-free anti-inflammatory meals

STEP #1
Plan for Just 30 Minutes

STEP #2
Keep Staple Foods and Ingredients Stocked

STEP #3
Utilize Minimally Processed Shortcuts

STEP #4
Prep 30 to 60 Minutes before the Week Starts

step #1
plan for 30 minutes each week

I've tried all kinds of ways to get around planning, but the reality is this: *You can't cook quick, healthy meals if you don't have a plan and ingredients on hand.* But how do you do that when you don't feel like you have the time or energy? My solution is holding myself accountable to 30 minutes of planning before I grocery shop at the start of the week. While this half-hour may seem minimal or even pointless, I promise it will set you up for smooth sailing in the kitchen all week.

the power of 30 minutes

A while back, I realized my tendency was to skip meal planning altogether if I didn't feel like I had enough time to do it "right." In those instances, I'd try to wing it, which often worked for a day or two before quickly going downhill and ending with me picking up takeout. I needed a solution, so I started making time— just 30 minutes—for planning at the start of the week.

Why 30 minutes? It's an amount of time so small that I knew I wouldn't easily let myself out of doing it. And as it turns out, a small amount of planning time is really all I usually need. Some Sundays, I do just the bare 30-minute minimum, but often I get caught up in perusing recipes (which can even be fun!), and it takes longer. The result is the same: I now have a plan I can use for shopping, so I'm fully prepared for the week ahead.

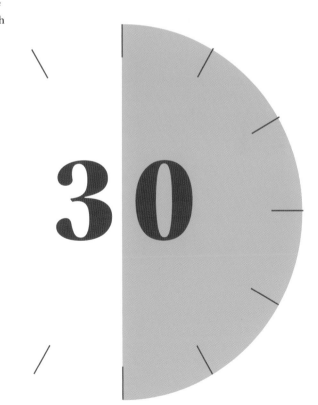

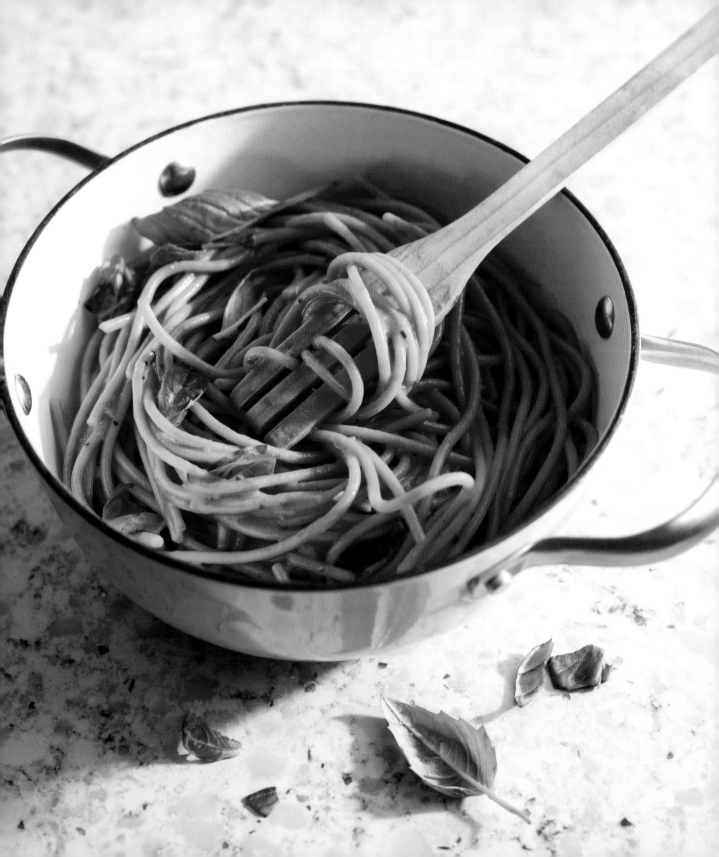

30-minute
planning & shopping checklist

☑ **WHAT'S GOING ON THIS WEEK?**

Look at the upcoming week and determine what nights you're cooking, eating leftovers, or eating out.

☑ **WHAT DO I NEED TO USE UP?**

Consider what perishables you have from the previous week (think refrigerated meat, seafood, and open condiments that have a limited shelf-life, as well as fresh herbs and produce). Don't forget about items you have in the freezer.

☑ **WHAT SHOULD YOU COOK?**

Identify recipes and dishes for the nights you're cooking. I like to plan a mix of tried-and-true dishes and new recipes. I tentatively identify what nights I'm planning to cook specific dishes. However, I recommend being flexible. The goal is getting something healthy on the table, and, some days, that may mean shifting your plan to cook on different days.

TRIED-AND-TRUE DISHES: These are recipes familiar to your family and that you know so well you can prepare them without a recipe (or maybe just a quick glance). Plan these for nights on busier days when you need a quick meal that you don't have to give too much thought to.

NEW RECIPES: Try to incorporate one to two new dishes a week and look for one-dish meals (like ones in this book) to minimize the prep, cooking, and cleanup. Make a note of the ones that are a hit, so you'll remember to plan for them in future weeks. Before you know it, these will become part of your tried-and-true repertoire.

☑ **CREATE YOUR SHOPPING LIST**

_____ What groceries do I need for the meals I planned?

_____ What staples in the pantry, fridge, or freezer are running low?

_____ What else do I need for the week?

_____ Consider breakfasts, snacks, lunches, side dishes, and beverages

_____ Identify any household or pet supplies that are running low

_____ Get input from others in the house—or not!

jump start:

PLAN A MEATLESS MONDAY

Research suggests that everyone benefits from eating more plant foods, and this includes plant-based proteins. This doesn't mean you have to write off animal proteins completely, but it's a good idea to slowly become more plant-forward in your eating approach by incorporating more protein-rich plant foods and reducing your reliance on animal proteins. Planning for Mondays to be meatless is one trick that's helped me get better about eating this way, but you can choose any day of the week.

If you're trying to slowly ease your family (or yourself) into eating meals with more plant-based protein, here are a few good ones to start with that are kid-approved and crowd-pleasers.

(1) Southwestern Caesar Salad (page 97)

(2) Spaghetti alla Vodka (page 195)

(3) White Cheddar–Pumpkin Mac and Cheese (page 196)

(4) Skillet Mexican Rice Casserole (page 205)

(5) Chana Masala (page 210)

(6) Southwestern Kale Salad (page 221, Meatless Main Variation)

(7) Garlic-Rosemary White Bean Soup (page 115)

(8) Chipotle-Lime Lentil Chili (page 119)

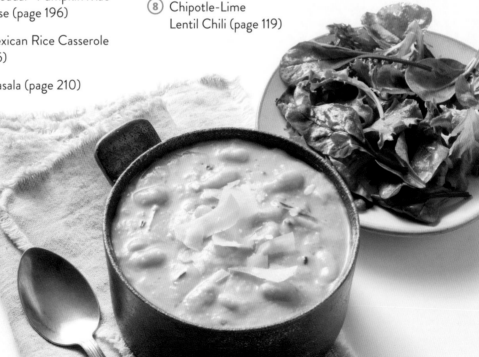

no-time-to-plan shopping list

Sometimes the weekend is so packed that even "just 30 minutes" of planning isn't happening. This is when I skip the planning (at least momentarily), and I use my **No-Time-to-Plan Shopping List**—what I refer to as my grocery list cheat sheet. Even though I haven't identified the recipes or meals that I plan to prepare over the next few days, this list guides me in purchasing smart ingredients that will allow me to plan and cook healthy meals once I do have the time. Think of it as reverse meal planning: Instead of planning meals and then identifying ingredient needs, you're strategically buying ingredients to plan meals around later.

☐ One to two lean proteins (animal or plant-based sources)

☐ One to two containers of leafy greens

☐ Two to three packages of fresh or frozen vegetables to roast or steam (such as broccoli, green beans, carrots)

☐ Two to three fresh fruit options

☐ Refrigerated products we use regularly that may be running low (such as yogurt, milk, eggs)

☐ Items needed for breakfasts, packed lunches, or snacks

☐ Meal shortcuts that may be running low (jarred marinara, tortillas, ready-to-heat grains)

☐ Ingredients for a meal that's quick and easy (such as tacos or breakfast for dinner)

☐ A good quality salad dressing if you aren't sure there's one in the fridge

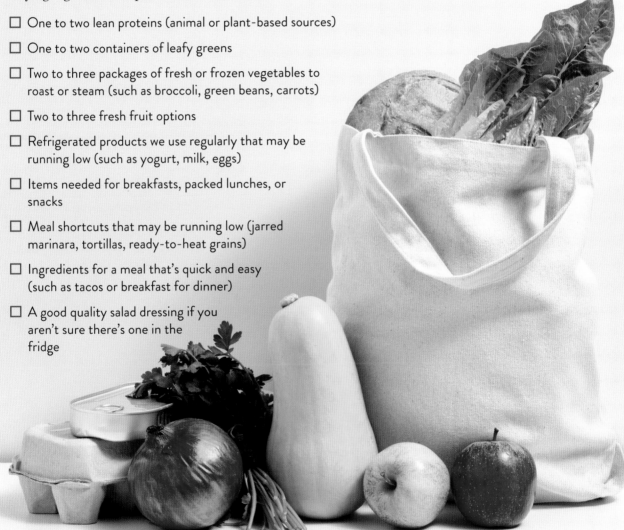

keep staple foods & ingredients stocked

Staple items stocked in the pantry, fridge, and freezer will keep you afloat. These shelf-stable or less perishable basics aren't the most exciting or flashy, but they ensure meal prep goes smoothly. They also provide you with the basics to throw together something quick with little planning.

PANTRY STAPLES

Almond flour	Sesame oil
Beans (all types)	Olives or capers
Broth and stock	Pesto*
Canned pumpkin	Roasted red peppers
Chiles in adobo sauce	Salsa*
Coconut milk	Salt and pepper
Cornstarch	Sriracha
Dijon mustard*	Soy sauce or tamari
Garlic cloves	Tomato products (paste, diced, stewed, whole)
Honey	
Maple syrup	Apple cider vinegar
Mayonnaise*	Red wine vinegar
Extra virgin olive oil	Balsamic or sherry vinegar
Avocado oil	Worcestershire sauce

GRAINS, PANTRY PROTEINS & READY-TO-HEAT OR COOK FOODS

Corn tortillas and taco shells	Whole grains and whole-grain products
Dried fruits	Dry grains (brown rice, oats, quinoa)
Green tea	Ready-to-heat whole grains
Jarred marinara or pasta sauce	Whole-grain or legume-based pastas
Nuts and nut butters	
Salmon or tuna pouches or cans	

Refrigerate after opening

REFRIGERATOR AND FREEZER BASICS	BAKING	DRIED SPICES, HERBS & BLENDS
Butter or ghee	Brown sugar	Cajun or Creole seasoning
Eggs	Baking soda	Chili powder
Fermented foods (see pages 32–33)	Baking powder	Curry powder
Kombucha	Coconut oil	Dried dill
Yogurt	Cream of tartar	Dried rosemary
Sauerkraut	Dark chocolate chips (vegan, if desired)	Gluten-free taco seasoning
Frozen berries	Gluten-free baking flour blend	Granulated garlic powder
Frozen vegetables	Granulated sugar	Greek seasoning
Good quality salad dressings	Pure vanilla extract	Ground cinnamon
Lemons or limes (actual fruit or bottled juice)	Turbinado sugar (optional)	Ground cloves
One hard cheese such as Parmesan and one soft such as goat or feta (optional)	Unsweetened cocoa powder	Ground cumin
		Red pepper flakes
		Smoked paprika
		Thyme

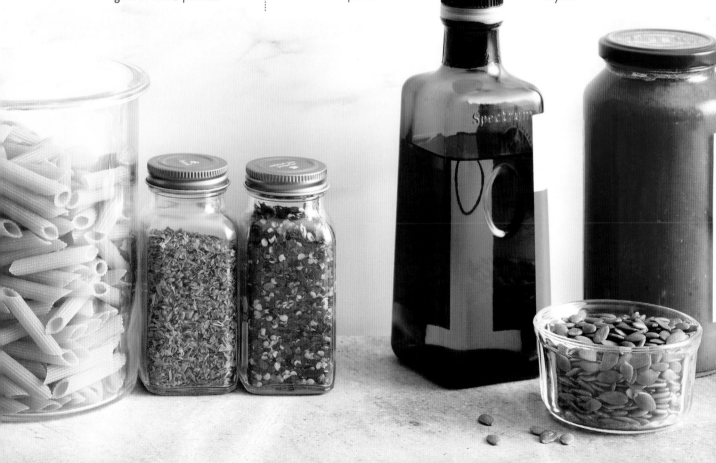

kitchen staples & gadgets

There's nothing more aggravating than kitchen equipment you don't use. But a few really good pieces can make cooking easier and quicker. This isn't meant to be a complete list, but it's a good start!

<table>
<tr><th>KITCHEN STAPLES I CAN'T LIVE WITHOUT</th><th>ONES THAT ARE NICE TO HAVE BUT NOT ESSENTIAL</th></tr>
<tr><td>Blender or food processor</td><td>Air fryer</td></tr>
<tr><td>Can opener</td><td>Immersion blender</td></tr>
<tr><td>Cast-iron skillet</td><td>Instant Pot</td></tr>
<tr><td>Ceramic-coated skillet</td><td>Microplane</td></tr>
<tr><td>Pots and pans (ceramic or stainless)</td><td></td></tr>
<tr><td>Cutting board</td><td></td></tr>
<tr><td>Glass and/or metal measuring cups and spoons</td><td></td></tr>
<tr><td>Good knives</td><td></td></tr>
<tr><td>Metal colander</td><td></td></tr>
<tr><td>Mixing bowls in several sizes</td><td></td></tr>
<tr><td>Reusable glass storage containers</td><td></td></tr>
<tr><td>Sturdy sheet pans</td><td></td></tr>
<tr><td>Twelve-cup muffin pan</td><td></td></tr>
<tr><td>Spiralizer</td><td></td></tr>
<tr><td>Wooden or metal cooking utensils with heat-protective handles</td><td></td></tr>
</table>

jump start:

ORGANIZE & UPDATE YOUR PANTRY TODAY

When's the last time you took a look at everything in your pantry? Here's the approach that I use. I try to do this quarterly or at least twice a year.

1. **ASSESS:** Check the expiration date on refrigerated items and open jars of sauces and condiments. Then check the expiration and use-by dates on dry goods and pantry items.

2. **PURGE:** Toss what is unsafe or past its prime. If it doesn't have a date and you can't recall when you bought it, go ahead and toss it. Going forward, keep a sharpie in a kitchen drawer to quickly note on the packaging or storage container the date that you open bags of dry goods or start to freeze items. Use small filing labels if you don't want to write on containers.

3. **CLEAN:** Wipe down shelves and organize a little while you have items pulled out. If you have multiple items of the same food (such as canned diced tomatoes or black beans), put the newest one at the back, so you'll use the ones you bought earlier first.

4. **RESTOCK:** What's running low and what's well-stocked? Make a list as you restock, so you can freshen up the pantry with nutrient-dense staples that help you pull a meal together quickly.

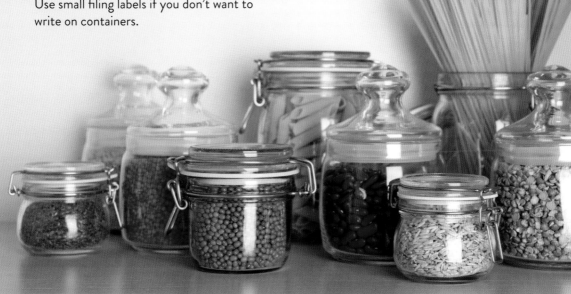

step #3
utilize minimally processed shortcuts

Here's something I cannot stress to you enough: *You do not have to cook everything from scratch to follow an anti-inflammatory eating approach.* In fact, if you visit my house, you will never find homemade almond milk, peanut butter, or yogurt—at least not a version that I made. This isn't to say that homemade isn't superior in quality or taste, but that level of preparation isn't doable (or of interest) for me at this stage in life. If you're in the same boat, that's okay! The good news is that there are lots of minimally processed foods and products on the market today that are close to homemade.

"bad" processed foods

Processed foods are a key inflammatory factor negatively impacting Americans' health. Not only are most people's diets composed primarily of processed foods and very little whole foods, but the processed foods that are the most readily available and inexpensive contain refined and higher-glycemic carbohydrates, added sugars, trans fats, less healthy vegetable oils, and additives like artificial colorings—all dietary inflamers. They also contribute to excess calorie and sodium intake. These processed foods are *not* minimally processed, so I don't suggest using them.

"good" processed foods

Anti-inflammatory eating should be centered around whole foods, so incorporating some processed foods to save time may seem contradictory. However, the term "processing" is broad; it encompasses things we typically think of as processing, like adding sugar and artificial colorings, as well as washing, cutting, and preserving produce. This means minimally processed foods like bagged salad greens, canned tomatoes, frozen berries, milk, and some nut butters can all be part of an anti-inflammatory eating approach. The healthier processed foods that I suggest here don't include any unnecessary or potentially harmful additions. Or, if they contain a small amount of one (such as an added sugar in a salad dressing), it serves a purpose, such as to balance acidic flavors.

MY #1 TIP FOR IDENTIFYING HEALTHIER SHORTCUT FOODS

look at the ingredient list

....

Would you be able to find all of the ingredients in a recipe IF you were making this food from scratch?

IF YES, you may have found a good one. Use the other tips below to help you determine if this is the case.

IF NO, or if the product has additional ingredients listed (particularly ones that you've never heard of or don't have in your kitchen), put it back.

OTHER TIPS FOR IDENTIFYING HEALTHIER PROCESSED FOODS

- For products that are primarily fat-based (such as salad dressing and mayonnaise), choose ones made with higher quality oils like extra virgin olive oil, expeller-pressed canola oil, or avocado oil when possible.

- Avoid products that have trans fats or any type of hydrogenated or partially hydrogenated oil.

- Keep an eye on added sugars per serving in the nutrition facts. Remember that more natural, less refined sugars like honey and maple syrup are still considered added sugars.

- Check the sodium amount and consider how it fits within a daily goal of 2300 mg or less.

- Don't assume labels like *natural, organic, gluten-free,* or *non-GMO* mean that the product is a good choice. Consider the overall quality and health value of the product.

MINIMALLY PROCESSED FOODS
I USE REGULARLY

These are processed foods I use and enjoy regularly, along with brands that I like. The products within each brand family can vary, so use the above tips for identifying healthier minimally processed foods.

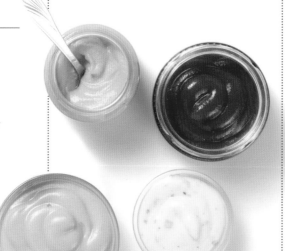

JARRED MARINARA OR PASTA SAUCE

Bertolli

Newman's Own

Primal Kitchen

Rao's Homemade

Simply Nature Organic by ALDI

Thrive Market
365 by Whole Foods

SALAD DRESSINGS

Briannas

Hak's

The New Primal

Primal Kitchen

Sir Kensington's

Newman's Own

Organic Girl

Tessemae's

Whole30

365 by Whole Foods

PEANUT & NUT BUTTERS

Crazy Richard's

MaraNatha

Peanut Butter and Co.

Santa Cruz

Smucker's Natural or Organic

Wild Friends

MAYONNAISE

Chosen Foods

Primal Kitchen

Sir Kensington's

Spectrum

Tessemae's

CONDIMENTS & SAUCES
such as ketchups, mustards & barbecue sauces

Annie's

The New Primal

Primal Kitchen

Tessemae's

365 by Whole Foods

FROZEN MASHED CAULIFLOWER & CAULIFLOWER RISOTTO

Alexia

Birds Eye

Green Giant

Kevin's

365 by Whole Foods

FROZEN VEGETABLES
like broccoli florets, riced cauliflower, green beans & mixed seasoning blends like chopped peppers & onions

No specific brand; choose organic when possible

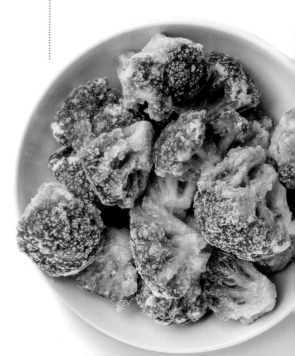

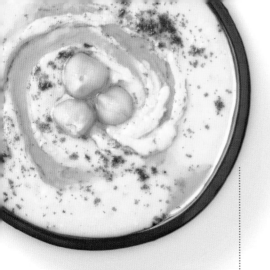

READY-TO-HEAT WHOLE GRAINS & WHOLE-GRAIN BLENDS

No specific brand; choose organic when possible

CORN TORTILLAS

No specific brand; choose organic and 100 percent corn when possible

ORGANIC TACO SEASONING

Primal Palate

Siete Foods

Simply Organic

Thrive Market

Wildtree

BAKING MIXES FOR THINGS LIKE PANCAKES, MUFFINS & PIZZA CRUSTS

Birch Benders

King Arthur Gluten-free

Kodiak Cakes

Krusteaz

Pamela's Baking and Pancake Mix

Purely Elizabeth

Simple Mills

Thrive Market

SALSA

No specific brand; choose organic when possible

HUMMUS & PREPARED GUACAMOLE

No specific brand

CRACKERS & SNACK FOODS

From the Ground Up

Kettle Brand

KIND

Late July

Lesser Evil

Newman's Own

Schär

Simple Mills

Thrive Market

365 by Whole Foods

BREAKFAST FOODS LIKE FROZEN WAFFLES & OATMEAL CUPS

Amy's Kitchen

Applegate Organics

Birch Benders

Bob's Red Mill

Good Food Made Simple

Purely Elizabeth

Van's

PREPARED MEALS OR ENTREES (REFRIGERATED OR FROZEN)

Amy's Kitchen

Blake's All Natural Foods

Cappello's Almond Flour Pasta

Deep Indian Kitchen

Evol

Frontera

Kevin's

Primal Kitchen

Realgood Foods Co.

Saffron Road

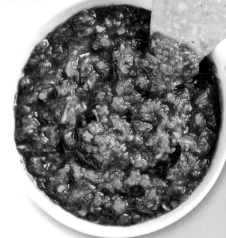

step #4
prep 45 to 60 minutes before the week starts

Being prepared is essential for making healthy food choices, but the concept of meal prepping is something I've never really liked. First, I didn't want to eat the same 1 to 2 dishes for an entire week. But on top of that, I didn't want to spend hours in the kitchen on Sundays.

My solution? I prep ingredients and meal components, not meals. I discovered that prepping a few key items at the start of the week gives me the jumpstart I need to make it even easier to get freshly cooked meals on the table. And, if needed, it also gives me the freedom to veer off plan because I have what I need to throw a quick meal together without a recipe (see **Quick Meals Using Prepped Ingredients and Kitchen Staples, page 83**). Think of it as ingredient prep, not meal prep.

how I prep for the week

I'll try to prepare (or make sure I have on hand) at least one quick protein, complex carb, and low-carb substitute. I also stock up veggies that I can eat raw or quickly cook before a meal. If I've got a little extra time, I'll roast some veggies and maybe even make a grain salad, chicken salad, or soup to have on hand for quick lunches. Any meals that I cook in advance I'll refrigerate in sealed containers. Then, I'll reheat as needed to add to main dishes, turn into a side dish, or create an impromptu grain bowl or salad. But if you're short on prep time, there are options where your only prep work is making sure you have them on hand!

- **A QUICK PROTEIN:** Season and cook one protein (outside of the recipes you're already planned) or make sure you have an extra protein on hand that cooks in 5 minutes or less (like shrimp, eggs, or beans) at the start of the week. While I don't recommend cooking fish in advance as part of meal prep, it's a great protein to keep on hand since it can quickly be cooked in the oven or skillet right before meals.

- **A COMPLEX CARB AND/OR LOW-CARB VEGGIE SUBSTITUTE:** Cook and refrigerate a whole-grain and/or a vegetable that can substitute as a lower-carb option for pasta or rice. Cooked whole grains keep well in the refrigerator for up to 7 days; cooked spaghetti squash strands refrigerate well for up to 3 days. Hold off cooking zucchini or butternut "noodles" and cauliflower "rice" until just before meals. Short on time? Stock up on ready-to-heat whole grains and frozen lower-carb substitutes.

	QUICK PROTEINS	COMPLEX CARBS OR LOW-CARB SUBSTITUTES	QUICK VEGGIES
Foods to cook and refrigerate	Chicken breasts or thighs (whole, shredded, or cut in pieces) Flank steak or other lean beef cut (thinly sliced) Pork tenderloin or loin (sliced or shredded)	Kid-friendly whole grains like brown rice, wild rice, and quinoa More adventurous whole grains like farro, amaranth, freekeh, and bulgur Spaghetti squash	Roasted vegetables (one vegetable or an assortment) Kid-friendly, lightly steamed and seasoned vegetables like broccoli, carrots, peas, and green beans
Foods to have on hand (and possibly thaw) that cook super-fast or don't need cooking	Canned beans Deli rotisserie chicken Eggs Fish (fresh or frozen) Frozen edamame Pouches or cans of salmon or tuna Shrimp (fresh or frozen) Tofu	Fresh cauliflower (florets or riced) Frozen riced cauliflower Frozen mashed cauliflower Frozen whole grains and whole-grain pilafs Ready-to-heat whole grains Zucchini or butternut squash (spirals or whole)	Baby carrots Cherry tomatoes Cucumbers Fresh or frozen broccoli, green beans, carrots, and sugar snap peas Prepared salad greens

soup and salad recipes that keep for 3 to 4 days

Consider preparing a salad or soup at the start of a busy week when you have extra prep time. Here are some recipes that hold or reheat well:

1. Chicken-Broccoli Slaw with Peanut Dressing (page 104)

2. Mediterranean Quinoa Salad (page 94)

3. Rosemary Chicken Salad (page 98)

4. Shaved Brussels Slaw (page 222)

5. Southwestern Kale Salad (page 221)

6. Tex-Mex Tuna Salad (page 101)

7. Tomato, Cucumber, and Chickpea Salad (page 225)

8. Chipotle-Lime Lentil Chili (page 119)

9. Creamy Buffalo Chicken Soup (page 122)

10. Creamy Southwestern Beef Soup (page 130)

11. Creamy Wild Rice and Chicken Soup (page 127)

12. Curried Butternut Soup with Spinach (page 116)

13. Garlic-Rosemary White Bean Soup (page 115)

14. Chile Verde with Shredded Pork (page 128)

15. Pesto Zoodle Chicken Soup (page 120)

16. Zuppa Toscano (page 124)

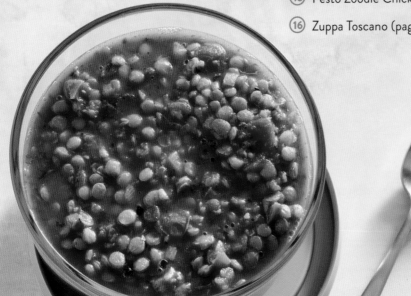

QUICK MEALS USING
PREPPED INGREDIENTS & KITCHEN STAPLES

Sometimes my best (and quickest) creations in the kitchen occur when I'm forced by necessity to find ways to combine staples in my pantry, fridge, and freezer. Here are some ideas for how to combine ingredients you may have on hand.

INGREDIENTS	ALMOST-INSTANT MEAL
Tofu + Frozen veggies + Brown or cauliflower rice + Soy sauce + Sesame oil	Tofu stir-fry
Eggs + Black beans + Cheese + Fresh veggies (like tomatoes, baby spinach) + Salsa	Southwestern scramble
Brown rice or quinoa + Leafy greens + Canned bean or protein + Nut or dried fruit + Bottled vinaigrette or sauce	Greens or grains bowl
Corn tortillas + Baby spinach + Black beans + Cheese + Salsa	Spinach and black bean quesadillas
Zucchini noodles (or pasta) + Frozen shrimp + Pesto + Cherry tomatoes + Shaved hard cheese	Pesto zoodles with shrimp
Spaghetti squash + Taco meat + Cherry tomatoes or salsa + Guacamole	Spaghetti squash taco bowl
Canned tuna + Brown rice + Soy sauce + Cherry tomatoes + Avocado + Scallions + Sesame seeds (if on hand)	Tuna poke bowl

nutrition information about these one-pot recipes

Most of the entrée recipes are designed to stand alone by providing adequate protein, fiber, and healthy fats to provide satiety and at least one serving of vegetables. Here are a few things to know when meal planning and preparing the recipes.

- **NUTRIENT VALUES:** Some nutrient values, such as calories, fat, and sodium, may be higher than "healthy" recipes from other sources, but this is because the nutrients per serving technically represent a whole meal, as opposed to an entrée that also has one to two side dishes served with it. Rather than focusing on individual numbers, consider how the meal will fit within a day, particularly when it comes to sodium. The goal for most is to keep sodium intake to less than 2300 mg per day, and all of the recipes can easily fit within this, leaving you a large window to accommodate other meals and snacks.

- **MEETING NUTRIENT NEEDS:** Adding a serving of fresh fruit, nuts, vegetables, whole grains, or salad greens is a great way to make meals more filling and help you meet nutrient needs. Nutrient-dense snacks are also great ways to boost produce intake and keep you satisfied between meals. Need some ideas for quick sides or snacks? Check out the sides and snacks listed in the meal plans on pages 85 to 91 that provide low-carb, moderate-carb, and vegetarian or vegan food options.

- **ALL RECIPES ARE GLUTEN-FREE:** All of the recipes are designed to be prepared gluten-free. If you follow a gluten-free diet, make sure you purchase certified gluten-free options for foods such as soy sauce and oats. It's also a good idea to check the allergen list (below the list of ingredients on the Nutrition Facts panel) to confirm there is no gluten or wheat in the food.

- **MOST RECIPES CAN BE PREPARED DAIRY-FREE:** The majority of the recipes are either dairy-free or provide a dairy-free variation. While I don't think I could ever completely give up cheese, I try to be very cognizant of the fact that many people may need to follow a dairy-free diet (my son included), so the usage of dairy products is very limited (I've only used it when the recipe just wasn't quite the same without it).

meal plans

How do you put the recipes and eating recommendations all together to create an anti-inflammatory eating diet on a daily and weekly basis? This is a question I often get, so I've created three sets of menu plans— Low-Carb, Moderate-Carb, and Vegetarian—to get you started. These plans will get you started and give you the practice to then create your own. Remember, there is no right or wrong way to do it as long as you're following the general recommendations for an anti-inflammatory diet.

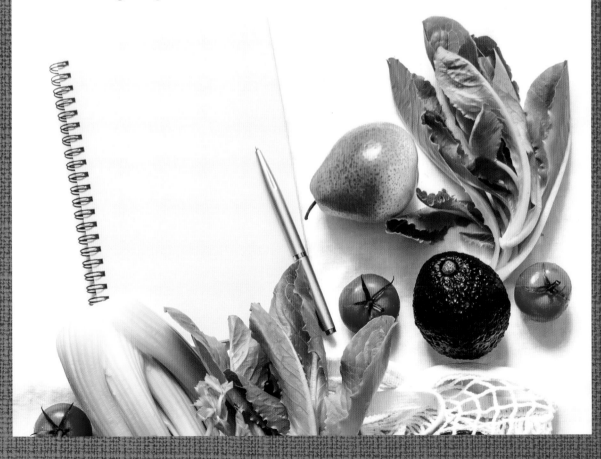

low-carb meal plan

This meal plan is designed to support lower-carbohydrate eating approaches, which vary in total carbohydrates or net carbohydrates (total carbohydrates less fiber) consumed each day. The daily menus include two meal ideas and one snack idea with daily totals that range from 16 to 26 grams net carbohydrates. But these menus are not designed to stand alone. Rather, they are designed to provide a solid foundation to which you can then add additional healthy sides, snacks, and/or breakfasts to meet your nutrient needs and fruit and vegetable goals, supporting intakes that may range from 30 to 65 grams daily net carbohydrates.

See pages 53–55 for information on Lower Carb Eating Approaches and tips for determining if this may be beneficial for you. The net carb value of each recipe and snack idea is provided within the menu plan. Ideas for additional sides and snacks are also provided.

	monday	tuesday
meal #1	Rosemary Chicken Salad, page 98 (NC: 3 g)	Easy Greek Frittata with Balsamic Tomatoes, page 102 (NC: 5 g)
meal #2	Fork-and-Knife Cauliflower Nachos, page 192 (NC: 13 g)	Hoisin Salmon with Warm Broccoli-Edamame Slaw, page 166 (NC: 10 g)
snack ideas	½ cup (46 g) sliced red pepper with 3 tablespoons hummus (NC: 7 g)	¼ cup (33 g) mixed nuts combined with 3 tablespoons unsweetened coconut chips or flakes (NC: 8 g)

side dish ideas
(≤8 g net carbs)

Cooked spaghetti squash
Frozen cauliflower rice or risotto
Frozen mashed cauliflower
Greens tossed with vinaigrette
Steamed or roasted vegetables (such as broccoli, brussels sprouts, green beans, summer squash, zucchini)
Zucchini spirals

NC: Net carbohydrates per serving

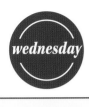 wednesday	thursday	friday	saturday	sunday
Avocado-Feta Shrimp Toss, page 109 (NC: 4 g)	Tex-Mex Tuna Salad, page 101 (NC: 13 g)	Chicken-Broccoli Slaw with Peanut Dressing, page 104 (NC: 10 g)	Thai-Inspired Beef Salad, page 110 (NC: 9 g)	Creamy Buffalo Chicken Soup, page 122 (NC: 10 g)
Sheet Pan Beef and Broccoli, page 149 (NC: 9 g)	Pan-Fried Chicken over Lemony Greens, page 136 (NC: 9 g)	Seared Tuna over Ginger-Soy Spinach and Avocado, page 170 (NC: 8 g)	Muffin Pan Pesto Turkey Meatloaves, page 145 (NC: 2 g)	Pork Piccata over Zoodles, page 159 (NC: 5 g)
⅔ cup (69 g) cucumber slices with ¼ cup (60 ml) yogurt-based tzatziki dip (NC: 6 g)	8 baby carrots with a single-serve (0.8 ounce/23 g) guacamole (NC: 4 g)	¼ cup (35 g) roasted almonds and a square (0.375 ounce/11g) of dark chocolate (NC: 7 g)	½ cup (45 g) toasted edamame (NC: 5 g)	⅔ cup (82 g) raspberries and a part-skim mozzarella stick (NC: 5 g)

snack dish ideas
(≤8 g net carbs)

Celery with almond or peanut butter

Cheese and nuts

Hard-boiled eggs

Lightly salted or seasoned nuts

Nut butters

Olives

side dish & snack recipes
(≤8 g net carbs)

Caprese Zoodles (page 229)

Charred Sriracha Green Beans (page 233)

Jalapeño Popper Zucchini Boats (page 242)

Lemony Arugula Salad with Parmesan (page 215)

Lima Bean Hummus with Cucumber Slices (page 248)

Marinated Feta-Veggie Skewers (page 252)

Roasted Parmesan Zucchini (page 230)

Rosemary-Parmesan Cauliflower Crisps (page 255)

Twice-Baked Cauliflower Casserole (page 241)

Wild Mushroom "Risotto" (page 234)

moderate-carb meal plan

This meal plan is designed to support an eating approach that is moderate in carbohydrate intake. It's substantially lower in carbohydrates than the average American diet yet still falls within the lower end of carbohydrate intake suggested by dietary guidelines. The daily menus include two meal ideas and one snack idea with daily totals that range from 42 to 52 grams net carbohydrates. But these menus are not designed to stand alone. Rather, they are designed to provide a solid foundation to which you can add additional healthy sides, snacks, and/or breakfasts to meet your nutrient needs and fruit and vegetable goals, supporting intakes that may range from 65 to 130 grams daily net carbohydrates. These menus can also be used as a foundation for those with higher carbohydrate needs who want to follow a lower-carb approach.

Low to moderate carbohydrate eating approaches vary greatly, and this is explained further on page 53. The net carb value of each recipe and snack idea is provided within the menu plan, and ideas for additional sides and snacks are listed below the meal plan.

	monday	tuesday
meal #1	Tomato, Cucumber, and Chickpea Salad, page 225 (Double portion, NC: 18 g)	Chicken-Broccoli Slaw with Peanut Dressing, page 104 (NC: 10 g)
meal #2	Balsamic-Rosemary Pork with Green Beans, page 156 (NC: 9 g)	Honey-Dijon Sheet Pan Salmon, page 169 (NC: 25 g)
snack ideas	½ large apple with 3 tablespoons almond butter (NC: 15 g)	½ cup (120 ml) low-sugar flavored Greek yogurt (such as Two Good) with ½ cup (74 g) blueberries (NC: 12 g)

side dish ideas
(9 to 20 g net carbs)

Cooked whole grains like quinoa

Fresh fruit

Greens tossed with vinaigrette and topped with fresh or dried fruit

Smashed or refried black beans

Sweet or small red potatoes

Sweet potato fries

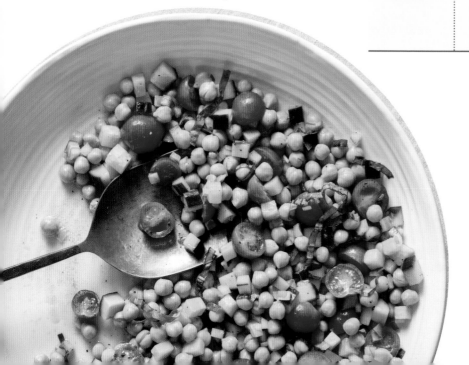

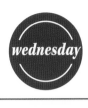wednesday	thursday	friday	saturday	sunday
Open-Faced Black Bean Burgers, page 202 (NC: 27 g)	Tex-Mex Tuna Salad, page 101 (NC: 13 g)	Zuppa Toscano, page 124 (NC: 16 g)	Southwestern Caesar Salad, page 97 (NC: 22 g)	Easy Greek Frittata with Balsamic Tomatoes, page 102 (NC: 5 g)
Pan-Fried Chicken over Lemony Greens, page 136 (NC: 9 g)	Chana Masala, page 210 (NC: 24 g)	Spaghetti Squash Pad Thai with Shrimp, page 174 (NC: 15 g)	Tzatziki "Rice" Bowls with Gyro Meatballs, page 154 (NC: 9 g)	Semi-Homemade Bolognese with Zoodles, page 146 (NC: 27 g)
⅓ cup (44 g) trail mix with ≤2 g of added sugar per serving (NC: 15 g)	A fruit and nut bar (such as KIND) with ≤5 g of added sugar (NC: 9 to 15 g)	A hard-boiled egg sprinkled with everything bagel seasoning and an orange (NC: 13 g)	¼ cup (35 g) toasted almonds and ½ cup (74 g) blueberries (NC: 12 g)	1 cup (240 ml) low-sodium vegetable soup with 8 grain-free crackers (NC: 15 g)

snack ideas
(9 to 20 g net carbs)

Air-popped popcorn

Berries, cantaloupe, and honeydew

Cherry tomatoes with fresh mozzarella

Grain-free crackers and cheese

Guacamole with gluten-free pretzels

Lightly salted nuts

Toasted edamame

Yogurt

side dish & snack recipes
(9 to 20 g net carbs)

Crispy Ranch Chickpeas (page 250)

Lower-Carb Mashed Potatoes (page 238)

Mango Salsa (page 247) with 100 percent corn or grain-free tortilla chips

Peanut Butter–Banana Smoothie (page 257)

Roasted Rosemary Butternut Squash (page 236)

Street Corn Salad (page 226)

Tomato, Cucumber, and Chickpea Salad (page 225)

Winter Greens with Maple-Cider Vinaigrette (page 218)

Also see the side and snack recipes suggested in the low-carb meal plan (page 87), which contain ≤8 g net carbs.

vegetarian meal plan

This meal plan is designed to support various types of vegetarian eating approaches by focusing on plant-based proteins for adequate nutrients. A few of the recipes contain dairy and/or eggs as written, but most provide dairy-free and/or vegan variations. For the side and snack ideas, make sure to check labels to ensure the product meets your specific vegetarian eating approach, as this can vary among brands.

The daily menus include two meal ideas and one snack idea. But these menus are not designed to stand alone. Rather, they are designed to provide a solid foundation to which you then add additional healthy sides, snacks, and/or breakfasts to meet your nutrient needs and fruit and vegetable goals.

	monday	**tuesday**
meal #1	Garlic-Rosemary White Bean Soup, page 115 (V)	Mediterranean Quinoa Salad, page 94 (V)
meal #2	Roasted Fall Vegetable Grain Bowl, page 199 (V)	Spaghetti alla Vodka, page 195 (V)
snack ideas	Hummus with baby carrots (V)	Frozen grapes and roasted almonds (V)

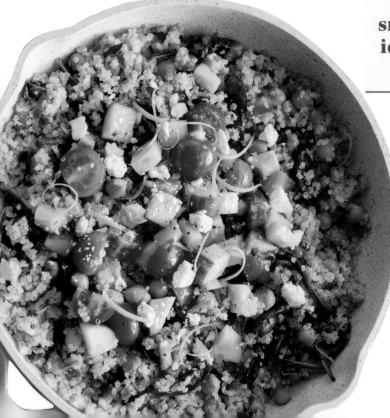

side dish ideas

Beans

Cooked whole grains

Fresh fruit

Frozen cauliflower rice

Greens tossed with vinaigrette and topped with nuts and/or fruit

Spaghetti squash

Steamed or roasted vegetables

Sweet or small red potatoes

Zucchini spirals

NC: Net carbohydrates per serving

DF: Indicates the recipe or food can be prepared or purchased dairy-free vegetarian

V: Indicates the recipe or food can be prepared or purchased containing no animal products and is vegan

wednesday	thursday	friday	saturday	sunday
Open-Faced Black Bean Burgers, page 202 (V)	Southwestern Kale Salad, page 221 (Meatless Main Variation, V)	Greek Fried Quinoa, page 200 (V)	Fork-and-Knife Cauliflower Nachos, page 192	Easy Greek Frittata with Balsamic Tomatoes, page 102 (DF)
Chipotle-Lime Lentil Chili, page 119 (V)	Instant Pot Hoppin' John, page 206 (V)	Wild Mushroom "Risotto," page 234 (double portion, DF) Lemony Arugula Salad with Parmesan, page 215 (DF or V)	Semi-Homemade Bolognese with Zoodles, page 146 (Vegetarian Option, V)	Chana Masala, page 210 (V)
Guacamole with gluten-free pretzels and blueberries (V)	Vanilla soy yogurt with walnuts and maple syrup drizzle (V)	Toasted edamame and a pear (V)	Small bowl of oatmeal with fruit and/or nuts (V)	An apple or pear with almond or nut butter (V)

snack ideas

Air-popped popcorn or grain-free crackers

Baked kale, cauliflower, or sweet potato chips

Fresh fruit

Fruit and nut bar with less than 5 g added sugar

Guacamole with gluten-free pretzels

Lightly salted or seasoned nuts

Small bowl of low-sodium vegetable or black bean soup

Small bowl of oatmeal with nuts and/or fruit

Soy or other dairy-free yogurt

Toasted edamame

vegetarian side dish & snack recipes

Charred Sriracha Green Beans (page 233)

Cold Brew Breakfast Smoothie (page 256)

Crispy Ranch Chickpeas (page 250)

Lemony Arugula Salad with Parmesan (page 215)

Lima Bean Hummus with baby carrots (page 248)

Lower-Carb Mashed Potatoes (page 238)

Mango Salsa (page 247) with tortilla chips

Peanut Butter–Banana Smoothie (page 257)

Roasted Rosemary Butternut Squash (page 236)

Shaved Brussels Slaw (page 222)

Southwestern Kale Salad (page 221)

Strawberry-Mango Green Smoothie (page 256)

Summer Salad with Lime-Basil Vinaigrette (page 217)

Tomato, Cucumber, and Chickpea Salad (page 225)

Winter Greens with Maple-Cider Vinaigrette (page 218)

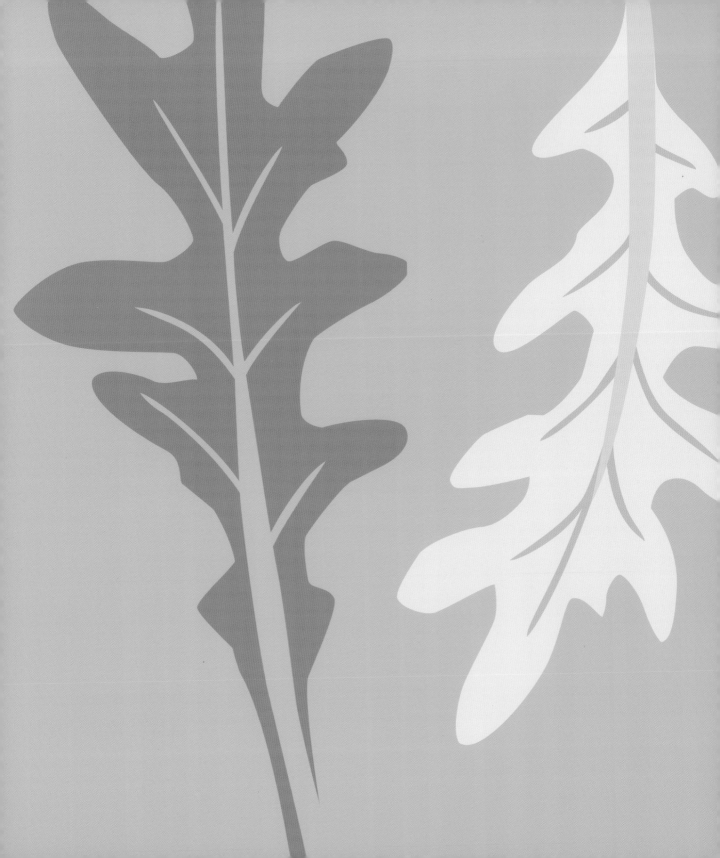

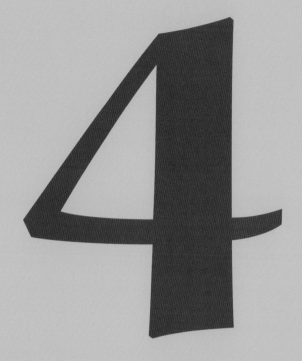

TOSS & GO MEALS

Gf
gluten-free

Ve
vegetarian

Df
dairy-free*

Nc
no cook

Pa
prep ahead

mediterranean quinoa salad

HANDS-ON: 15 MINUTES :: TOTAL: 15 MINUTES :: SERVES 5

The flavor of this salad gets better each day, so using a hearty whole grain like quinoa is key since it will hold its shape and texture if you want to prep ahead. And since the serving options for this salad are endless, these leftovers are far from boring. Serve it over crisp lettuce for a filling plant-based meal. Or top it with leftover grilled shrimp or chicken or stir in drained canned tuna for a little more protein.

1 Combine the quinoa, chickpeas, tomatoes, cucumber, onion, basil, salt, and pepper in a large bowl, tossing to combine.

2 In a small bowl, whisk together the vinaigrette and lemon juice. Add the dressing and cheese to the quinoa, tossing gently to combine all ingredients.

3 Store in an airtight container in the refrigerator for up to five days. Serve over a bed of chopped romaine lettuce.

NUTRITION FACTS (SERVING SIZE: 1½ CUPS/289 G): CALORIES 335; FAT 14 G (SAT 3 G); PROTEIN 11 G; CARB 40 G; FIBER 7 G; SUGARS 4 G (ADDED SUGARS 0 G); SODIUM 397 MG

TIP You can cook a batch of quinoa at the start of the week and then refrigerate it to use in a quick whole-grain salad like this one or serve as a warm side dish. No time to cook a batch in advance? Pick up a pouch of ready-to-heat quinoa instead of cooking! Microwave the pouch according to package directions; then, allow the quinoa to cool to room temperature before adding it to the salad.

DAIRY-FREE/VEGAN OPTION Omit the feta cheese. Before serving, gently fold in ½ cup (74 g) diced avocado.

Ingredients

3 cups (555 g) cooked quinoa, chilled

One 15-ounce (425 g) can no-salt-added chickpeas, rinsed and drained

1 cup (149 g) cherry tomatoes, quartered

1 cup (133 g) diced cucumber

¼ cup (40 g) finely chopped red onion

⅓ cup (14 g) chopped fresh basil

½ teaspoon salt

½ teaspoon black pepper

⅓ cup (80 ml) bottled olive oil vinaigrette

1 tablespoon lemon juice

⅓ cup (50 g) crumbled feta

Chopped romaine lettuce

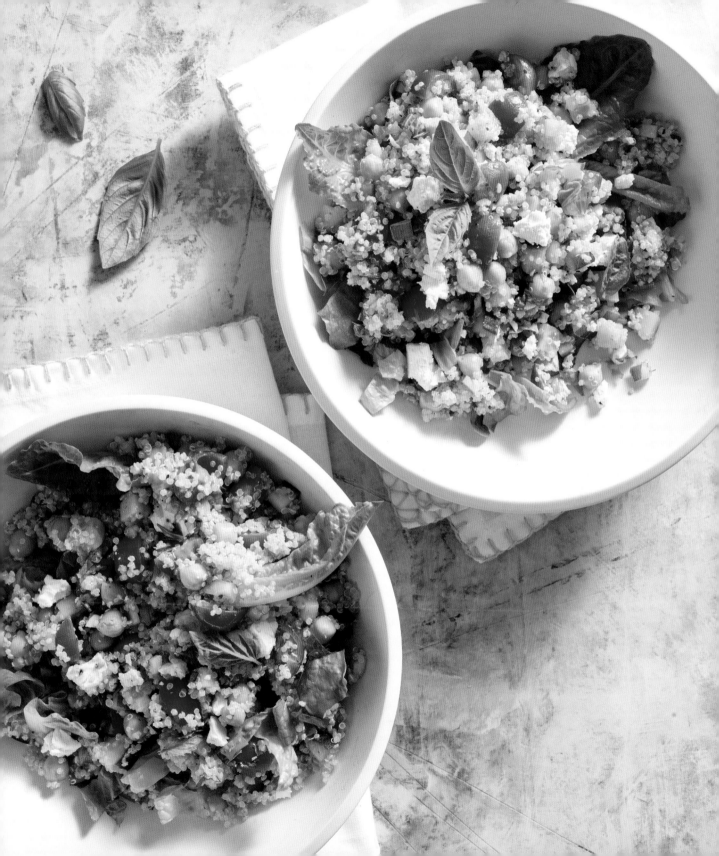

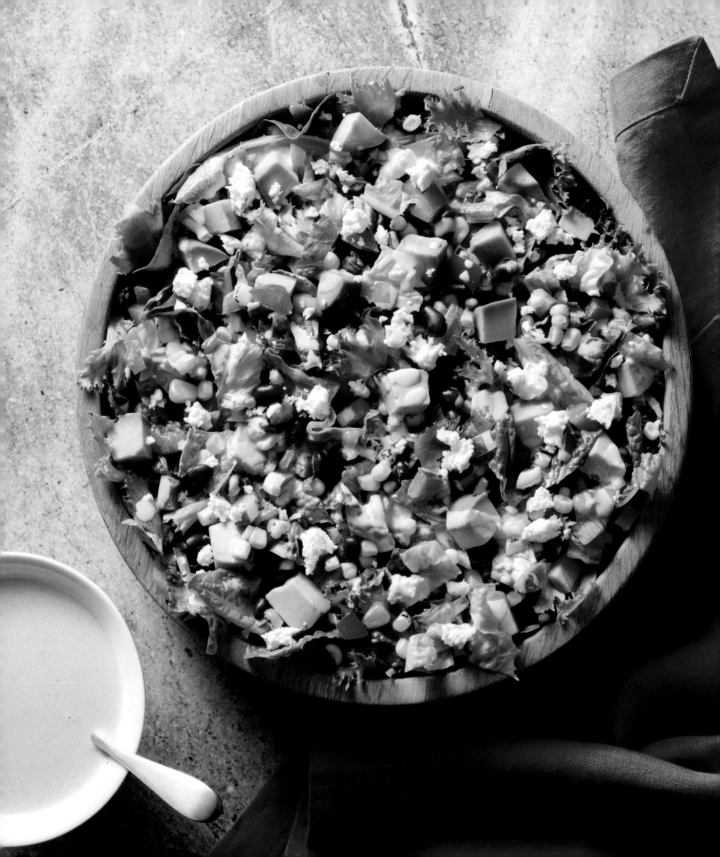

southwestern caesar salad

HANDS-ON: 15 MINUTES :: TOTAL: 15 MINUTES :: SERVES 4

Chipotle chile peppers in adobo sauce are a great way to add smoky depth and a subtle spicy-sweet flavor to sauces, marinades, dressings, and dishes. Recipes rarely call for the whole can, so there are a few ways to store the leftover to prevent it from going to waste. You can freeze whatever's left in a freezer-safe container. Then, thaw before using. Or puree the peppers with the sauce in a small food processor or blender to create a paste. Then, dollop the paste by tablespoons onto a small sheet pan lined with parchment paper and freeze. Once frozen, place the dollops into a freezer-safe container.

1 Combine the yogurt, mayonnaise, vinegar, soy sauce, chipotle sauce, and honey in a small bowl. Cover and refrigerate until ready to use.

2 Assemble the salad by combining the lettuce, black beans, corn, red pepper, onion, and cheese. To serve, add the avocado and dressing, tossing gently to combine. Serve immediately.

NUTRITION FACTS (SERVING SIZE: ¼ OF SALAD): CALORIES 308; FAT 16 G (SAT 3.5 G); PROTEIN 12 G; CARB 31 G; FIBER 9 G; SUGARS 7 G (ADDED SUGARS 1 G); SODIUM 432 MG

TIP Roasting or lightly charring corn kernels in a skillet adds color and flavor, and frozen roasted corn kernels are readily available in the freezer section at most grocery stores. Using a frozen version is an easy way to save time, but it's also easy to roast your own! Lightly coat a skillet with cooking spray, then place over medium-high heat; add fresh corn kernels or thawed frozen corn kernels. Cook, stirring frequently, until browned and beginning to char, 3 to 5 minutes.

DAIRY-FREE OPTION Use an equivalent amount of a plain nondairy yogurt alternative made with almond, cashew, or other plant-based milk in place of the Greek yogurt. Omit the cheese and sprinkle the salad with ¼ cup (30 g) toasted pepitas (pumpkin seeds) before serving.

¼ cup (61 g) low-fat plain Greek yogurt

¼ cup (60 g) olive or avocado oil-based mayonnaise

2 tablespoons rice vinegar

1 tablespoon lower-sodium soy sauce or tamari

1 tablespoon sauce from chipotle chiles in adobo

1 teaspoon honey

4 cups (188 g) chopped romaine lettuce

One 15-ounce (425 g) can black beans, rinsed and drained

1 cup (145 g) frozenroasted corn kernels, thawed

½ cup (75 g) diced red bell pepper

⅓ cup (53 g) diced red onion

½ cup (61 g) crumbled cotija or feta

1 avocado, diced

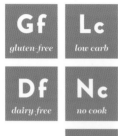

Gf gluten-free **Lc** low carb

Df dairy free **Nc** no cook

 Pa prep ahead

rosemary chicken salad

HANDS-ON: 12 MINUTES :: TOTAL: 12 MINUTES :: SERVES 5

Rosemary Chicken Salad is one of my favorite meals to prep before heading into a busy week. Quickly warming the rosemary in a little olive oil before adding it to the dressing is my secret trick for giving this salad an amazing depth of fresh herb flavor. It also keeps well in the refrigerator for up to three days.

1 Combine the oil and rosemary in a small microwave-safe bowl. Microwave on high for 30 seconds, stirring after 15 seconds.

2 In a large bowl, stir together the mayonnaise, lemon juice, garlic powder, and rosemary oil. Add the chicken, stirring to coat with the mayonnaise mixture. Add the grapes, onions, and almonds, mixing to combine well. Refrigerate, covered, until ready to serve.

NUTRITION FACTS (SERVING SIZE: ½ CUP/97 G): CALORIES 192; FAT 11 G (SAT 1.5 G); PROTEIN 18 G; CARB 4 G; FIBER 1 G; SUGARS 3 G (ADDED SUGARS 0 G); SODIUM 234 MG

TIP A rotisserie chicken is an easy way to get 3 to 4 cups (420 to 560 g) of chopped cooked chicken breast fast! Remove the skin before shredding or chopping, and store extra in the refrigerator for another meal or to use in Chicken-Broccoli Slaw with Peanut Dressing (page 104) or Cheesy Chicken, Broccoli, and "Rice" Casserole (page 134).

1 tablespoon extra virgin olive oil

2 teaspoons chopped fresh rosemary

¼ cup (60 g) olive or avocado oil-based mayonnaise

2 teaspoons lemon juice

¼ teaspoon garlic powder

2 cups (280 g) chopped cooked chicken breast

½ cup (76 g) seedless red grapes, halved

¼ cup (25 g) chopped scallions

3 tablespoons sliced almonds, toasted

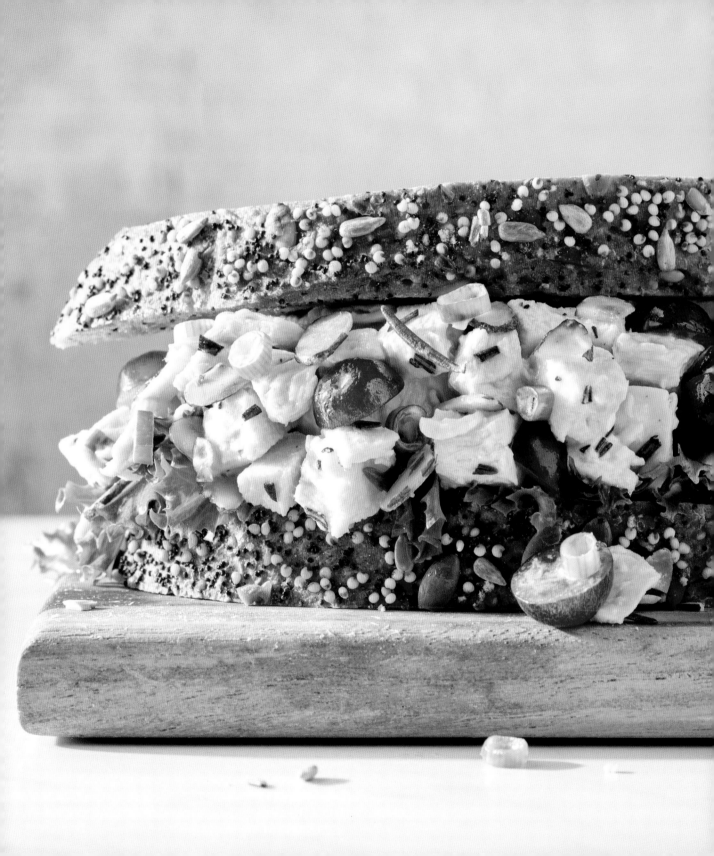

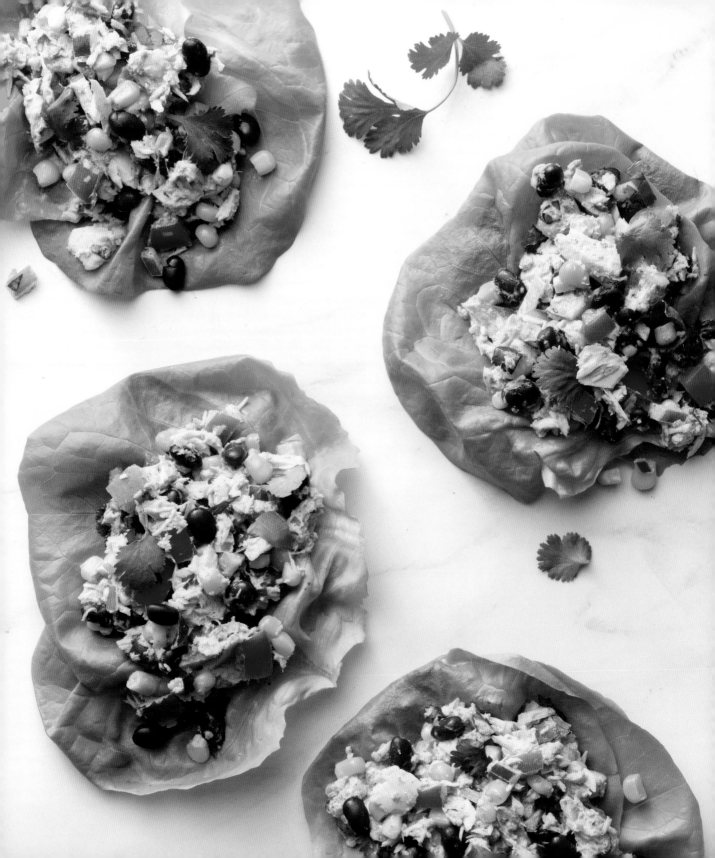

tex-mex tuna salad

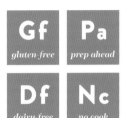

A little lime juice, taco seasoning, and olive oil mayonnaise are all that's needed to create a quick Southwestern-inspired dressing. For an added kick of flavor and spice, use a chipotle-flavored mayonnaise and decrease the amount of taco seasoning to 1 ½ teaspoons. I've found that chipotle mayonnaises vary greatly in their seasoning levels, so you can always add more seasoning later if needed. Serve over salad greens or as a filling for crisp romaine lettuce wraps.

1 Combine the tuna, beans, corn, tomato, avocado, onion, and cilantro in a large bowl.

2 In a small bowl, whisk together the mayonnaise, lime juice, and taco seasoning. Add to the tuna mixture and toss gently to fully combine.

NUTRITION FACTS (SERVING SIZE: ABOUT 1 CUP/227 G): CALORIES 260; FAT 13 G (SAT 1.5 G); PROTEIN 19 G; CARB 18 G; FIBER 5 G; SUGARS 3 G (ADDED SUGARS 0 G); SODIUM 388 MG

TIP If prepping this salad ahead, hold off on adding the avocado until just before serving.

Three 5-ounce (142 g) cans lower-sodium chunk light tuna, drained

One 15-ounce can (425 g) no-salt-added black beans, rinsed and drained

1 cup (145 g) fresh or thawed frozen corn kernels

2 Roma tomatoes, diced

1 small avocado, diced

⅓ cup (48 g) diced red onion

3 tablespoons chopped cilantro

½ cup (120 g) olive or avocado oil-based mayonnaise

3 tablespoons lime juice

1 tablespoon lower-sodium taco seasoning

Lime wedges (optional)

Gf *gluten-free*

Ve *vegetarian*

Lc *low carb*

Df *dairy-free**

St *stovetop*

3 large eggs

3 large egg whites

½ teaspoon Greek seasoning

¼ teaspoon black pepper

1 teaspoon avocado oil

4 cups (227 g) packed baby spinach leaves, torn into small pieces

¼ teaspoon garlic powder

⅛ teaspoon salt

3 tablespoons crumbled feta

1½ cups (224 g) cherry tomatoes

1 tablespoon bottled balsamic vinaigrette

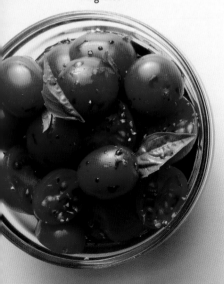

easy greek frittata with balsamic tomatoes

HANDS-ON: 12 MINUTES :: TOTAL: 12 MINUTES :: SERVES 2

This quick skillet meal is perfect any time of day, but I'm a big fan of making it for lunch on days I work from home. With minimal effort and in less than 15 minutes, I can cook a hot meal from scratch. Feel free to add in other vegetables, like chopped onion or bell pepper. To do this, I recommend sautéing them in the skillet in the oil first. When almost tender, add the spinach to the skillet to wilt.

1 Preheat the broiler to high.

2 Whisk together the eggs, egg whites, Greek seasoning, and pepper in a small bowl. Set aside.

3 Heat the oil in an 8-inch (20 cm) cast-iron or other small oven-proof skillet over medium-high heat. Add the spinach and cook, stirring frequently, until beginning to wilt, 2 minutes. Sprinkle with garlic powder and salt.

4 Spread the wilted spinach evenly across the bottom of the skillet. Pour the egg mixture over the spinach, then sprinkle with the cheese. Cook until the egg mixture starts to appear set, about 2 minutes. (Do not stir.)

5 Place the skillet in the oven. Broil for 2 to 3 minutes until the frittata is puffy and golden.

6 While the frittata broils, combine the tomatoes and vinaigrette in a small bowl. Slice the frittata into wedges and serve the tomatoes over the top or on the side.

NUTRITION FACTS (SERVING SIZE: ½ OF FRITTATA AND TOMATOES): CALORIES 250; FAT 13 G (SAT 3.5 G); PROTEIN 20 G; CARB 9 G; FIBER 4 G; SUGARS 4 G (ADDED SUGARS 0 G); SODIUM 546 MG

DAIRY-FREE OPTION Omit the feta cheese.

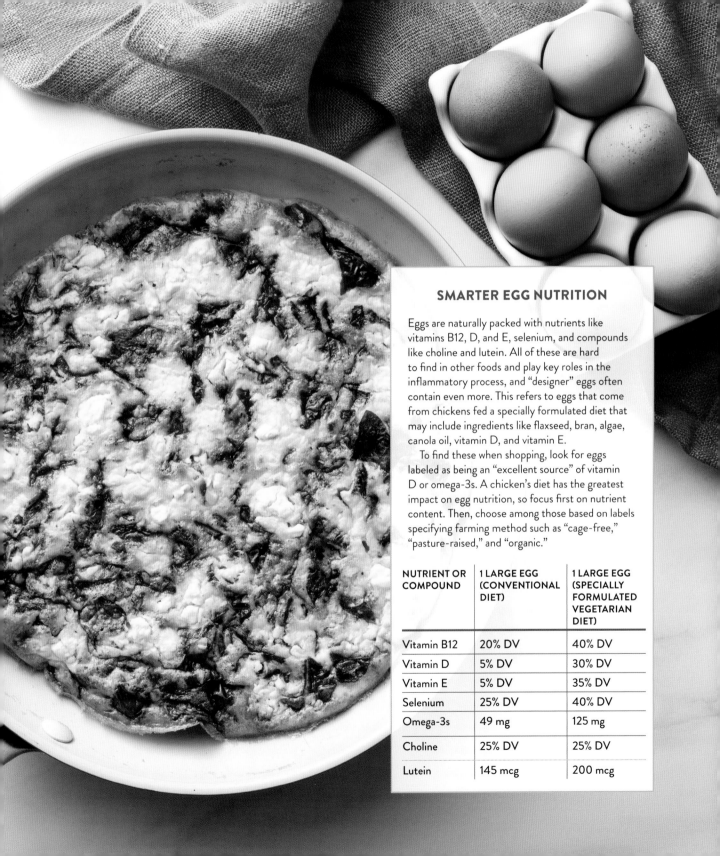

SMARTER EGG NUTRITION

Eggs are naturally packed with nutrients like vitamins B12, D, and E, selenium, and compounds like choline and lutein. All of these are hard to find in other foods and play key roles in the inflammatory process, and "designer" eggs often contain even more. This refers to eggs that come from chickens fed a specially formulated diet that may include ingredients like flaxseed, bran, algae, canola oil, vitamin D, and vitamin E.

To find these when shopping, look for eggs labeled as being an "excellent source" of vitamin D or omega-3s. A chicken's diet has the greatest impact on egg nutrition, so focus first on nutrient content. Then, choose among those based on labels specifying farming method such as "cage-free," "pasture-raised," and "organic."

NUTRIENT OR COMPOUND	1 LARGE EGG (CONVENTIONAL DIET)	1 LARGE EGG (SPECIALLY FORMULATED VEGETARIAN DIET)
Vitamin B12	20% DV	40% DV
Vitamin D	5% DV	30% DV
Vitamin E	5% DV	35% DV
Selenium	25% DV	40% DV
Omega-3s	49 mg	125 mg
Choline	25% DV	25% DV
Lutein	145 mcg	200 mcg

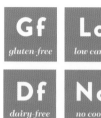

Gf
gluten-free

Lc
low carb

Df
dairy-free

Nc
no cook

Pa
prep ahead

chicken-broccoli slaw with peanut dressing

HANDS-ON: 15 MINUTES :: TOTAL: 15 MINUTES :: SERVES 4

This is one of my favorite lunches to make in advance of a busy week. It can be made in just a few minutes thanks to a bag of broccoli slaw and a rotisserie chicken, and the flavors actually get better as it chills! Almond or sunflower butter can be substituted for peanut butter, if desired. If you're following a gluten-free diet, be sure to check your soy sauce and fish sauce to ensure that they are gluten-free, as some brands may contain gluten.

¼ cup (64 g) peanut butter

2 tablespoons lower-sodium soy sauce or tamari

1 tablespoon lime juice

1 tablespoon rice vinegar

2 teaspoons fish sauce

2 teaspoons honey

1 10-ounce (284 g) package broccoli slaw

2 cups (280 g) chopped cooked skinless chicken breast

½ cup (59 g) frozen shelled edamame, thawed

Chopped peanuts or cashews, cilantro, and scallions (optional)

1 Whisk together the peanut butter, soy sauce, lime juice, vinegar, fish sauce, and honey in a small bowl.

2 Place the broccoli slaw, chicken, and edamame in a large bowl or container with a lid. Add the peanut butter mixture. Stir well to fully coat the slaw.

3 Refrigerate for 1 to 2 hours before serving. If desired, top each serving with chopped peanuts, cashews, cilantro, or scallions.

NUTRITION FACTS (SERVING SIZE: ¼ OF SLAW): CALORIES 301; FAT 12 G (SAT 2 G); PROTEIN 34 G; CARB 12 G; FIBER 2 G; SUGARS 6 G (ADDED SUGARS 3 G); SODIUM 623 MG

TIP The peanut butter mixture for the dressing is thick, so I recommend making it in a small container with a lid, if possible. Combine the dressing ingredients (peanut butter through honey), cover, and shake well to combine.

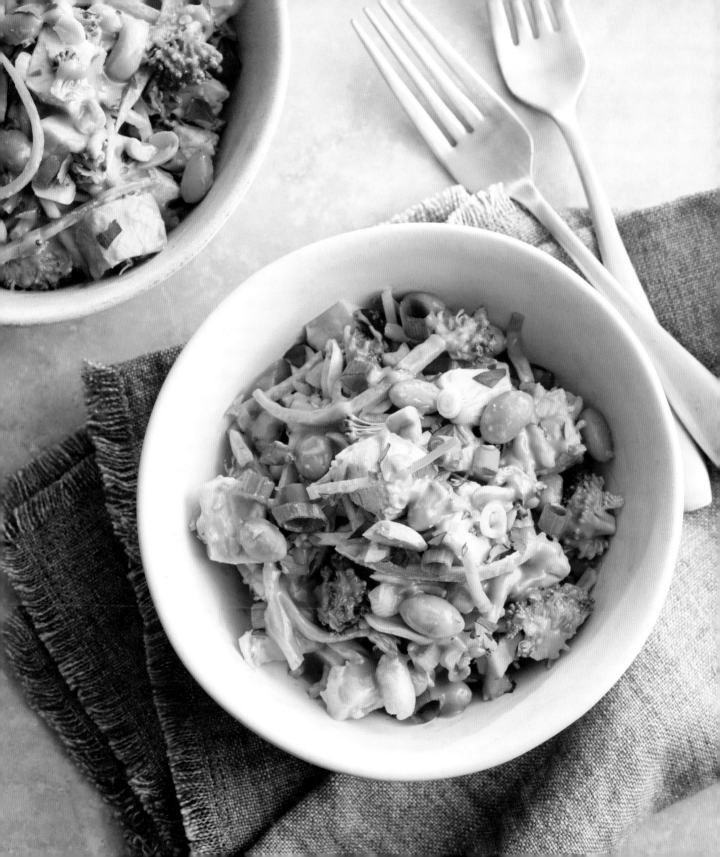

Gf *gluten-free*

 Pa *prep ahead*

 Df *dairy-free*

 Nc *no cook*

tuna, edamame, and rice bowl

HANDS-ON: 10 MINUTES :: TOTAL: 10 MINUTES :: SERVES 2

Three 2.6-ounce (74 g) pouches lower-sodium chunk light tuna, drained

½ cup (78 g) frozen shelled edamame, thawed

2 tablespoons chopped cilantro

3 tablespoons bottled sesame-ginger dressing

3 cups (128 g) mixed greens

1 cup (195 g) cooked brown rice

½ cup (75 g) diced avocado

½ cup (75 g) cherry tomatoes, quartered

½ cup (55 g) grated carrot

Selenium is an antioxidant that helps to regulate excessive inflammatory responses, which can curtail or minimize chronic inflammation. Top food sources of selenium are seafood, lean beef, eggs, and some nuts and whole grains. Thanks to this filling one-dish meal, you get 200 percent of the daily value of selenium in one bowl.

1 Combine the tuna, edamame, cilantro, and dressing in a bowl; toss gently to combine. Cover, and refrigerate until ready to serve.

2 To assemble and serve, divide the greens among 2 bowls. Top each bowl evenly with the tuna mixture, rice, avocado, tomatoes, and carrot.

NUTRITION FACTS (SERVING SIZE: 1 BOWL): CALORIES 432; FAT 16 G (SAT 2 G); PROTEIN 37 G; CARB 39 G; FIBER 9 G; SUGARS 4 G (ADDED SUGARS 2 G); SODIUM 485 MG

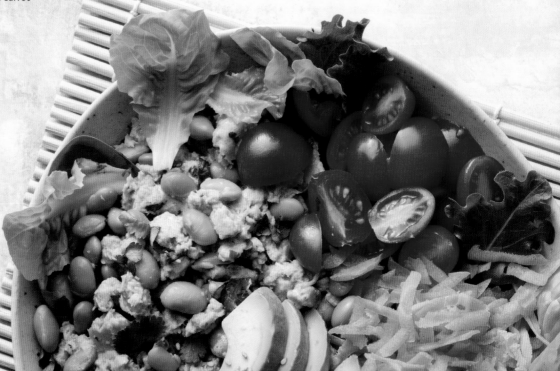

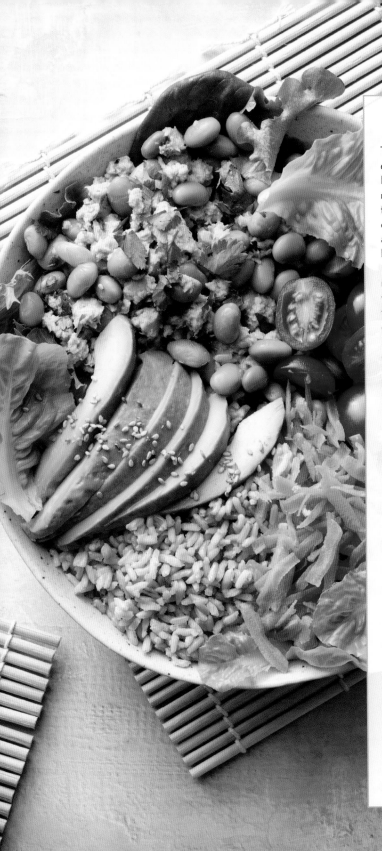

WHAT TUNA IS HEALTHIEST?

The latest dietary guidelines recommend that adults eat at least 8 ounces (225 g) of seafood per week. Keeping shelf-stable tuna on hand in your pantry makes it easier to reach this goal, and the first step is figuring out what type of tuna to buy. But this can get overwhelming because there are more tuna varieties available than ever, as well as seemingly conflicting health information.

Here's what you need to know: All tunas contain mercury, as well as omega-3s, and choosing the tuna with the lowest mercury levels is the most important factor to consider. Mercury is an environmental contaminant that, when consumed in excess, triggers inflammation. In addition, research links mercury consumption to autoimmunity, an early malfunction in the immune system that can potentially lead to the development of an autoimmune condition down the road. However, the decision to purchase tuna in cans or pouches or tuna packed in oil or water is up to you, though many people opt for water-packed because it's lower in calories and fat.

HEALTHIEST CHOICE: Chunk or Solid Light Tuna

Tuna labeled "light" is considered the healthiest option, according to both the FDA and the EPA, since it has the lowest mercury levels. The difference between "chunk" and "solid" is the flake size, and chunk is usually the preferred option for tuna salads because it has smaller pieces. It's healthy to eat 2 to 3 servings per week of seafood from the FDA's "Best Choices" list, which includes canned light tuna. (See page 185 for more information on choices.)

OKAY CHOICE: Chunk or Solid White Tuna, Albacore Tuna, or Yellowfin Tuna

It's easy to assume that "light" and "white" on food labels would be comparable. However, "white" tuna has higher levels of mercury compared to "light" tuna. Tunas labeled albacore or yellowfin also contain higher amounts than white. It's healthy to eat 1 serving per week of seafood from the FDA's "Good Choices" list, which includes these types of canned tuna.

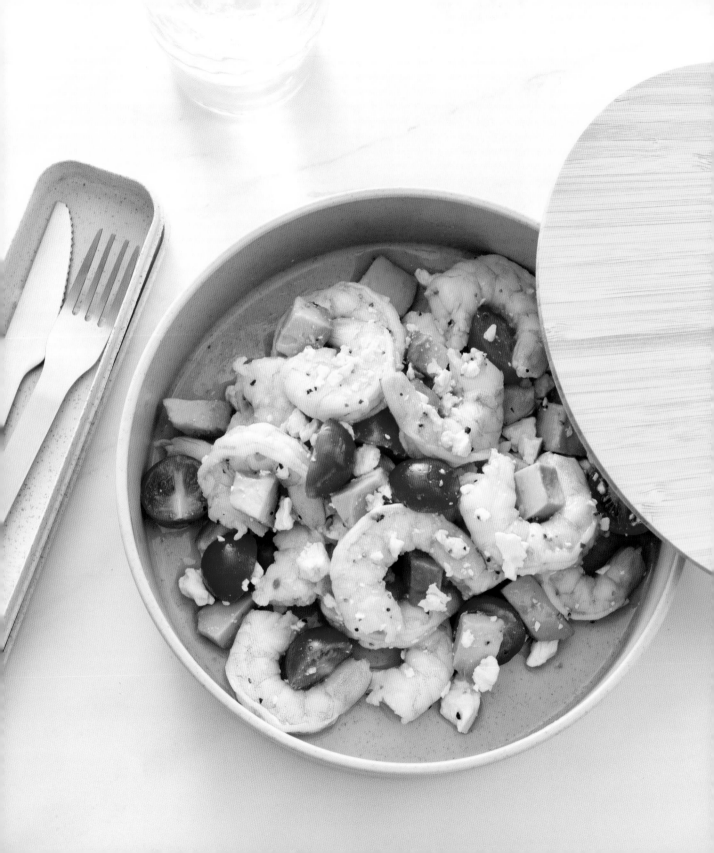

avocado-feta shrimp toss

HANDS-ON: 10 MINUTES :: TOTAL: 10 MINUTES :: SERVES 2

This low-calorie, low-carb meal is super satisfying, thanks to healthy amounts of protein and fiber, which help to fill you up and keep you feeling full. You can prepare this salad two to three hours in advance by combining all of the ingredients except for the cheese and avocado. Refrigerate and, when ready to serve, add them in.

1 Remove the tails from the shrimp and discard. Combine the shrimp and tomatoes in a medium bowl.

2 In a small bowl, whisk together the vinegar, oil, garlic powder, salt, and pepper. Add to the shrimp mixture, stirring to combine. Gently fold in the feta and avocado.

NUTRITION FACTS (SERVING SIZE: ABOUT 1½ CUPS/304 G): CALORIES 265; FAT 14 G (SAT 3 G); PROTEIN 27 G; CARB 9 G; FIBER 5 G; SUGARS 3 G (ADDED SUGARS 0 G); SODIUM 520 MG

TIP See if your grocery store seafood counter will steam raw, peeled, and deveined shrimp while you wait. Most offer this service, and it usually takes less than 5 minutes. Store the cooked shrimp for up to 3 days in the refrigerator until ready to use.

½ pound (227 g) cooked, peeled, and deveined shrimp

1½ cups (224 g) cherry tomatoes, halved

1½ tablespoons red wine vinegar

1½ teaspoons extra virgin olive oil

¼ teaspoon garlic powder

¼ teaspoon salt

¼ teaspoon black pepper

¼ cup (28 g) crumbled feta

1 small avocado, diced

Gf *gluten-free*

Lc *low carb*

Df *dairy-free*

Nc *no cook*

Pa *prep ahead*

thai-inspired beef salad

HANDS-ON: 10 MINUTES :: TOTAL: 10 MINUTES :: SERVES 2

A copycat version of my favorite salad at my local Thai restaurant, this salad is crisp and refreshing, but it's also an excellent source of zinc, containing almost 50 percent of the daily value per serving. This is important since zinc is essential for proper immune system functioning and tamping down inflammation. In fact, a lack of zinc can actually amplify the body's inflammatory response. Research also suggests that many people, particularly older individuals, may not regularly consume adequate amounts of zinc. This salad is the solution!

1 cup (133 g) chopped English cucumber

½ cup (75 g) cherry tomatoes, halved

¼ cup (6 g) chopped fresh mint leaves

¼ cup (4 g) chopped cilantro leaves

¼ cup (29 g) thinly sliced red onion

1½ tablespoons sesame or grapeseed oil

1½ tablespoons lower-sodium soy sauce or tamari

1 tablespoon lime juice

1½ teaspoons honey

½ teaspoon garlic powder

6 ounces (170 g) cooked lean flank or top sirloin steak, thinly sliced against the grain

2 cups (94 g) chopped romaine lettuce

1 Combine the cucumber, tomato, mint, cilantro, and onion in a large bowl.

2 In a small bowl, whisk together the oil, soy sauce, lime juice, honey, and garlic powder. Pour over the cucumber mixture, tossing to combine. Refrigerate, covered, until ready to serve and up to 24 hours in advance.

3 To serve, add the beef and lettuce to the cucumber mixture; toss well. Divide evenly among two plates.

NUTRITION FACTS (SERVING SIZE: 1 SALAD): CALORIES 305; FAT 15 G (SAT 3.5 G); PROTEIN 29 G; CARB 12 G; FIBER 3 G; SUGARS 8 G (ADDED SUGARS 4 G); SODIUM 496 MG

TIP Lean flank or top sirloin steak only takes about 10 minutes to cook, but it's also a great protein to prep ahead and refrigerate for dishes like this. See page 80 for best ways to do this.

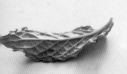

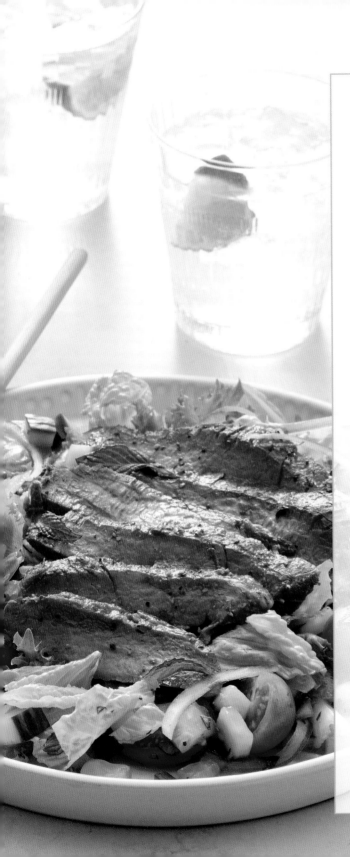

HOW TO PURCHASE A HEALTHIER SALAD DRESSING

Until a few years ago, it was hard to find bottled salad dressings that could not only rival the flavor and taste of homemade versions but also the nutritional quality. There's been a slow shift in the bottled dressing industry, as some companies have started to place more emphasis on both. This is great news for those who need the convenience of a bottled dressing, but it's important to know how to identify those brands and varieties. Use this mental checklist to select a healthier bottled dressing.

Step 1: What's in the Ingredient List?

Do you recognize all the ingredients? Are they ones that you might find in a recipe for a dressing in a cookbook? Dressings are typically composed of an oil and an acid. This may be a single oil and acid (such as vinegars or citrus juices) or a combination of oil(s) and acid(s). Other ingredients to expect are seasonings (such as garlic, ginger, herbs, and spices) and possibly an emulsifier, an ingredient that helps the oil and acid components stay blended. The most common emulsifiers used are mustards and egg yolks. There isn't much need for a dressing, even a bottled one, to contain more than this. If you are able to identify these components on a label, then move on to step 2.

Step 2: What's the Primary Fat or Oil Used?

The fat or oil listed first in the ingredient list is the primary oil in the dressing, and the healthiest bets are those whose primary oil is extra virgin olive oil, flaxseed oil, avocado oil, or a nut oil, like walnut. Often, dressings will contain more than one fat or oil source. If this is the case, the first two fats or oils listed should be a combination of olive, flaxseed, avocado, nut, or canola oils, or a fat source, like avocado. Avoid vegetable oil and seed oils (see page 16 for recommendations) when possible, and always steer clear of hydrogenated or partially hydrogenated oils.

Step 3: How Much Added Sugar and Sodium Does it Contain?

Salad dressings often need a touch of sweetness to balance acidic flavors, so a little sugar is okay. Look for a dressing that keeps added sugars to a minimum (ideally less than 2 g of sugars per 2 tablespoons) and skip ones that contain more than that. Keep tabs on sodium since bottled dressings tend to be higher than homemade. A good rule of thumb is to find a dressing with less than 300 mg of sodium per 2 tablespoons.

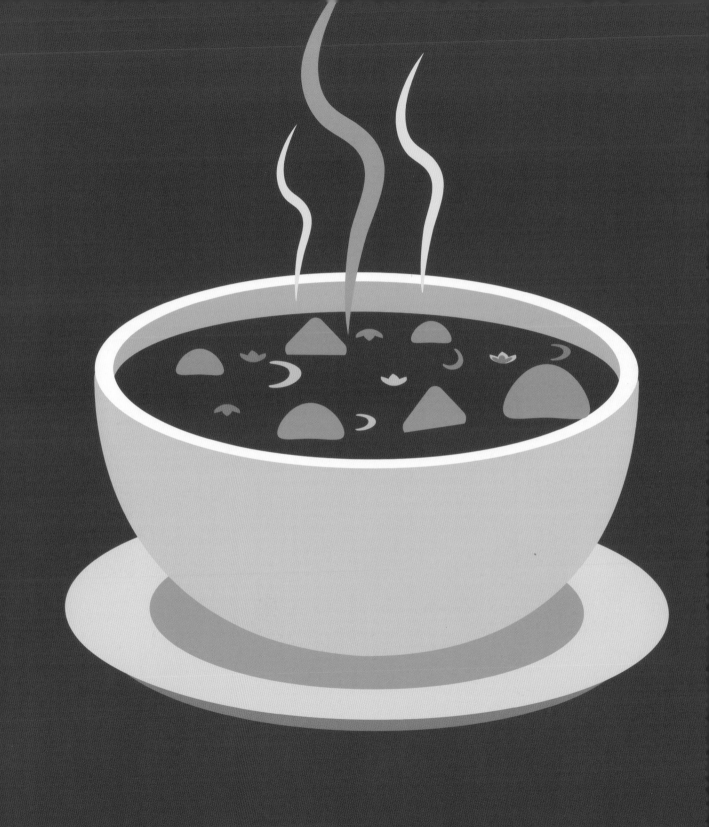

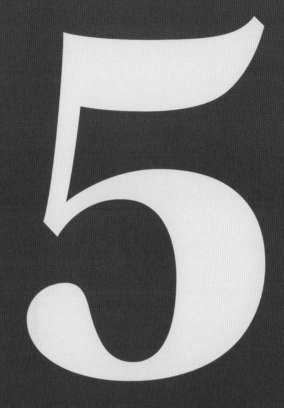

5

: : : : : : : : : : : : : :

SOUPS & STEWS

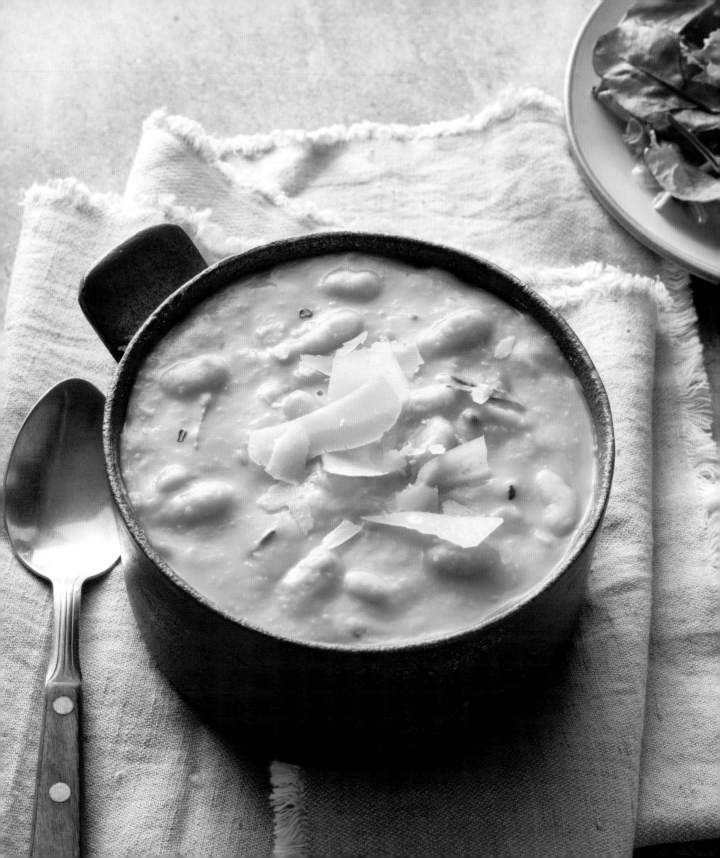

garlic-rosemary white bean soup

HANDS-ON: 6 MINUTES :: TOTAL: 30 MINUTES :: SERVES 4

This recipe's short ingredient list allows for simple prep and makes it one of the most inexpensive in this book. But that's where the minimalism ends because this is one of the most satisfying, flavorful vegetarian soups I've ever made. Pureeing some of the beans gives it a creamy texture that pairs perfectly with fresh greens dressed with a light lemony vinaigrette. Or you can truly make it a one-bowl meal by stirring in fresh kale or spinach, just until it wilts, toward the end of the cooking process.

1 Heat the oil in a small saucepan over medium heat. Cook the shallot until it begins to soften, 3 minutes, stirring occasionally. Add the garlic and sauté until fragrant, 30 seconds.

2 Stir in the beans, broth, rosemary, salt, and pepper flakes, and increase the heat to medium-high. Bring to a boil. Cover and reduce the heat to medium-low. Simmer until slightly thickened and hot throughout, 10 minutes.

3 Remove and discard the rosemary. Carefully ladle ⅓ of the soup into a blender and puree until smooth. Return the pureed soup to the pan, stirring to combine. Serve, topped with freshly grated Parmesan, if desired.

NUTRITION FACTS (SERVING SIZE: 1¼ CUPS/360 G): CALORIES 250; FAT 8 G (SAT 1 G); PROTEIN 11 G; CARB 34 G; FIBER 9 G; SUGARS 4 G (ADDED SUGARS 0 G); SODIUM 493 MG

NOTE This recipe can easily be doubled or tripled by preparing it in a Dutch oven or large saucepan.

2 tablespoons olive oil

1 chopped shallot

4 garlic cloves, minced

Two 15-ounce (425 g) cans no-salt-added cannellini beans, rinsed and drained

2 cups (480 ml) low-sodium vegetable broth

1 rosemary sprig

¾ teaspoon salt

½ teaspoon crushed red pepper flakes

Freshly grated Parmesan (optional)

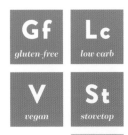

Gf *gluten-free* **Lc** *low carb*

V *vegan* **St** *stovetop*

Df *dairy-free*

curried butternut soup with spinach

HANDS-ON: 12 MINUTES :: TOTAL: 20 MINUTES :: SERVES 5

Coconut milk and pureed butternut squash give this quick soup a velvety rich texture without excessive fat or the addition of dairy. Add in a little curry paste, lime juice, and baby spinach, and you've got soup that's not only hearty and flavorful but also healthy.

1 tablespoon olive oil

1 large onion, chopped

4 garlic cloves, minced

1 to 2 teaspoons yellow curry paste

Two 12-ounce (340 g) packages frozen pureed butternut squash, thawed

One 14.5-ounce (411 g) can no-salt-added fire-roasted diced tomatoes

One 32-ounce (960 ml) carton lower-sodium chicken or vegetable broth

One 13.5-ounce (383 g) can light coconut milk

1 tablespoon lime juice

1 teaspoon salt

4 cups (227 g) baby spinach, torn into small pieces

1 Heat the oil in a large saucepan over medium heat. Cook the onion in the hot oil until just tender, 5 minutes, stirring frequently. Add the garlic and curry paste. Sauté until fragrant, 30 seconds.

2 Add the squash, tomatoes, broth, coconut milk, lime juice, and salt, stirring to combine. Increase the heat to medium-high. Bring to a simmer and cook until slightly thickened, 10 minutes, reducing the heat as needed to prevent the mixture from coming to a boil.

3 Reduce the heat to medium. Add the spinach and cook until just wilted, stirring frequently, 1 to 2 minutes.

NUTRITION FACTS (SERVING SIZE: 1¼ CUPS/557 G): CALORIES 181; FAT 6 G (SAT 3 G); PROTEIN 6 G; CARB 28 G; FIBER 4 G; SUGARS 7 G (ADDED SUGARS 0 G); SODIUM 377 MG

TIP You can steam and puree fresh or frozen butternut squash cubes instead of using store-bought frozen puree.

SHRIMP VARIATION In step 2, stir in 1 pound (454 g) of peeled and deveined, medium raw shrimp during the last 2 minutes of cooking.

NUTRITION FACTS (SERVING SIZE: 1⅓ CUPS/648 G): CALORIES 258; FAT 6 G (SAT 3 G); PROTEIN 24 G; CARB 28 G; FIBER 4 G; SUGARS 7 G (ADDED SUGARS 0 G); SODIUM 485 MG

CHICKEN VARIATION In step 3, stir in 2 cups (280 g) of chopped cooked chicken breast before adding the spinach. Cook until the chicken is warm throughout and the spinach is wilted.

NUTRITION FACTS (SERVING SIZE: 1½ CUPS/613 G): CALORIES 273; FAT 8 G (SAT 3.5 G); PROTEIN 23 G; CARB 28 G; FIBER 4 G; SUGARS 7 G (ADDED SUGARS 0 G); SODIUM 418 MG

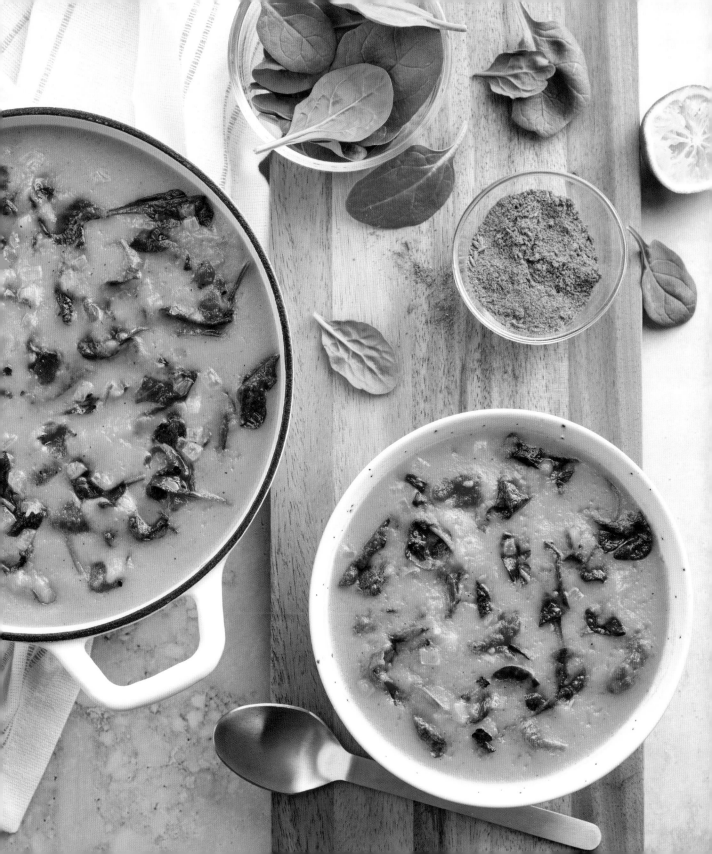

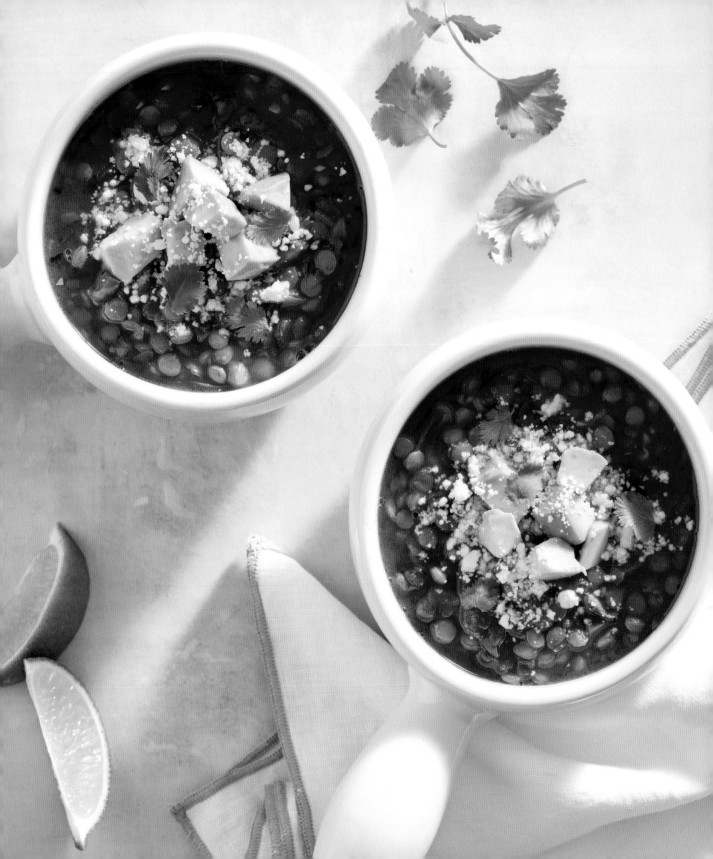

chipotle-lime lentil chili

HANDS-ON: 10 MINUTES :: TOTAL: 40 MINUTES :: SERVES 7

Lentils are part of the legume family, which includes beans and peas. This means they're packed with fiber and plant-based protein. However, unlike beans and peas, they require significantly less cooking time and no overnight soaking because of their tiny size. And because brown lentils keep their shape and texture when cooked, they're a perfect substitute for meat in chilis and hearty stews.

1 Add the oil to the pressure cooker and press the SAUTÉ button. Cook the onion and bell pepper in the hot oil until the edges of the vegetables are beginning to soften, 2 minutes. Add the garlic, chili powder, cumin, and salt. Sauté until fragrant, 1 minute. Press the KEEP WARM/CANCEL button.

2 Add the broth, tomatoes, lentils, and chipotles, gently stirring to combine. Secure the lid, making sure the pressure valve is secured. Press the SOUP button and cook for 12 minutes.

3 Manually release the pressure and open the pressure cooker. Stir in the cilantro and lime juice. Top each serving with any desired toppings.

NUTRITION FACTS (SERVING SIZE: 1⅓ CUPS/354 G): CALORIES 272; FAT 4 G (SAT 0.5 G); PROTEIN 15 G; CARB 46 G; FIBER 9 G; SUGARS 4 G (ADDED SUGARS 0 G); SODIUM 531 MG

TIP If you want to turn up the heat, add a seeded and diced jalapeño in step 2. Not sure what to do with the leftovers in a can of chipotle chiles? See page 97 for tricks on how to save and use them later.

STOVETOP OPTION

1 Heat the oil in a large stockpot over medium heat. Cook the onion and bell pepper in the hot oil until the edges of the vegetables begin to soften, about 2 minutes. Add the garlic, chili powder, cumin, and salt. Sauté until fragrant, 1 minute.

2 Add the broth, tomatoes, lentils, and chipotles, gently stirring to combine. Increase the heat to medium-high and bring to a boil. Reduce the heat slightly to maintain a simmer. Cover and cook until the lentils are tender, 38 to 45 minutes.

3 Remove from the heat. Stir in the cilantro and lime juice. Top each serving with any desired toppings.

1 tablespoon avocado oil

1 small onion, diced

1 green bell pepper, cored and diced

2 tablespoons minced garlic

2 tablespoons chili powder

1 teaspoon ground cumin

1 teaspoon salt

One 32-ounce carton (960 ml) low-sodium vegetable broth

Two 14.5-ounce (411 g) cans no-salt-added diced tomatoes

2 cups (384 g) brown lentils, rinsed and drained

3 chipotles in adobo sauce, chopped

¼ cup (4 g) chopped fresh cilantro

3 tablespoons lime juice

Lime wedges, avocado slices, Greek yogurt, cotija (optional)

Gf gluten-free

Lc low carb

Df dairy-free*

St stovetop

6 cups (1440 ml) chicken bone broth or unsalted chicken stock

2½ cups (284 g) shredded, cooked skinless chicken breasts

⅓ cup (83 g) pesto

1 teaspoon garlic powder

One 10-ounce (284 g) package zucchini spirals

½ teaspoon salt

¼ teaspoon black pepper

2 teaspoons lemon juice

Freshly grated Parmesan (optional)

pesto zoodle chicken soup

HANDS-ON: 5 MINUTES :: TOTAL: 15 MINUTES :: SERVES 5

Shredded chicken and zucchini spirals are simmered in a pesto-seasoned broth to create a delicious low-carb version of chicken noodle soup. Thanks to convenience products like prepared pesto, packaged zucchini noodles, deli rotisserie chicken, and canned broth, the soup is ready in 15 minutes—proof that healthy doesn't require making everything from scratch!

1 Place the broth in a Dutch oven or large saucepan over medium-high heat. Bring to a low boil. Add the chicken, pesto, and garlic powder, stirring to combine. Reduce the heat to medium and simmer until the liquid is slightly reduced and hot throughout, 5 minutes.

2 Stir in the zucchini, salt, and pepper. Cook until the zucchini is just tender, 2 minutes. Remove from the heat and stir in the lemon juice. Top with Parmesan, if desired.

NUTRITION FACTS (SERVING SIZE: ABOUT 1½ CUPS/423 G): CALORIES 221; FAT 9 G (SAT 1.5 G); PROTEIN 30 G; CARB 5 G; FIBER 1 G; SUGARS 2 G (ADDED SUGARS 0 G); SODIUM 523 MG

TIP Use kitchen shears or a knife to cut the zucchini noodles into 1-inch (2.5 cm) pieces before adding to the broth. One 10-ounce (284 g) package of fresh zucchini spirals contains about 3 cups. If you prefer to make your own spirals, purchase 1 pound (431 g) of whole zucchini.

DAIRY-FREE OPTION Substitute an equivalent amount of dairy-free or vegan pesto.

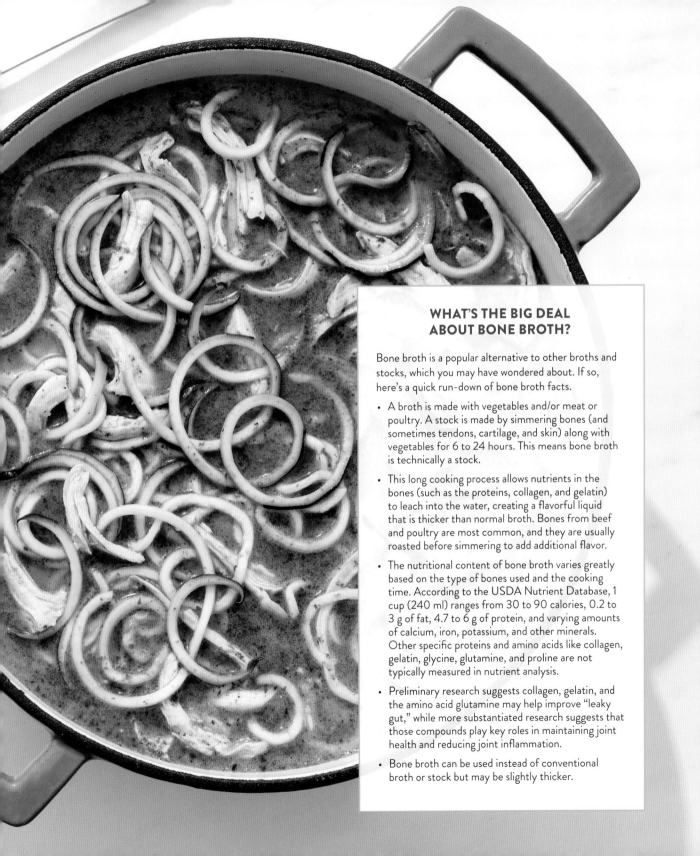

WHAT'S THE BIG DEAL ABOUT BONE BROTH?

Bone broth is a popular alternative to other broths and stocks, which you may have wondered about. If so, here's a quick run-down of bone broth facts.

- A broth is made with vegetables and/or meat or poultry. A stock is made by simmering bones (and sometimes tendons, cartilage, and skin) along with vegetables for 6 to 24 hours. This means bone broth is technically a stock.

- This long cooking process allows nutrients in the bones (such as the proteins, collagen, and gelatin) to leach into the water, creating a flavorful liquid that is thicker than normal broth. Bones from beef and poultry are most common, and they are usually roasted before simmering to add additional flavor.

- The nutritional content of bone broth varies greatly based on the type of bones used and the cooking time. According to the USDA Nutrient Database, 1 cup (240 ml) ranges from 30 to 90 calories, 0.2 to 3 g of fat, 4.7 to 6 g of protein, and varying amounts of calcium, iron, potassium, and other minerals. Other specific proteins and amino acids like collagen, gelatin, glycine, glutamine, and proline are not typically measured in nutrient analysis.

- Preliminary research suggests collagen, gelatin, and the amino acid glutamine may help improve "leaky gut," while more substantiated research suggests that those compounds play key roles in maintaining joint health and reducing joint inflammation.

- Bone broth can be used instead of conventional broth or stock but may be slightly thicker.

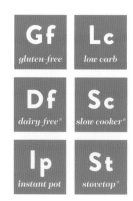

creamy buffalo chicken soup

HANDS-ON: 12 MINUTES :: TOTAL: 35 MINUTES :: SERVES 8

This crowd-pleaser is perfect for a football-watching party, but it's also simple enough to make for a weeknight family dinner. Instead of using heavy cream, I use coconut milk to add dairy-free creaminess. You'd never know since the bold flavors in the buffalo sauce and ranch mix mask most of the coconut milk's natural sweetness and flavor. You can also add a squeeze of lime juice to cut the coconut flavor a little more.

1 tablespoon olive oil

1 cup (160 g) chopped onion

4 cups (428 g) cauliflower florets

3 cups (720 ml) lower-sodium chicken broth or bone broth

One 14.5-ounce (411 g) can no-salt-added fire-roasted tomatoes

⅓ cup (80 ml) buffalo sauce

2 tablespoons dry ranch dressing mix

½ teaspoon garlic powder

1 pound (454 g) boneless, skinless chicken breasts

1 cup (240 ml) canned coconut milk or half-and-half

Extra buffalo sauce, chopped scallions (optional)

1 Add the oil to the pressure cooker and press the SAUTÉ button. Cook the onion and cauliflower in the hot oil until the onion is just starting to soften, 4 minutes. Press the KEEP WARM/CANCEL button.

2 Add the broth, tomatoes, buffalo sauce, ranch mix, and garlic powder, gently stirring to combine. Nestle the chicken in the broth mixture. Secure the lid, making sure the pressure valve is secured. Press the SOUP button and cook for 20 minutes.

3 Manually release the pressure valve and open the pressure cooker. Carefully remove the chicken breasts and let cool slightly. Puree the soup in a blender, in batches, and return to the pressure cooker. Shred the chicken with two forks.

4 Press the SAUTÉ button. Add the shredded chicken and coconut milk to the soup. Cook, stirring frequently, until slightly thickened and warm throughout, 2 minutes. Ladle into bowls to serve. Top with extra buffalo sauce and scallions, if desired.

NUTRITION FACTS (SERVING SIZE: 1⅔ CUPS/420 G): CALORIES 254; FAT 13 G (SAT 8 G); PROTEIN 21 G; CARB 13 G; FIBER 3 G; SUGARS 4 G (ADDED SUGARS 0 G); SODIUM 653 MG

DAIRY-FREE OPTION Use 2 tablespoons of dairy-free ranch dressing mix, if available. If not, make your own mix by combining 1 tablespoon of dried parsley; 1 teaspoon each of dried chives, dried dill, garlic powder, and onion powder; ½ teaspoon of salt, and ¼ teaspoon of black pepper in a small bowl and use in place of the 2 tablespoons of store-bought mix.

SLOW COOKER OPTION Heat the oil in a large skillet over medium heat; add the onion and cauliflower. Cook for 4 minutes, or until vegetables are just beginning to soften on the edges. (Note: The vegetables will not be done.) Transfer to a slow cooker, and add the broth, tomatoes, buffalo sauce, ranch mix, and garlic powder. Stir gently to combine. Nestle the chicken breasts into the mixture. Cover, and cook on LOW for 6 to 8 hours or HIGH for 4 hours. Remove the chicken breasts and let cool slightly; shred with two forks and set aside. Puree the soup in a blender in batches, then return the soup to the slow cooker. Add the shredded chicken and coconut milk. Cook, stirring frequently, until slightly thickened and warm throughout, 5 minutes.

STOVETOP OPTION Heat the oil in a Dutch oven over medium heat. Add the chicken breasts and cook, 3 to 5 minutes on each side until the outside is browned and the center is no longer pink. Remove from the pot and set aside to cool. Add the onion and cauliflower to the Dutch oven and cook until onion is just starting to soften, stirring frequently, 4 minutes. Add the broth, tomatoes, buffalo sauce, ranch mix, and garlic powder, gently stirring to combine. Increase the heat to medium-high and bring to a boil. Reduce the heat to medium, cover, and cook until the cauliflower is very tender, 25 to 30 minutes. Puree the soup in a blender in batches, then return the soup to the pot. Shred the cooked chicken using two forks. Add the shredded chicken and coconut milk to the soup. Cook, stirring frequently, until slightly thickened and warm throughout, 5 minutes.

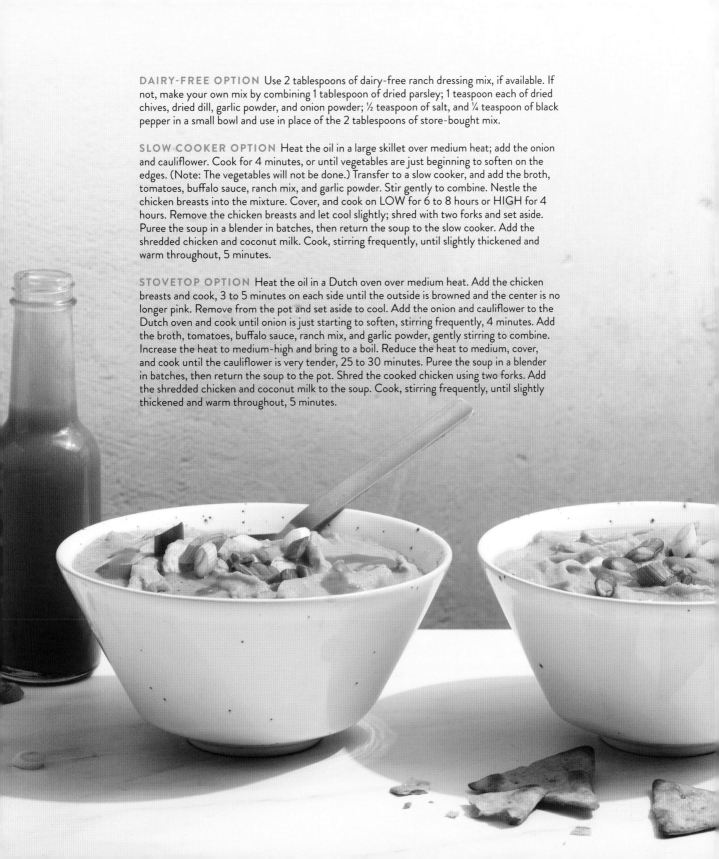

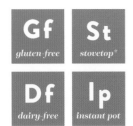

Gf *gluten-free* **St** *stovetop**

Df *dairy-free* **Ip** *instant pot*

¾ pound (340 g) Italian turkey sausage

4 uncured bacon slices, diced

1 small yellow onion, diced

5 garlic cloves, minced

2 tablespoons gluten-free baking mix or arrowroot flour

One 32-ounce (960 ml) carton unsalted chicken stock

One 15-ounce (425 g) can no-salt-added white beans, rinsed and drained

One 14.5-ounce (411 g) can no-salt-added fire-roasted diced tomatoes

3 carrots, sliced

1 tablespoon Italian seasoning

4 cups (64 g) chopped kale

¾ cup (170 g) plain Greek yogurt

Fresh parsley, red pepper flakes (optional)

zuppa toscano

HANDS-ON: 15 MINUTES :: TOTAL: 50 MINUTES :: SERVES 6

Zuppa Toscana is a popular menu choice at a large Italian chain restaurant, and even though there are lots of recipe variations, it typically contains some assortment of kale, potatoes, sausage, bacon, cannellini beans, carrots, zucchini, olive oil, broth, and cream. The end product is a bowl of hearty comfort food that also tends to be high in sodium and saturated fat. To create a healthier version that's just as delicious, I kept the key players needed for flavor, opting for a slightly smaller amount of bacon and using alternatives like Italian turkey sausage, unsalted stock, and Greek yogurt.

1 Press the SAUTÉ button on the pressure cooker. Cook the sausage until browned, 5 minutes, stirring to crumble. Drain the sausage to remove excess fat; set aside.

2 Add the bacon. Cook, stirring frequently, until the bacon pieces are starting to crisp, 3 minutes. Remove the bacon from the pot to drain, reserving the drippings in the pressure cooker.

3 Add the onion and garlic to the drippings. Sauté until fragrant, 1 minute. Sprinkle the baking mix over the vegetables. Cook, stirring constantly, until the baking mix is golden, 1 minute. Slowly whisk in the stock. Cook until slightly thickened, 2 minutes. Add the beans, tomatoes, carrots, and seasoning. Cancel the SAUTÉ mode, lock in the lid, and set to MANUAL high pressure for 10 minutes.

4 Manually release the pressure valve and open the pressure cooker. Press the SAUTÉ button. Stir in the kale, yogurt, sausage, and bacon. Cook until hot throughout, stirring occasionally, 5 minutes.

NUTRITION FACTS (SERVING SIZE: 1½ CUPS/287 G): CALORIES 273; FAT 10 G (SAT 3.5 G); PROTEIN 22 G; CARB 21 G; FIBER 5 G; SUGARS 5 G (ADDED SUGARS 0 G); SODIUM 650 MG

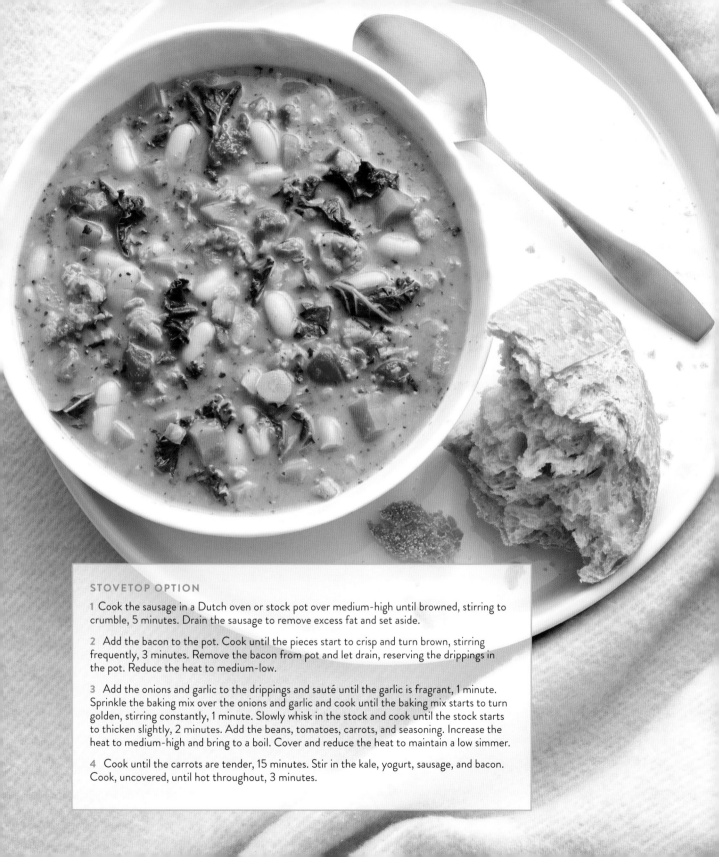

STOVETOP OPTION

1 Cook the sausage in a Dutch oven or stock pot over medium-high until browned, stirring to crumble, 5 minutes. Drain the sausage to remove excess fat and set aside.

2 Add the bacon to the pot. Cook until the pieces start to crisp and turn brown, stirring frequently, 3 minutes. Remove the bacon from pot and let drain, reserving the drippings in the pot. Reduce the heat to medium-low.

3 Add the onions and garlic to the drippings and sauté until the garlic is fragrant, 1 minute. Sprinkle the baking mix over the onions and garlic and cook until the baking mix starts to turn golden, stirring constantly, 1 minute. Slowly whisk in the stock and cook until the stock starts to thicken slightly, 2 minutes. Add the beans, tomatoes, carrots, and seasoning. Increase the heat to medium-high and bring to a boil. Cover and reduce the heat to maintain a low simmer.

4 Cook until the carrots are tender, 15 minutes. Stir in the kale, yogurt, sausage, and bacon. Cook, uncovered, until hot throughout, 3 minutes.

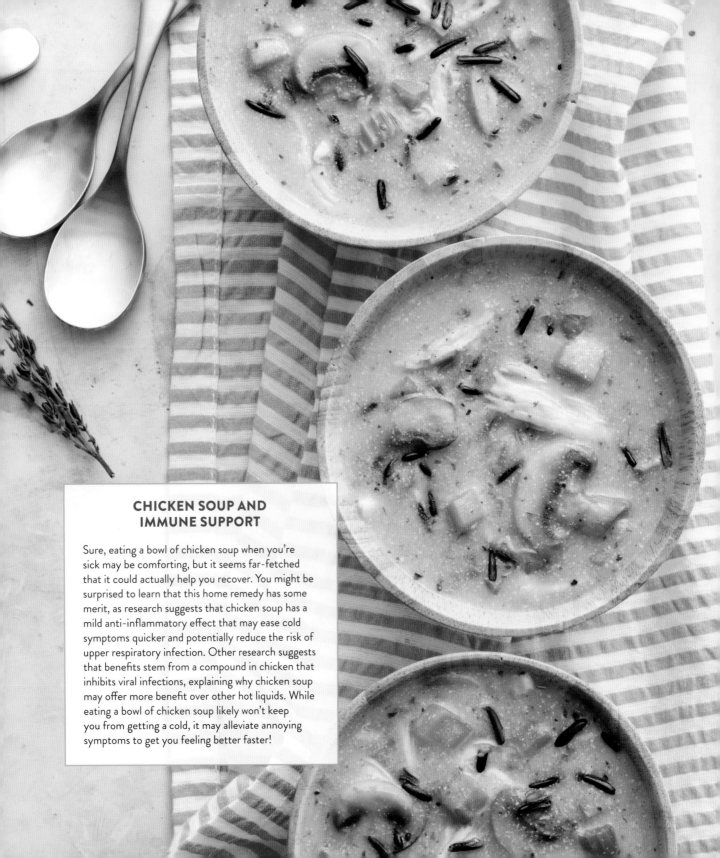

CHICKEN SOUP AND IMMUNE SUPPORT

Sure, eating a bowl of chicken soup when you're sick may be comforting, but it seems far-fetched that it could actually help you recover. You might be surprised to learn that this home remedy has some merit, as research suggests that chicken soup has a mild anti-inflammatory effect that may ease cold symptoms quicker and potentially reduce the risk of upper respiratory infection. Other research suggests that benefits stem from a compound in chicken that inhibits viral infections, explaining why chicken soup may offer more benefit over other hot liquids. While eating a bowl of chicken soup likely won't keep you from getting a cold, it may alleviate annoying symptoms to get you feeling better faster!

creamy wild rice and chicken soup

HANDS-ON: 10 MINUTES :: TOTAL: 25 MINUTES :: SERVES 8

This soup's secret ingredient is extra-creamy oat milk, which is thicker than other plant-based milks. In fact, its consistency rivals that of coconut milk, but it has a much milder flavor. This allows the flavors of the herbs, vegetables, wild rice, and chicken to take center stage. For best results, look for an oat milk labeled "extra-creamy" that has 7 to 9 grams of fat per 1-cup (240 ml) serving.

1   Heat the oil in a large Dutch oven over medium-high heat. Sauté the onion, celery, and carrot in the hot oil until the vegetables are beginning to soften, 4 minutes. Add the mushrooms and garlic; cook until the edges of the mushrooms are beginning to soften, stirring frequently, 2 minutes.

2   Stir in the baking mix. Gradually add the broth, stirring to combine. Stir in the seasoning, salt, pepper, rosemary, and thyme. Bring to a simmer.

3   Add the chicken, rice, and milk. Reduce the heat to low. Cook until hot throughout and slightly thickened, 8 to 10 minutes. Remove the rosemary and thyme sprigs before serving.

NUTRITION FACTS (SERVING SIZE: 1½ CUPS/356 G): CALORIES 258; FAT 9 G (SAT 1 G); PROTEIN 23 G; CARB 23 G; FIBER 2 G; SUGARS 3 G (ADDED SUGARS 0 G); SODIUM 459 MG

TIP Use a blend of cooked wild and brown rice, if desired. To save time, look for ready-to-heat pouches of wild and brown rice. Each pouch typically contains 2 cups (328 g) of cooked rice.

1 tablespoon avocado oil

1 onion, chopped

2 stalks celery, chopped

1 carrot, chopped

One 8-ounce (227 g) package sliced mushrooms

4 garlic cloves, minced

2 tablespoons gluten-free baking mix or arrowroot flour

One 32-ounce (960 ml) carton lower-sodium chicken broth

1 tablespoon Italian herb seasoning

1 teaspoon salt

½ teaspoon black pepper

1 rosemary sprig

1 thyme sprig

3 cups (420 g) shredded cooked skinless chicken breast

3 cups (492 g) cooked wild rice

2 cups (480 ml) plain extra-creamy oat milk

chile verde with shredded pork

Gf *gluten-free*

Lc *low carb*

Df *dairy-free*

St *stovetop**

Ip *instant pot*

HANDS-ON: 15 MINUTES　　TOTAL: 65 MINUTES　　SERVES 7

If you're a fan of tortilla soup and looking for a change, then you'll love this green chile pork stew. Traditionally, chile verde is made by slowly simmering a pork shoulder in a broth made with roasted tomatillos and green chiles. This shortcut variation uses canned chiles and a prepared salsa verde to shave work time down to 15 minutes while a pressure cooker speeds up the simmering process.

One 2-pound (907 g) lean boneless pork shoulder, trimmed

2 teaspoons ground cumin

½ teaspoon salt

½ teaspoon black pepper

1 tablespoon avocado oil

One 32-ounce (960 ml) carton low-sodium chicken broth

1½ cups (360 ml) refrigerated salsa verde

One 4-ounce (113 g) can diced green chiles

1 onion, chopped

4 garlic cloves, minced

3 tablespoons cornmeal

¼ cup (4 g) chopped cilantro, plus more for serving

1 tablespoon lime juice

1 Cut the pork into 5 or 6 pieces and season with the cumin, salt, and pepper.

2 Add the oil to the pressure cooker and press the SAUTÉ button. Cook the pork in the hot oil, turning occasionally to lightly brown both sides, 3 minutes. (Note: The pork will not be fully cooked.)

3 Press the KEEP WARM/CANCEL button. Add the broth, salsa, chiles, onion, and garlic, gently stirring to combine. Secure the lid, making sure the pressure valve is secured. Press the SOUP button and cook for 20 minutes.

4 Manually release the pressure valve and open the pressure cooker. Carefully remove the pork and let cool slightly. Then, shred the pork with two forks. Place ⅓ cup (80 ml) of the broth in a small bowl. Whisk the cornmeal into the broth until smooth.

5 Press the SAUTÉ button. Add the pork, broth-cornmeal mixture, cilantro, and lime juice to the pot, stirring to combine. Cook until slightly thickened and hot throughout, 5 minutes. Serve, topped with additional chopped cilantro, if desired.

NUTRITION FACTS (SERVING SIZE: 1½ CUPS/353 G): CALORIES 229; FAT 7 G (SAT 2 G); PROTEIN 29 G; CARB 9 G; FIBER 2 G; SUGARS 3 G (ADDED SUGARS 0 G); SODIUM 572 MG

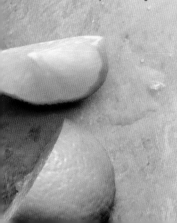

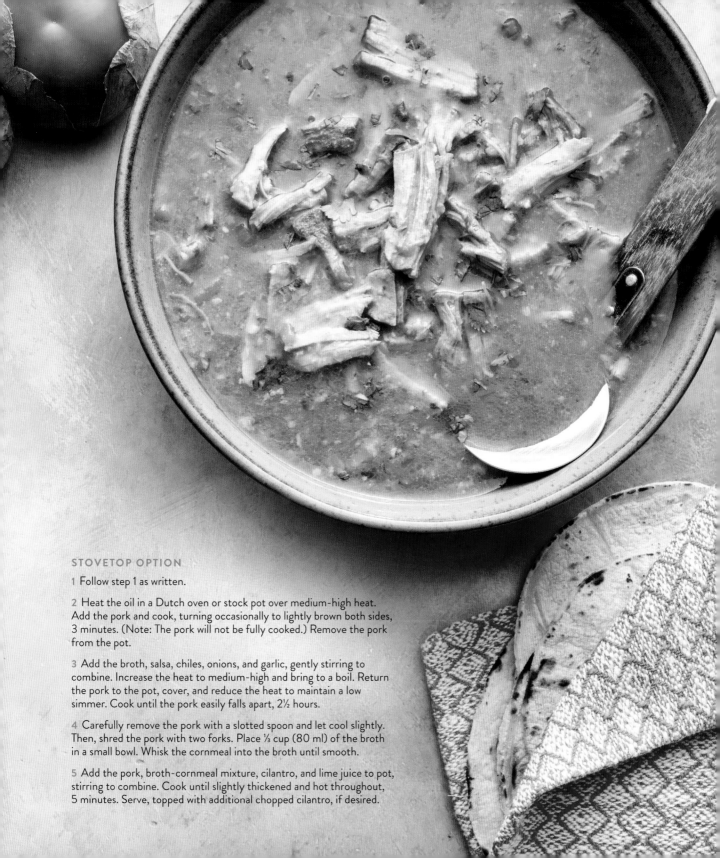

STOVETOP OPTION

1 Follow step 1 as written.

2 Heat the oil in a Dutch oven or stock pot over medium-high heat. Add the pork and cook, turning occasionally to lightly brown both sides, 3 minutes. (Note: The pork will not be fully cooked.) Remove the pork from the pot.

3 Add the broth, salsa, chiles, onions, and garlic, gently stirring to combine. Increase the heat to medium-high and bring to a boil. Return the pork to the pot, cover, and reduce the heat to maintain a low simmer. Cook until the pork easily falls apart, 2½ hours.

4 Carefully remove the pork with a slotted spoon and let cool slightly. Then, shred the pork with two forks. Place ⅓ cup (80 ml) of the broth in a small bowl. Whisk the cornmeal into the broth until smooth.

5 Add the pork, broth-cornmeal mixture, cilantro, and lime juice to pot, stirring to combine. Cook until slightly thickened and hot throughout, 5 minutes. Serve, topped with additional chopped cilantro, if desired.

Gf
gluten-free

Ip
instant pot

V
vegan*

St
stovetop*

Df
dairy-free

creamy southwestern beef soup

HANDS-ON: 15 MINUTES :: TOTAL: 52 MINUTES :: SERVES 7

What happens when you combine a brothy taco soup with a creamy tortilla soup? You get this hearty, comforting dish that incorporates the best components from each: lean ground beef, tomatoes, chiles, and black beans. A touch of lime juice cuts the coconut milk's prominent flavor, so this dairy-free soup has a rich, dairy-like taste.

1½ pounds (680 g) lean ground beef

2 bell peppers, chopped

1 onion, chopped

2 garlic cloves, minced

One 14.5-ounce (411 g) can no-salt-added fire-roasted tomatoes

One 14-ounce (397 g) can no-salt-added black beans

One 4-ounce (113 g) can diced green chiles

One 1-ounce (28 g) envelope fajita seasoning

One 32-ounce (960 ml) carton lower-sodium beef or chicken broth

One 13.5-ounce (383 g) can light coconut milk, chilled

¼ cup (4 g) chopped cilantro

2 tablespoons lime juice

Lime wedges, tortilla chips, queso fresco, chopped cilantro, or diced avocado (optional)

1 Press the SAUTÉ button on the pressure cooker. Cook the beef until browned and fully cooked through, stirring to crumble, 5 minutes. Drain the beef to remove excess fat; set aside.

2 Add the peppers and onion to the pressure cooker and cook until just beginning to soften, 2 minutes. Add the garlic and sauté until fragrant, 30 seconds. Press the KEEP WARM/CANCEL button.

3 Add the tomatoes, beans, chiles, seasoning, beef, and broth, gently stirring to combine. Secure the lid, making sure the pressure valve is secured. Press the SOUP button and cook for 15 minutes.

4 While the soup cooks, open the chilled coconut milk. Remove the coconut cream at the top of the can with a spoon to fill a ½-cup (120 ml) measuring cup. Reserve the remaining coconut milk for another use.

5 Manually release the pressure valve and open the pressure cooker. Press the SAUTÉ button. Add the coconut cream, cilantro, and lime juice. Cook until slightly thickened and warm throughout, stirring frequently, 3 minutes. Serve with toppings of choice, if desired.

NUTRITION FACTS (SERVING SIZE: 1⅓ CUPS/374 G): CALORIES 228; FAT 8 G (SAT 3 G); PROTEIN 22 G; CARB 17 G; FIBER 4 G; SUGARS 3 G (ADDED SUGARS 0 G); SODIUM 516 MG

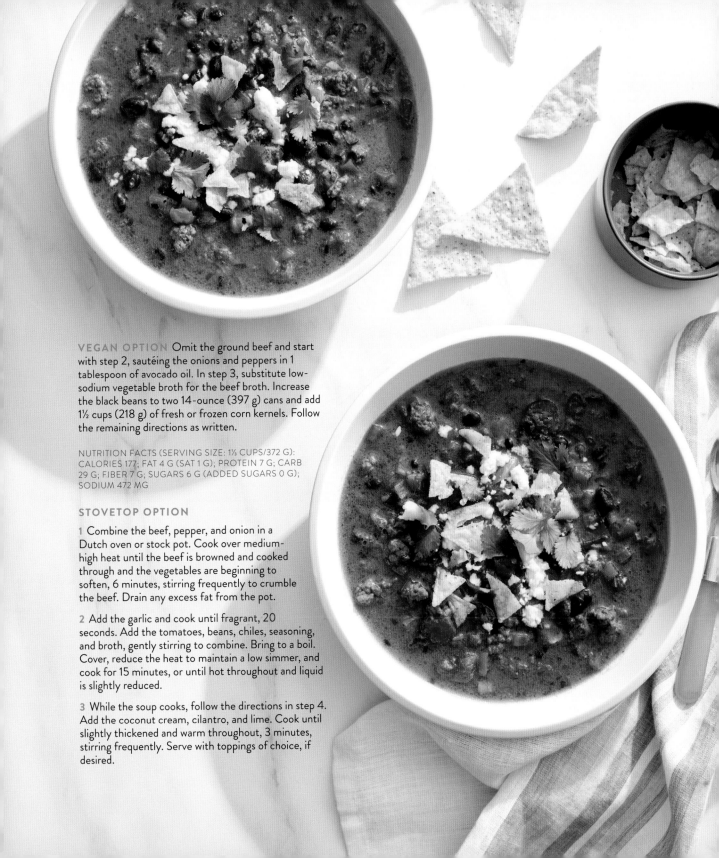

VEGAN OPTION Omit the ground beef and start with step 2, sautéing the onions and peppers in 1 tablespoon of avocado oil. In step 3, substitute low-sodium vegetable broth for the beef broth. Increase the black beans to two 14-ounce (397 g) cans and add 1½ cups (218 g) of fresh or frozen corn kernels. Follow the remaining directions as written.

NUTRITION FACTS (SERVING SIZE: 1⅓ CUPS/372 G): CALORIES 177; FAT 4 G (SAT 1 G); PROTEIN 7 G; CARB 29 G; FIBER 7 G; SUGARS 6 G (ADDED SUGARS 0 G); SODIUM 472 MG

STOVETOP OPTION

1 Combine the beef, pepper, and onion in a Dutch oven or stock pot. Cook over medium-high heat until the beef is browned and cooked through and the vegetables are beginning to soften, 6 minutes, stirring frequently to crumble the beef. Drain any excess fat from the pot.

2 Add the garlic and cook until fragrant, 20 seconds. Add the tomatoes, beans, chiles, seasoning, and broth, gently stirring to combine. Bring to a boil. Cover, reduce the heat to maintain a low simmer, and cook for 15 minutes, or until hot throughout and liquid is slightly reduced.

3 While the soup cooks, follow the directions in step 4. Add the coconut cream, cilantro, and lime. Cook until slightly thickened and warm throughout, 3 minutes, stirring frequently. Serve with toppings of choice, if desired.

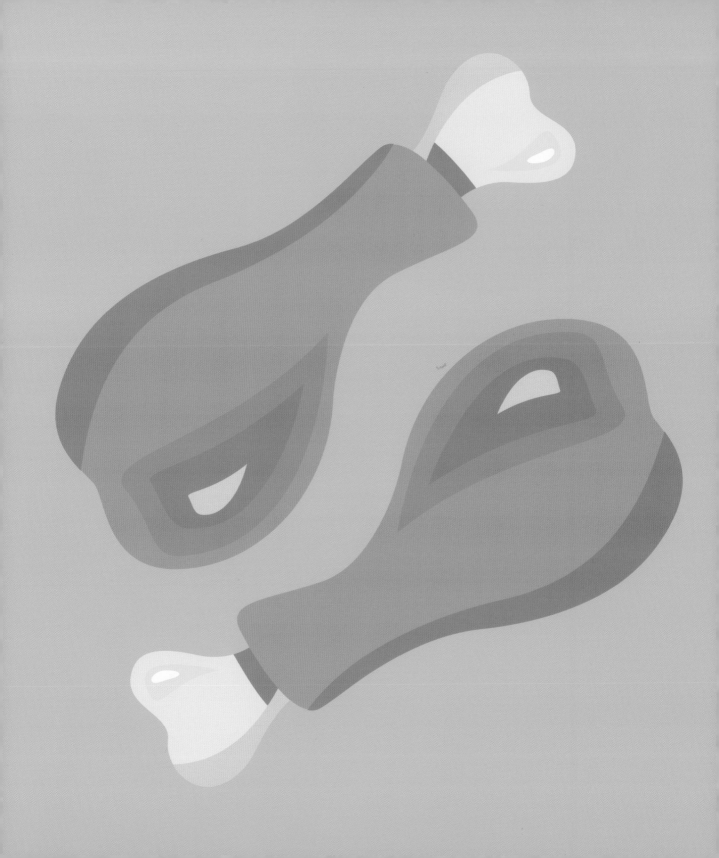

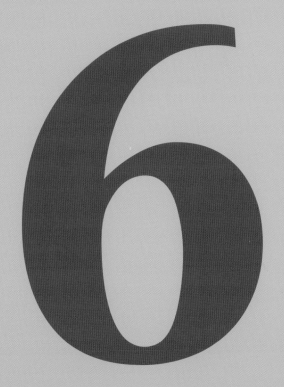

6

MEAT & POULTRY

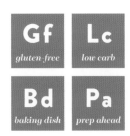

Gf gluten-free

Lc low carb

Bd baking dish

Pa prep ahead

One 20-ounce (567 g) package
frozen riced cauliflower, thawed

One 10-ounce (284 g) package
frozen broccoli florets, thawed

Cooking spray

1 tablespoon olive oil

1 small yellow onion, chopped

One 8-ounce (227 g) package
sliced mushrooms

2 teaspoons minced garlic

1 tablespoon gluten-free baking
mix or arrowroot flour

1½ cups (360 ml) low-fat milk

One 8-ounce (227 g) package
shredded reduced-fat sharp
cheddar

½ cup (40 g) freshly grated
Parmesan

1 teaspoon dry mustard

¾ teaspoon salt

½ teaspoon black pepper

3 cups (420 g) chopped or
shredded cooked skinless
chicken breast

cheesy chicken, broccoli, and "rice" casserole

HANDS-ON: 15 MINUTES   ::   TOTAL: 45 MINUTES   ::   SERVES 8

Everyone loves a cheesy casserole, and this is a family-friendly one that you can feel good about serving and eating. Riced cauliflower has a mild flavor and a grain-like texture, making it the perfect lower-carb substitute for rice in casseroles. The hearty dish can easily stand alone, but you could also pair it with a quick green salad, roasted green beans, or fresh fruit. When putting leftovers away, I like to store them in individual serving containers for an easy-to-grab lunch to reheat later in the week.

1 Spread the cauliflower and broccoli across clean kitchen or paper towels. Let stand for 10 minutes to drain any excess moisture.

2 Preheat the oven to 375°F (190°C). Lightly coat a 9 x 13-inch (23 x 33 cm) or 2-quart (1.9 L) baking dish with cooking spray.

3 Heat the oil in a Dutch oven or large saucepan over medium heat. Add the onion, mushrooms, and garlic; sauté until the mushrooms begin to soften, 3 minutes.

4 Sprinkle the flour over the onions and mushrooms. Cook, stirring constantly, until the flour begins to turn golden, 1 minute. Slowly whisk in the milk. Continue to stir until the mixture starts to thicken, 3 minutes. Add 1 cup (113 g) of the cheddar and the Parmesan, dry mustard, salt, and pepper. Cook, stirring constantly, until the cheeses are melted, stirring constantly, 1 minute. Remove from the heat.

5 Add the cauliflower, broccoli, and chicken to the cheese sauce, gently stirring to combine. Spoon into the prepared baking dish, then sprinkle with the remaining cheddar. Bake at 375°F (190°C) for 25 minutes, or until the cheese is beginning to brown on the edges and the casserole is hot throughout and bubbly.

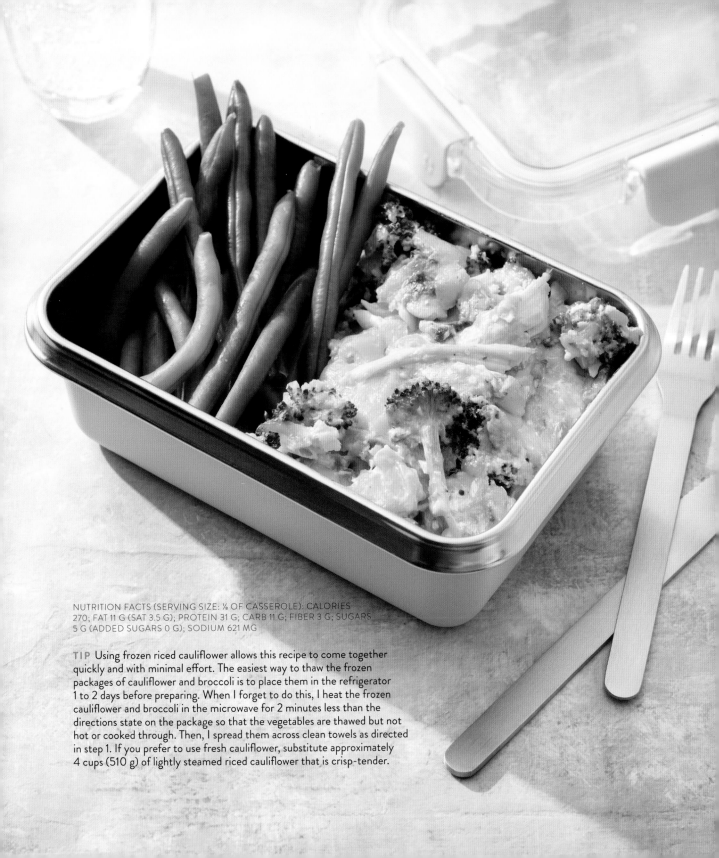

NUTRITION FACTS (SERVING SIZE: ⅛ OF CASSEROLE): CALORIES
270; FAT 11 G (SAT 3.5 G); PROTEIN 31 G; CARB 11 G; FIBER 3 G; SUGARS
5 G (ADDED SUGARS 0 G); SODIUM 621 MG

TIP Using frozen riced cauliflower allows this recipe to come together
quickly and with minimal effort. The easiest way to thaw the frozen
packages of cauliflower and broccoli is to place them in the refrigerator
1 to 2 days before preparing. When I forget to do this, I heat the frozen
cauliflower and broccoli in the microwave for 2 minutes less than the
directions state on the package so that the vegetables are thawed but not
hot or cooked through. Then, I spread them across clean towels as directed
in step 1. If you prefer to use fresh cauliflower, substitute approximately
4 cups (510 g) of lightly steamed riced cauliflower that is crisp-tender.

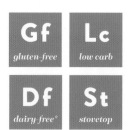

Gf — gluten-free
Lc — low carb
Df — dairy-free*
St — stovetop

1 pound (454 g) boneless, skinless chicken cutlets

2 tablespoons gluten-free baking mix

½ teaspoon salt

½ teaspoon black pepper

1 large egg

⅓ cup (40 g) gluten-free panko or bread crumbs

¼ cup (20 g) freshly grated Parmesan

¼ teaspoon garlic powder

1 tablespoon butter or ghee

One 5-ounce (142 g) container arugula and spring mix blend

¼ cup (60 ml) bottled olive oil vinaigrette

1 tablespoon lemon juice

pan-fried chicken over lemony greens

HANDS-ON: 15 MINUTES :: TOTAL: 25 MINUTES :: SERVES 4

"Mom's famous chicken" is how my kids refer to this dish, and I have to admit that it's a good one! The secret is browning the chicken in a little butter or ghee to create a golden crust with a rich, slightly decadent flavor. Finishing off the cooking process in the oven keeps the crust crisp and the chicken tender. Thanks to a vinaigrette that gets a squeeze of lemon, the lightly dressed greens perfectly complement the crispy, decadent-tasting chicken.

1 Preheat the oven to 375°F (190°C).

2 Place the chicken on a large cutting board or platter; sprinkle with the baking mix and ¼ teaspoon each of salt and pepper, turning to lightly season both sides.

3 Place the egg and 2 tablespoons of water in a shallow bowl; whisk to combine. In a separate shallow dish, combine the panko, Parmesan, garlic powder, and ¼ teaspoon each of salt and pepper. Dip one chicken breast in the egg mixture, turning to coat. Allow the excess to drip off; then place in the panko mixture, turning to lightly coat both sides. Place the coated chicken on the cutting board. Repeat with the remaining chicken breasts, egg mixture, and panko mixture.

4 Heat the butter in a large cast-iron or oven-proof skillet over medium-high heat. Cook the chicken in the hot butter until starting to turn golden, 3 minutes on each side. (Note: The chicken will not be fully cooked.) Remove the skillet from the stovetop and place in the preheated oven. Bake for 8 minutes, or until the chicken is cooked through and the outside is crispy and golden.

5 Place the arugula in a large bowl. Add the vinaigrette and lemon juice; toss well. Divide the arugula evenly among 4 plates. Top each with a chicken breast.

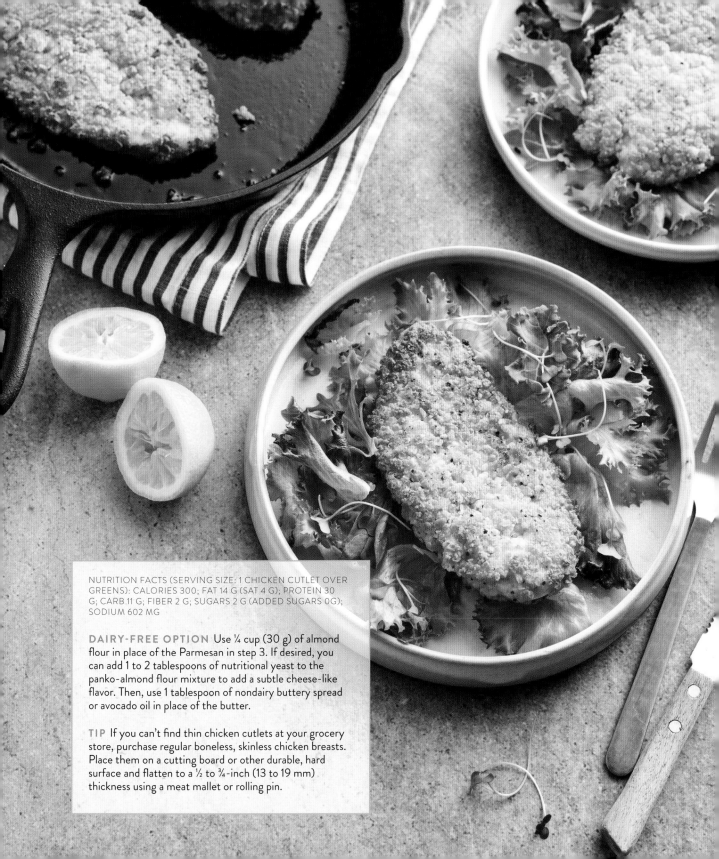

NUTRITION FACTS (SERVING SIZE: 1 CHICKEN CUTLET OVER GREENS): CALORIES 300; FAT 14 G (SAT 4 G); PROTEIN 30 G; CARB 11 G; FIBER 2 G; SUGARS 2 G (ADDED SUGARS 0G); SODIUM 602 MG

DAIRY-FREE OPTION Use ¼ cup (30 g) of almond flour in place of the Parmesan in step 3. If desired, you can add 1 to 2 tablespoons of nutritional yeast to the panko-almond flour mixture to add a subtle cheese-like flavor. Then, use 1 tablespoon of nondairy buttery spread or avocado oil in place of the butter.

TIP If you can't find thin chicken cutlets at your grocery store, purchase regular boneless, skinless chicken breasts. Place them on a cutting board or other durable, hard surface and flatten to a ½ to ¾-inch (13 to 19 mm) thickness using a meat mallet or rolling pin.

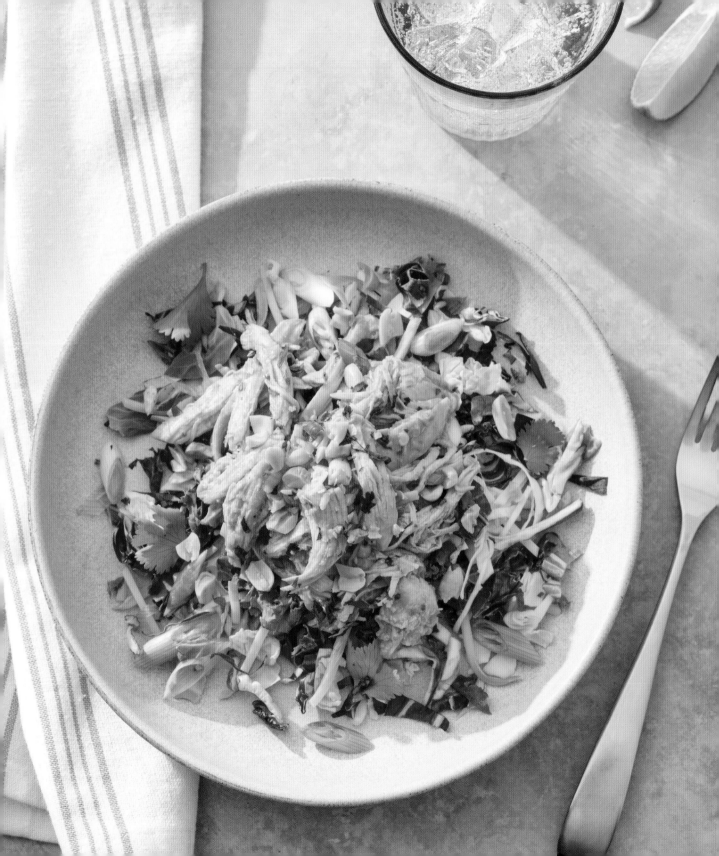

saucy peanut-coconut chicken

HANDS-ON: 10 MINUTES :: TOTAL: 20 MINUTES :: SERVES 8

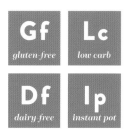

Even though they're often associated with Thai cuisine, creamy peanut sauces originated in Indonesia as an accompaniment to satay or grilled meat skewers, according to food historians. I've always loved satays served with peanut dipping sauces, and I created this instant pot version as a nod to the flavors in that dish. Saucy Peanut-Coconut Chicken is a perfect cold-weather, healthy comfort food that can be served over rice, riced cauliflower, or finely shredded napa cabbage for a little crunch and texture. And it's even better reheated the next day for lunch.

2 teaspoons avocado oil

2 pounds (1089 g) boneless, skinless chicken breasts

⅓ cup (80 ml) low-sodium chicken broth

¼ cup (60 ml) chili-garlic sauce

¼ cup (60 ml) lower-sodium soy sauce or tamari

2 tablespoons peanut butter

1½ tablespoons minced garlic

1½ tablespoons minced ginger

2 teaspoons lime juice

⅓ cup (80 ml) canned coconut milk

Chopped cilantro (optional)

1 Add the oil to the pressure cooker and press the SAUTÉ button. Cook the chicken in the hot oil until lightly browned, 2 minutes on each side. Press the KEEP WARM/CANCEL button.

2 In a small bowl, whisk together the broth, chili sauce, soy sauce, peanut butter, garlic, ginger, and lime juice. Pour over the chicken in the pressure cooker, turning to coat all sides. Secure the lid, making sure the pressure valve is secured. Press the POULTRY button and cook for 7 minutes. Then manually release the pressure valve and open the pressure cooker.

3 Remove the chicken breasts using a slotted spoon. Let cool slightly, then shred the chicken with two forks. Add the chicken and coconut milk back to the pressure cooker, stirring to combine.

NUTRITION FACTS (SERVING SIZE: ½ CUP/159 G CHICKEN IN SAUCE): CALORIES 215; FAT 9 G (SAT 2.5 G); PROTEIN 28 G; CARB 4 G; FIBER 0 G; SUGARS 2 G (ADDED SUGARS 0 G); SODIUM 507 MG

TIP If difficult to whisk, heat the broth mixture in the microwave for 10 to 15 seconds. This will soften the peanut butter so that the mixture is easier to combine.

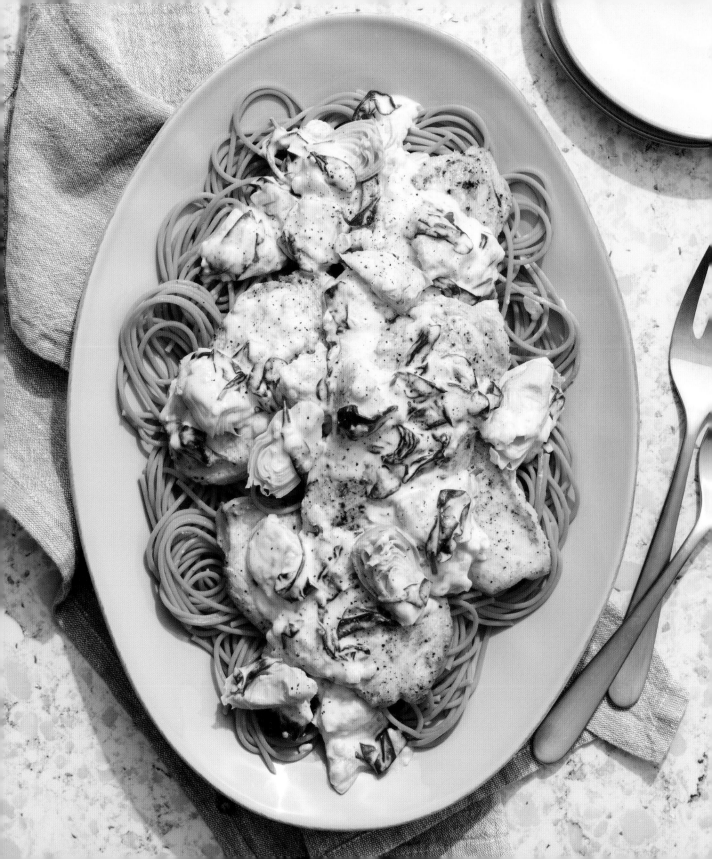

creamy spinach-artichoke chicken

HANDS-ON: 15 MINUTES :: TOTAL: 25 MINUTES :: SERVES 5

Warm spinach-artichoke dip gets turned into a cheesy skillet dinner using chicken cutlets. A quick, homemade cream sauce keeps nutrition in check, even providing 20 percent of the daily value for calcium and 15 percent of the daily value for potassium, thanks to the sauce's vegetables. This dish is delicious served by itself, as well as over spaghetti squash strands, whole-grain or chickpea pasta, or brown rice.

1 Season the chicken breasts on both sides with the garlic powder and ¼ teaspoon each of salt and pepper.

2 Heat the oil in a large skillet over medium heat. Cook the chicken until cooked through, 3 minutes on each side. Remove from the pan; set aside and keep warm.

3 Add the butter, onion, and garlic to the skillet. Sauté until fragrant, 1 to 2 minutes. Sprinkle the baking mix over the onion. Cook, stirring constantly, until the mix begins to turn golden, 1 minute.

4 Slowly whisk in the milk. Cook, stirring constantly, until the mixture starts to thicken, 2 minutes. Add the Parmesan and the remaining ¼ teaspoon of salt and pepper. Cook, stirring constantly, until the cheese is melted, 1 to 2 minutes.

5 Reduce the heat to low. Add the artichoke hearts, spinach, and chicken to the skillet. Cook until the spinach is beginning to wilt and the chicken is hot, 1 to 2 minutes.

NUTRITION FACTS (SERVING SIZE: ⅕ OF SKILLET): CALORIES 319; FAT 12 G (SAT 4 G); PROTEIN 38 G; CARB 13 G; FIBER 4 G; SUGARS 4 G (ADDED SUGARS 0 G); SODIUM 560 MG

1½ pounds (680 g) chicken breast cutlets

2 teaspoons garlic powder

½ teaspoon salt

½ teaspoon black pepper

1 tablespoon avocado oil

1½ teaspoons butter

1 small yellow onion, diced

4 garlic cloves, minced

2 tablespoons gluten-free baking mix or arrowroot flour

1¼ cups (300 ml) low-fat milk

⅔ cup (53 g) freshly grated Parmesan

One 9-ounce (255 g) package frozen artichoke hearts, thawed and chopped

3 cups (90 g) packed baby spinach

Gf gluten-free

Lc low carb

Df dairy-free*

St stovetop

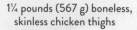

- 1¼ pounds (567 g) boneless, skinless chicken thighs
- ¼ teaspoon salt
- ¼ teaspoon black pepper
- 1½ tablespoons butter or ghee
- ¾ cup (180 ml) low-sodium chicken broth
- 1 tablespoon lemon juice
- 1 tablespoon minced garlic
- 2 teaspoons cornstarch or arrowroot flour
- 2 teaspoons chopped fresh rosemary

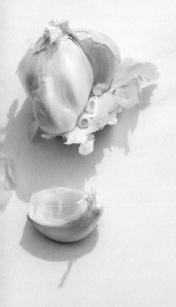

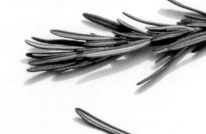

lemon-garlic chicken thighs

HANDS-ON: 15 MINUTES :: TOTAL: 15 MINUTES :: SERVES 4

Chicken thighs have been overshadowed by chicken breasts for years. The lighter breast meat was often seen as healthier, but the opposite is closer to reality. The darker meat in chicken thighs only has an additional 1.5 grams of fat when you compare a 4-ounce (115 g) thigh to a breast. Some think this makes thighs more satiating, but thighs also have more than double the iron, zinc, and vitamin B12 compared to breasts. In this quick dinner, the chicken is seared and then finished at a lower temperature to keep it tender and juicy. Brown bits from the searing process then get incorporated into a simple but flavorful butter sauce that features lemon juice and rosemary.

1 Sprinkle the chicken with the salt and pepper. Heat 1 tablespoon of the butter in a large cast-iron or other heavy skillet over medium-high heat. Cook the chicken until lightly browned on one side, 3 minutes. Turn the chicken and cook until the other side is lightly browned, 2 minutes. Reduce the heat to medium. Cook 2 to 3 minutes, until cooked through and no longer pink in the middle. Remove the chicken from the skillet and keep warm.

2 Add the broth, lemon juice, garlic, and the remaining ½ tablespoon of butter to the skillet. Reduce the heat to low; cook, stirring occasionally to loosen browned bits of chicken from bottom of skillet, until the butter is melted, 1 minute.

3 Add the cornstarch and rosemary. Cook, stirring frequently, until slightly thickened, 1 minute. Return the chicken to the skillet; remove from the heat. Spoon the sauce over the chicken and serve.

NUTRITION FACTS (SERVING SIZE: ¼ OF CHICKEN): CALORIES 230; FAT 11 G (SAT 4 G); PROTEIN 28 G; CARB 2 G; FIBER 0 G; SUGARS 0 G (ADDED SUGARS 0 G); SODIUM 302 MG

DAIRY-FREE OPTION Use 1 tablespoon of avocado oil in step 1 and ½ tablespoon of nondairy buttery spread in place of the butter.

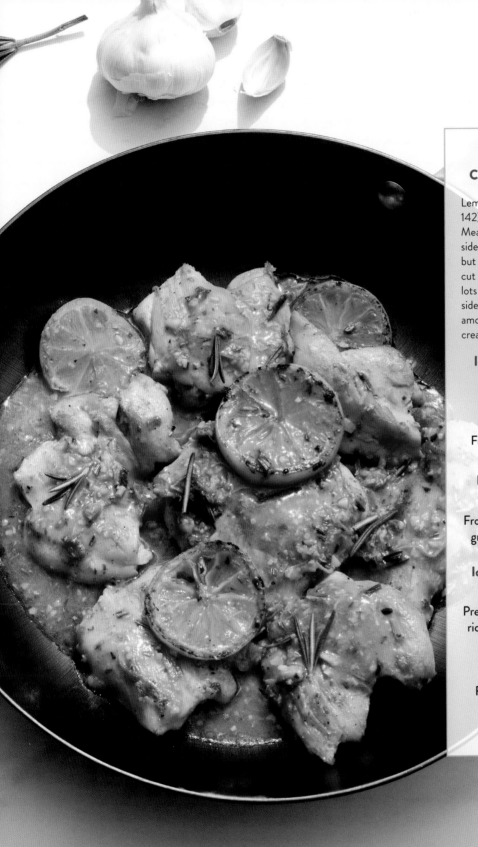

PERSONALIZED CARBOHYDRATE MEALS

Lemon-Garlic Chicken Thighs (page 142) and Muffin Pan Pesto Turkey Meatloaves (page 145) need a quick side to make them a satisfying meal, but this requires additional cooking. To cut down on cooking time, there are lots of ready-to-heat or almost-instant sides (with varying carbohydrate amounts to suit any goal) that I use to create a well-rounded meal.

Ideas for Low-Carbohydrate Meals

Frozen prepared mashed cauliflower

Frozen cauliflower or butternut squash risotto

Leafy or mixed greens tossed with a vinaigrette

Frozen steam-in-the-bag broccoli, green beans, or other vegetable

Ideas for Moderate to Higher Carbohydrate Meals

Precooked or ready-to-heat brown rice, quinoa, or other whole grain

Frozen prepared mashed sweet potatoes

Frozen seasoned sweet potato or wedges

Fresh fruit

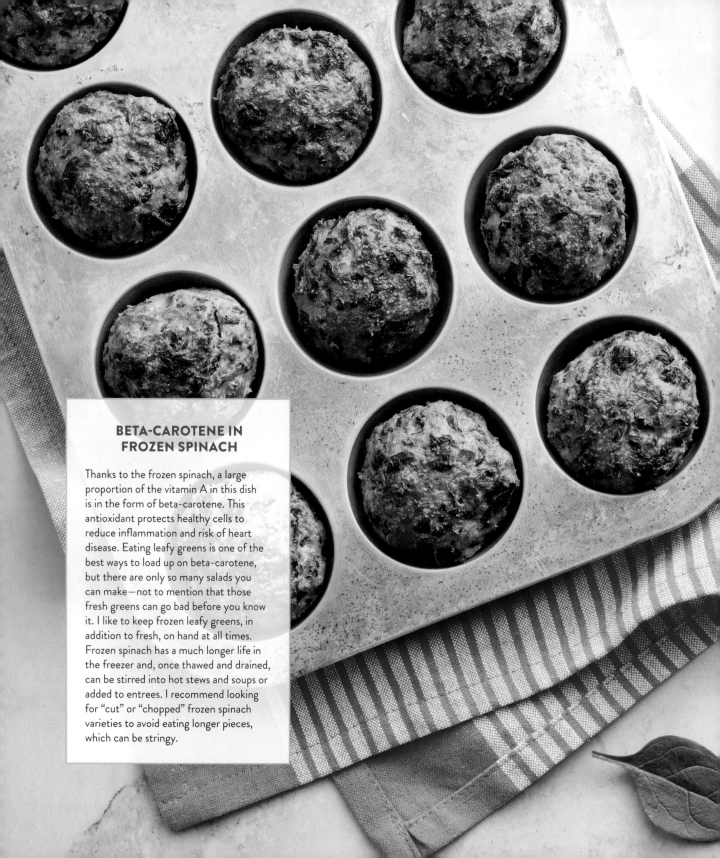

BETA-CAROTENE IN FROZEN SPINACH

Thanks to the frozen spinach, a large proportion of the vitamin A in this dish is in the form of beta-carotene. This antioxidant protects healthy cells to reduce inflammation and risk of heart disease. Eating leafy greens is one of the best ways to load up on beta-carotene, but there are only so many salads you can make—not to mention that those fresh greens can go bad before you know it. I like to keep frozen leafy greens, in addition to fresh, on hand at all times. Frozen spinach has a much longer life in the freezer and, once thawed and drained, can be stirred into hot stews and soups or added to entrees. I recommend looking for "cut" or "chopped" frozen spinach varieties to avoid eating longer pieces, which can be stringy.

muffin pan pesto turkey meatloaves

HANDS-ON: 15 MINUTES :: TOTAL: 35 MINUTES :: SERVES 5

I've never been a fan of meatloaf, but I can't get enough of this muffin pan variation! Instead of ketchup and ground beef, this one uses ground turkey, jarred pesto, garlic, and chopped spinach. The result is not only delicious and a favorite among my kids but is also low-carb and a great source of vitamin A (over 35 percent of the daily value per serving). These mini-meatloaves can stand alone, but I often pair them with some of the ready-to-heat sides listed for the Lemon-Garlic Chicken Thighs (page 142).

Cooking spray

One 10-ounce package (82 g) frozen chopped spinach, thawed

1 large egg

1 pound (454 g) ground turkey

⅓ cup (32 g) almond flour

2 tablespoons pesto

2 teaspoons minced garlic

½ teaspoon salt

1 Preheat the oven to 350°F (180°C). Lightly grease a 12-cup muffin pan with cooking spray.

2 Place the spinach on clean kitchen or paper towels. Squeeze out the excess water.

3 Whisk the egg in a medium bowl. Add the drained spinach, turkey, almond flour, pesto, garlic, and salt. Mix the ingredients using clean hands until well combined. Divide the turkey mixture evenly among 10 muffin cups (about ¼ cup/60 ml in each).

4 Bake for 18 to 20 minutes, until the turkey registers 160°F (71°C). Let stand 5 minutes before serving.

NUTRITION FACTS (SERVING SIZE: 2 MEATLOAVES): CALORIES 212; FAT 10 G (SAT 1.5 G); PROTEIN 28 G; CARB 5 G; FIBER 3 G; SUGARS 1 G (ADDED SUGARS 0 G); SODIUM 472 MG

DAIRY-FREE OPTION Substitute an equivalent amount of a dairy-free or vegan pesto for traditional pesto.

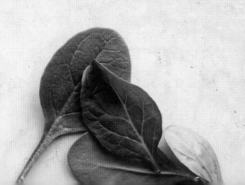
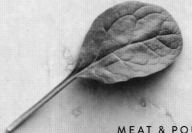

Gf gluten-free

Ma make ahead

V vegan*

St stovetop

Df dairy-free

semi-homemade bolognese with zoodles

HANDS-ON: 15 MINUTES :: TOTAL: 25 MINUTES :: SERVES 6

Eating five or more servings of fruits and vegetables each day is a key dietary habit that's associated with lower levels of chronic inflammation and reduces the risk of heart disease and high blood pressure. It can be a challenge, but swapping starches like rice and pasta for veggie noodles is an easy way to get closer to this goal. This recipe uses zucchini "noodles" in place of pasta to lower calories and carbohydrates; they also help to boost potassium to provide 30 percent of the daily value.

1 tablespoon avocado oil

½ cup (80 g) chopped yellow onion

2 teaspoons minced garlic

1 pound (454 g) Italian turkey sausage

One 24-ounce (680 g) jar lower-sodium marinara sauce

Two 14.5-ounce (411 g) cans no-salt-added diced fire-roasted tomatoes

¼ cup (11 g) torn fresh basil

4½ cups (646 g) zucchini spirals

1 Heat the oil in a Dutch oven or large saucepan over medium-high heat. Add the onion. Cook, stirring frequently, until beginning to soften, 4 minutes. Add the garlic and sausage. Cook until the sausage is browned, stirring to crumble, 6 minutes.

2 Stir in the marinara sauce, tomatoes, and basil, and bring to a simmer. Reduce the heat to medium-low, cover, and cook until hot and bubbly, 10 minutes.

3 Add the zucchini noodles, stirring to combine. Cook until warmed through, 2 minutes.

NUTRITION FACTS (SERVING SIZE: ABOUT 1⅔ CUPS/452 G): CALORIES 298; FAT 11 G (SAT 1.5 G); PROTEIN 21 G; CARB 30 G; FIBER 3 G; SUGARS 11 G (ADDED SUGARS 0 G); SODIUM 627 MG

VEGAN OPTION Substitute one 13.5-ounce (383 g) package of Italian sausage veggie crumbles in place of the turkey sausage in step 1.

TIP I recommend purchasing fresh zucchini spirals from the produce section or 2 to 3 whole zucchini to create your own fresh spirals; 1½ pounds (680 g) of zucchini will yield the amount of spirals needed for this recipe.

NOTE This is a great dish to prep ahead. Prepare the sauce in advance and refrigerate. When ready to use, heat the sauce in a skillet over medium heat until hot throughout. Then, add the zucchini spirals as directed in step 3.

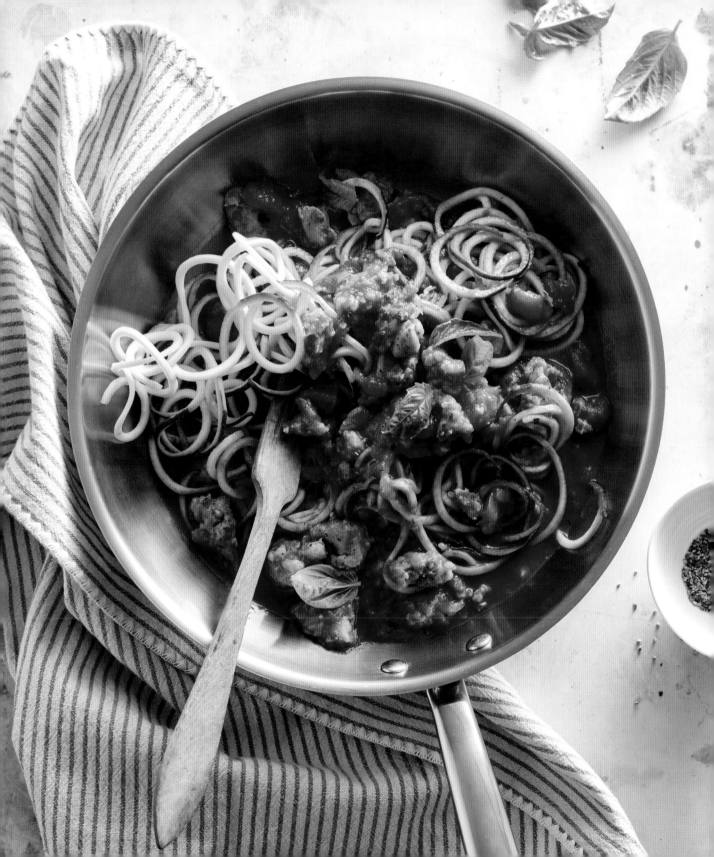

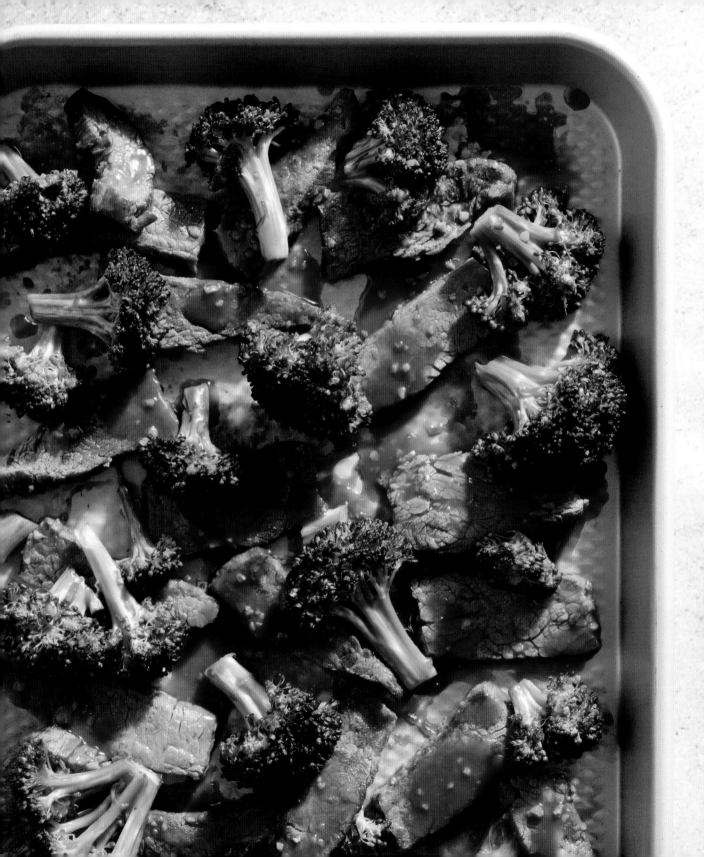

sheet pan beef and broccoli

HANDS-ON: 15 MINUTES :: TOTAL: 45 MINUTES :: SERVES 4

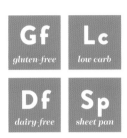

Not only is it quick and easy, but this sheet pan spin on a popular American Chinese-inspired dish is also a crowd-pleaser. The marinade is so flavorful that the beef only needs to spend a few minutes soaking it up. Use quick-cooking boil-in-bag brown rice or ready-to-heat brown rice pouches to keep the rest of dinner as simple as the entrée.

1 Cut the steak against the grain into ¼-inch (6 mm) thick slices. Cut each slice into three pieces.

2 Combine the soy sauce, garlic, ginger, vinegar, oil, and sugar in a large bowl; whisk to combine. Place 2 tablespoons in a small separate bowl for later use. Add the steak pieces to the mixture in the large bowl, stirring to make sure all of the pieces are covered. Let the steak marinate for 15 minutes.

3 Preheat the oven to 425°F (215°C). Place a large sheet pan in the oven until hot.

4 Place the broccoli in a separate bowl or shallow dish. Drizzle with the reserved 2 tablespoons of soy sauce mixture; toss to combine.

5 Remove the steak from the marinade and drain well; discard the marinade. Remove the hot sheet pan from the oven and lightly coat with cooking spray. Spread the steak evenly across the sheet pan, then top with the broccoli. Bake for 10 minutes, or until the steak reaches the desired degree of doneness and the broccoli is crisp-tender.

6 Pour the juices from the sheet pan into a small skillet over medium-high heat. Add the cornstarch, whisking to combine. Cook, stirring frequently, until thickened, 1 to 2 minutes. Pour over the steak and broccoli.

1 pound (454 g) flank steak

⅓ cup (80 ml) lower-sodium soy sauce or tamari

1 tablespoon minced garlic

1 tablespoon minced ginger or ginger paste

1 tablespoon rice wine vinegar

1 tablespoon sesame oil

1 tablespoon brown sugar

One 12-ounce (340 g) package steam-in-the-bag broccoli

Cooking spray

2 teaspoons cornstarch

NUTRITION FACTS (SERVING SIZE: ¼ OF SHEET PAN): CALORIES 247; FAT 9 G (SAT 3 G); PROTEIN 29 G; CARB 11 G; FIBER 2 G; SUGARS 6 G (ADDED SUGARS 3 G); SODIUM 516 MG

Gf gluten-free

Lc low carb

Df dairy-free

Sp sheet pan

1 pound (453 g) flank steak, trimmed

2 tablespoons taco seasoning

4 cups (227 g) chopped romaine lettuce

1½ cups (231 g) frozen roasted corn kernels, thawed

1 cup (149 g) cherry tomatoes, halved

2 tablespoons extra virgin olive oil

2 tablespoons lime juice

1 teaspoon honey

1 avocado, diced

southwestern flank steak salad

HANDS-ON: 15 MINUTES :: TOTAL: 15 MINUTES :: SERVES 4

Pro tip: Turn the broiler on while you prep the steak and slip your pan in the oven so it gets nice and hot before you cook the meat. This will help you get an even better sear on the outside. When the steak is done, let it rest for a few minutes—this makes it easier to cut it into thin slices. Make the dressing and toss the rest of the salad ingredients while you wait. Serve with fresh salsa and a few tortilla chips, if desired.

1 Preheat the broiler.

2 Score the steak diagonally against the grain on both sides. Rub both sides of the steak with 1 tablespoon plus 2 teaspoons of the taco seasoning and place on a broiler pan or in a ceramic or metal baking dish. Broil the steak for 6 minutes on each side, or until desired degree of doneness. Remove the steak from the oven; let stand 5 minutes.

3 Place the lettuce, corn, and tomatoes in a large bowl. Whisk together the oil, lime juice, honey, and the remaining 1 teaspoon of the taco seasoning in a small bowl. Pour over the salad and toss well to combine.

4 Divide the salad among four plates. Slice the steak into thin strips. Top each salad evenly with steak slices and avocado.

NUTRITION FACTS (SERVING SIZE: 1 SALAD): CALORIES 360; FAT 18 G (SAT 4 G); PROTEIN 28 G; CARB 21 G; FIBER 5 G; SUGARS 7 G (ADDED SUGARS 1 G); SODIUM 467 MG

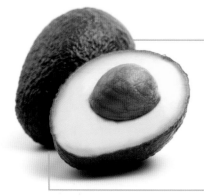

AVOCADO HEALTH BENEFITS

Avocados are full of nutrient and bioactive compounds like monounsaturated fats, vitamin E, fiber, and carotenoids that work together to soothe inflammation in the body. Research suggests that this combination may even help to counteract inflammation triggered by less healthy foods containing saturated fats. And if you're worried about the fat and calories in this creamy fruit, don't be. Those who eat avocado regularly, even daily, tend to have lower body weights in comparison to those who rarely eat avocado.

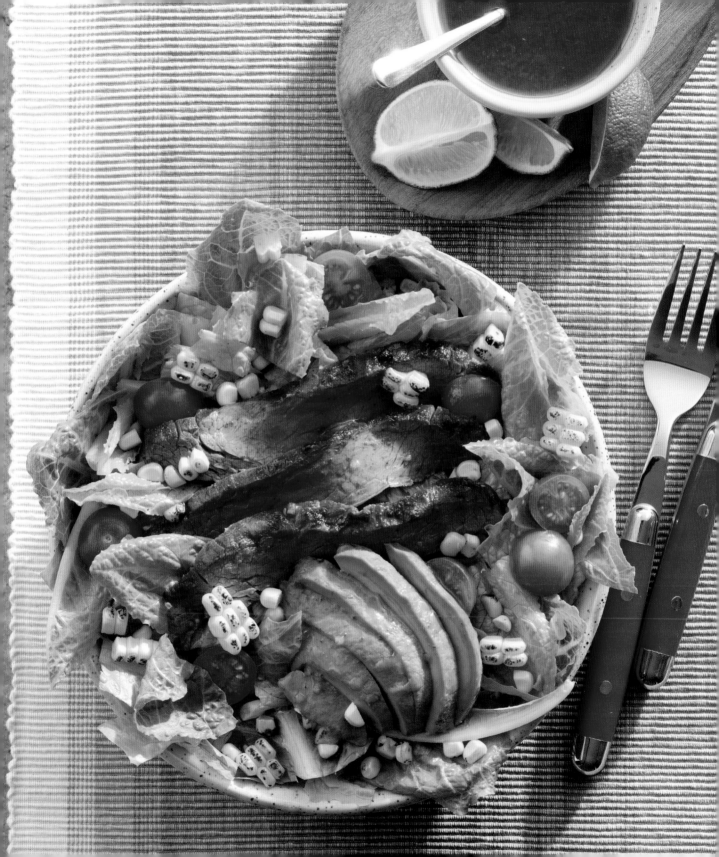

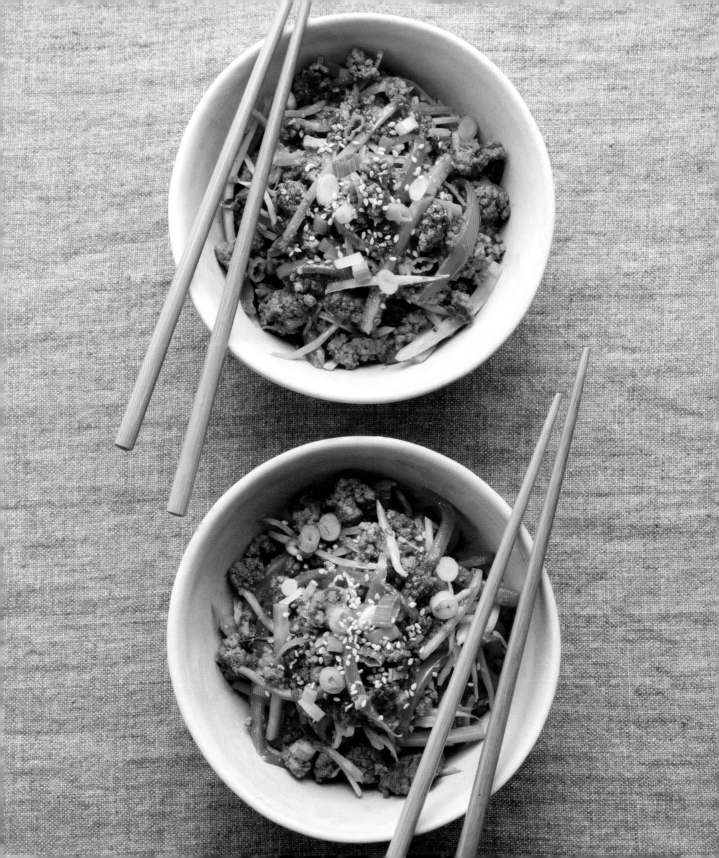

beef bulgogi skillet

HANDS-ON: 15 MINUTES :: TOTAL: 20 MINUTES :: SERVES 5

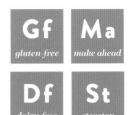

Beef bulgogi is a Korean dish in which thin slices of beef are marinated in a savory, slightly sweet, umami sauce and then grilled or seared. It's typically eaten over steamed rice or used as a filling for lettuce wraps. Beef bulgogi was the inspiration for this spin-off dish that streamlines prep by using ground beef to create a one-dish dinner. Serve the beef and cabbage mixture as is or on top of hot riced cauliflower or brown rice.

1 Heat 1 tablespoon of the oil over medium heat in a large cast-iron or heavy skillet. Sauté the coleslaw in the hot oil until beginning to soften but still crisp, 3 minutes. Add the scallions and 1 tablespoon each of the soy sauce and vinegar. Cook until hot throughout, 1 minute. Remove from the skillet; set aside and keep warm.

2 Heat the remaining 1 tablespoon oil in the skillet over medium heat. Cook the beef in the hot oil until browned, stirring to crumble, 6 minutes.

3 Return the coleslaw to the skillet. Whisk together the remaining 3 tablespoons of soy sauce, 1 tablespoon of vinegar, brown sugar, garlic, and ginger in a small bowl. Add to the skillet and cook until hot throughout, 2 minutes, stirring to combine.

NUTRITION FACTS (SERVING SIZE: ABOUT ¾ CUP/253 G): CALORIES 229; FAT 12 G (SAT 3 G); PROTEIN 21 G; CARB 8 G; FIBER 2 G; SUGARS 5 G (ADDED SUGARS 3 G); SODIUM 418 MG

NOTE This skillet dinner only takes 20 minutes, but it can be made in advance so that you have a hot meal even quicker. To do this, refrigerate both the slaw and the beef mixture. Reheat in the microwave or in a skillet over medium heat until hot.

2 tablespoons sesame oil

One 10-ounce (284) package tri-color coleslaw or vegetable slaw

½ cup (50 g) chopped scallions

¼ cup (60 ml) lower-sodium soy sauce or tamari

2 tablespoons rice wine vinegar

1 pound (454 g) lean ground beef

1 tablespoon brown sugar

2 teaspoons minced garlic

1 teaspoon minced ginger (or ½ teaspoon ground ginger)

Toasted sesame seeds and scallions (optional)

Gf
gluten-free

Lc
low carb

Sp
sheet pan

Cooking spray

1 large egg

½ pound (226 g) lean ground beef

½ pound (226 g) lean ground lamb

¼ cup (40 g) minced red onion

1 tablespoon Greek seasoning

¾ teaspoon salt

½ teaspoon garlic powder

½ teaspoon black pepper

Two 12-ounce (340 g) packages frozen riced cauliflower

1½ cups (200 g) diced cucumber

1 cup (149 g) cherry tomatoes, quartered

2 tablespoons crumbled feta

2 tablespoons bottled Greek or red wine vinaigrette

½ cup (120 ml) yogurt-based tzatziki

tzatziki "rice" bowls with gyro meatballs

HANDS-ON: 15 MINUTES :: TOTAL: 30 MINUTES :: SERVES 4

Greek seasoning, red onion, and a combination of ground beef and lamb create juicy, flavorful meatballs. Baking them in the oven saves you hands-on time and lets you prep the rest of the meal while they cook. Or make them in advance and reheat them when you're ready to assemble the bowls. If you're feeding picky eaters, place the different ingredients in serving dishes and let everyone assemble their own bowls.

1 Preheat the oven to 400°F (200°C). Line a baking sheet with foil and lightly coat with cooking spray.

2 Gently whisk the egg in a large bowl. Add the beef, lamb, onion, Greek seasoning, ½ teaspoon of salt, garlic powder, and ¼ teaspoon of pepper. Mix the ingredients using clean hands until combined well. Roll the mixture into approximately twenty-eight 1½-inch (3.8 cm) meatballs and place on the baking sheet. Bake for 15 minutes, or until browned on the outside and cooked through on the inside.

3 Heat the cauliflower in the microwave according to package directions. While the cauliflower heats, combine the cucumber, tomatoes, and feta in a medium bowl. Add the vinaigrette; toss gently to combine.

4 Place the cauliflower in a separate bowl or serving dish. Stir in ¼ teaspoon each of salt and pepper, then divide the cauliflower evenly among four bowls. Add the cucumber mixture to one side of each bowl. Place the meatballs on the other side of each bowl. Dollop each bowl with 2 tablespoons of tzatziki.

NUTRITION FACTS (SERVING SIZE: 1 BOWL): CALORIES 307; FAT 15 G (SAT 5.5 G); PROTEIN 30 G; CARB 14 G; FIBER 5 G; SUGARS 8 G (ADDED SUGARS 0 G); SODIUM 641 MG

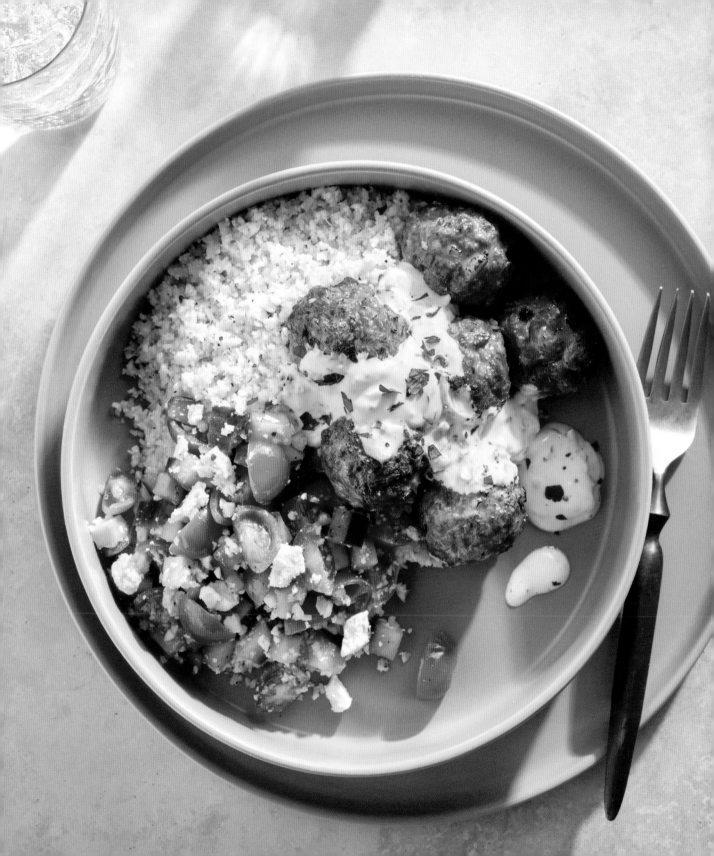

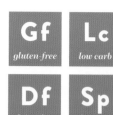

½ cup (120 ml) lower-sodium soy
sauce or tamari

¼ cup (60 ml) avocado oil

¼ cup (60 ml) balsamic vinegar

2 tablespoons brown sugar or
maple syrup

1½ tablespoons crushed dried
rosemary

2 teaspoons minced garlic

1½ teaspoons ground ginger

¾ teaspoon dry mustard

1½ pounds (646 g) pork
tenderloin

Cooking spray

One 12-ounce (299 g) bag
trimmed green beans

¼ teaspoon salt

¼ teaspoon black pepper

balsamic-rosemary pork with green beans

HANDS-ON: 12 MINUTES :: TOTAL: 2 HOURS 45 MINUTES :: SERVES 5

Prep and refrigerate this early in the day so that dinner only requires heating the oven and popping in a sheet pan. The pork tenderloin's flavors are amplified the longer it marinates. Pork is an excellent source of several B vitamins and minerals. In fact, one serving of this recipe provides over 60 percent of the daily value of B6 and selenium. This is important since adequate B6 is needed to maintain immune and nervous system health, and selenium is key to thyroid functioning. Selenium is also an antioxidant that protects cells from damage that can potentially lead to new inflammation.

1 Place the soy sauce, oil, vinegar, brown sugar, rosemary, garlic, ginger, and dry mustard in a small bowl, whisking to combine. Reserve ¼ cup (60 ml) of the mixture in a small bowl and cover for later use in step 5.

2 Place the pork in a shallow dish or sealable bag. Pour over the remaining marinade, then cover the dish or seal the bag. Marinate in the refrigerator for at least 2 hours and up to 36, turning once or twice.

3 Preheat the oven to 400°F (200°C) and place a sheet pan in the oven to heat.

4 Remove the pork from the marinade; discard the marinade. Remove the hot sheet pan from the oven and lightly coat with cooking spray. Place the pork on one side of the sheet pan and bake for 20 minutes.

5 Coat the green beans with cooking spray and sprinkle with salt and pepper. Spread the green beans across the other side of the sheet pan.

6 Bake for 15 to 20 minutes, until the pork is lightly browned and cooked through and the beans are crisp-tender and browned on the edges. Warm the reserved marinade in the microwave for 15 to 20 seconds. Drizzle over the pork and serve.

NUTRITION FACTS (SERVING SIZE: ⅕ OF PORK AND GREEN BEANS): CALORIES 251; FAT 10 G (SAT 1.5 G); PROTEIN 29 G; CARB 11 G; FIBER 2 G; SUGARS 8 G (ADDED SUGARS 3 G); SODIUM 546 MG

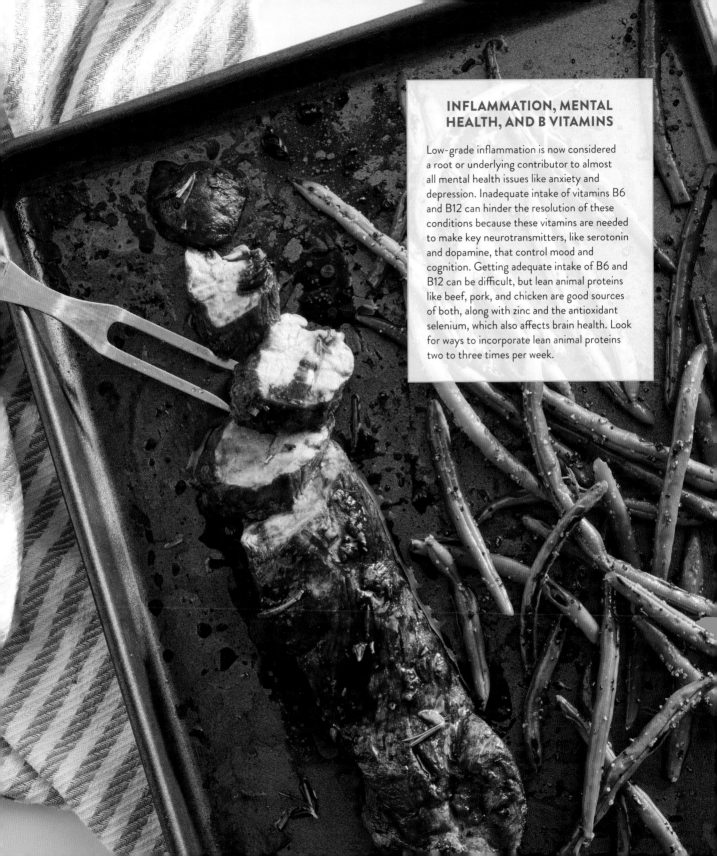

INFLAMMATION, MENTAL HEALTH, AND B VITAMINS

Low-grade inflammation is now considered a root or underlying contributor to almost all mental health issues like anxiety and depression. Inadequate intake of vitamins B6 and B12 can hinder the resolution of these conditions because these vitamins are needed to make key neurotransmitters, like serotonin and dopamine, that control mood and cognition. Getting adequate intake of B6 and B12 can be difficult, but lean animal proteins like beef, pork, and chicken are good sources of both, along with zinc and the antioxidant selenium, which also affects brain health. Look for ways to incorporate lean animal proteins two to three times per week.

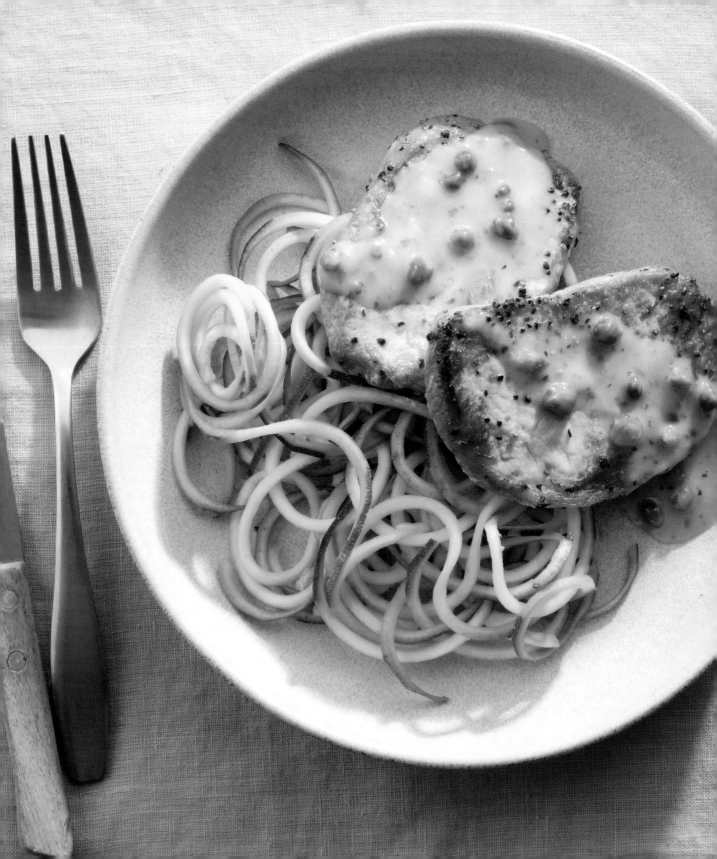

pork piccata over zoodles

HANDS-ON: 15 MINUTES :: TOTAL: 25 MINUTES :: SERVES 4

"Piccata" refers to a dish where meat, poultry, or seafood is sautéed and then served in a butter sauce with capers and lemon juice. The meat is typically pounded thin, which helps to keep it tender and its cook time minimal. This dish can also be served over whole-grain or legume-based pasta if you'd prefer that to zoodles.

1 Season the pork with salt and pepper. Heat the oil in a large skillet over medium-high heat. Cook the pork in the hot oil until golden brown and cooked through, 3 minutes per side. Transfer to a plate and keep warm.

2 Add the broth, wine, capers, lemon juice, and cornstarch to the skillet and bring to a simmer. Cook until the liquid is slightly reduced, 1 to 2 minutes. Remove from the heat and add the butter, stirring until melted. Pour the broth mixture into a small bowl and set aside.

3 Add the zucchini noodles to the skillet. Sauté until crisp-tender, 1 to 2 minutes. (For more cooked, tender zucchini noodles, remove the skillet from the heat. Cover and let stand for 2 to 3 minutes.) Add the pork and drizzle with the broth mixture.

NUTRITION FACTS (SERVING SIZE: ¼ OF PORK AND ZUCCHINI): CALORIES 282; FAT 13 G (SAT 5 G); PROTEIN 35 G; CARB 7 G; FIBER 2 G; SUGARS 4 G (ADDED SUGARS 0 G); SODIUM 427 MG

DAIRY-FREE OPTION Use a nondairy buttery spread in place of the butter.

TIP Substitute additional broth in place of the white wine, if desired.

Ingredients

- 1¼ pounds (437 g) boneless pork cutlets, pounded to ½-inch (13 mm) thick
- ¼ teaspoon salt
- ¼ teaspoon black pepper
- 1 tablespoon avocado oil
- ½ cup (120 ml) low-sodium chicken broth
- ¼ cup (60 ml) white wine
- 3 tablespoons drained capers
- 2 tablespoons lemon juice
- 1½ teaspoons cornstarch
- 2½ tablespoons butter or ghee, cubed
- 1½ pounds (646 g) zucchini spirals
- Chopped fresh flat-leaf parsley, lemon wedges (optional)

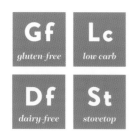

Gf *gluten-free* **Lc** *low carb*

Df *dairy-free* **St** *stovetop*

Two 12-ounce (340 g) packages steam-in-the-bag broccoli

1½ pounds (680 g) bone-in, center-cut pork chops

¼ teaspoon salt

¼ teaspoon black pepper

1 tablespoon avocado oil

6 garlic cloves, minced

¼ cup (60 ml) low-sodium chicken broth or water

¼ cup (60 ml) chili-garlic sauce

2½ tablespoons apple cider vinegar

1 tablespoon honey

1 teaspoon cornstarch

Fresh chopped parsley (optional)

chile-garlic pork chops and broccoli

HANDS-ON: 12 MINUTES :: TOTAL: 25 MINUTES :: SERVES 4

Chili-garlic sauce serves as the base for this saucy pork glaze and imparts both a touch of sweetness and a little heat. The flavors are reminiscent of a sweet-and-sour pork or chicken dish with a subtle hint of spice. On the shelf, sweet red chili sauce looks very similar to chili-garlic sauce. However, sweet red chili sauce is loaded with added sugars, while chili-garlic sauce has no added sugars, only a few grams of natural sugar.

1 Cook the broccoli in the microwave according to the package directions.

2 Season the pork with salt and pepper. Heat the oil in a large cast-iron or heavy skillet over medium-high heat. Cook the pork chops in the hot oil until lightly browned and cooked through, 4 minutes on each side. Transfer to a plate; keep warm.

3 Reduce the heat to medium. Add the garlic and sauté until fragrant, 30 seconds. Add the broth, chili-garlic sauce, vinegar, honey, and cornstarch, whisking to combine and to scrape up any browned bits from the bottom of the skillet. Cook, stirring frequently, until the sauce begins to thicken, 1 minute.

4 Add the pork back to the skillet. Serve the pork with the steamed broccoli, drizzling both with the skillet sauce. Garnish with parsley, if desired.

NUTRITION FACTS (SERVING SIZE: ¼ OF PORK AND BROCCOLI): CALORIES 301; FAT 11 G (SAT 3 G); PROTEIN 33 G; CARB 15 G; FIBER 6 G; SUGARS 8 G (ADDED SUGARS 4 G); SODIUM 511 MG

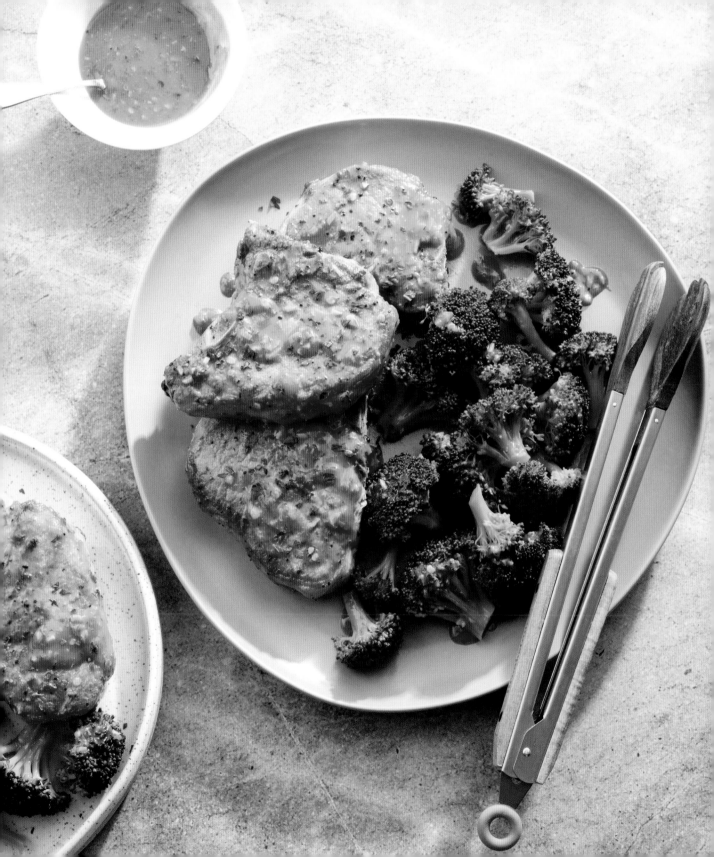

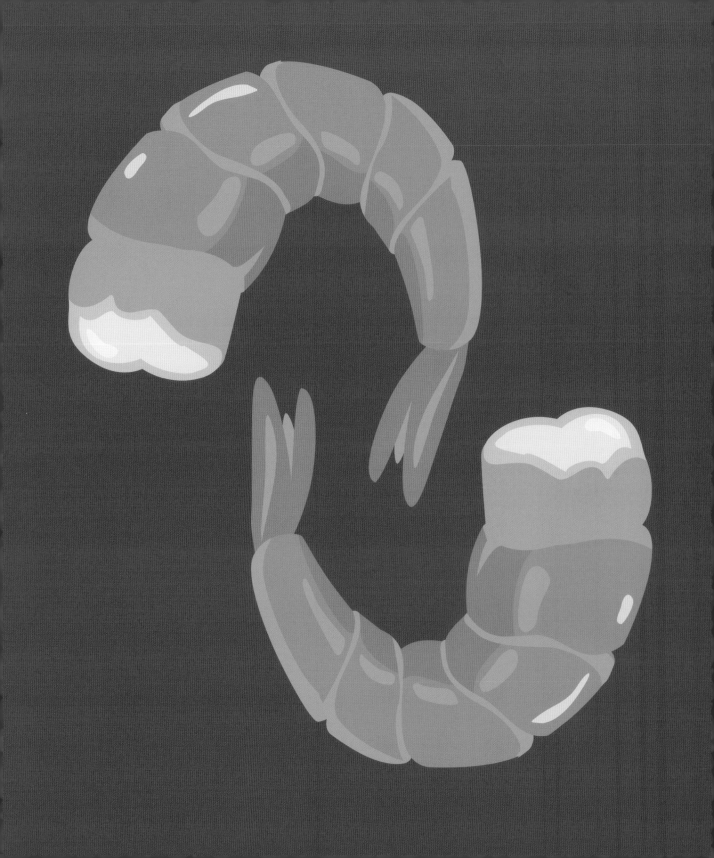

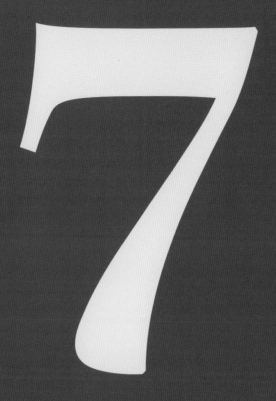

7

. . . .

FISH & SEAFOOD

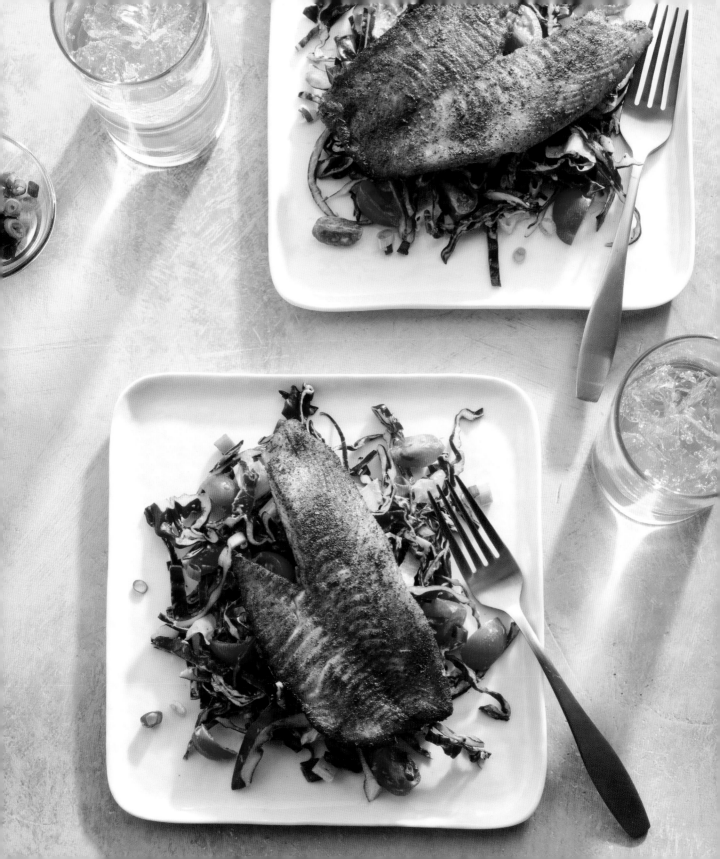

blackened fish over avocado-lime slaw

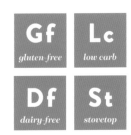

HANDS-ON: 15 MINUTES :: TOTAL: 15 MINUTES :: SERVES 4

Deconstructed fish tacos are the best way to describe this dish, which highlights the flavors of blackened fish, avocado, and lime juice. It's a filling, low-carb meal on its own, but you can also serve the fish and slaw in warm corn tortillas. Make the slaw ahead, cover, and refrigerate for up to two hours before serving. Don't have a food processor? Coarsely mash the avocado with the back of a spoon or fork. Add the lime juice, stirring to combine, and mash the avocado further. Then, add the mayonnaise, cumin, garlic powder, and salt.

1 Combine the cabbage, tomatoes, and scallions in a large mixing bowl. Place the avocado, mayonnaise, lime juice, cumin, garlic powder, and salt in the bowl of a food processor. Secure the top and process until blended, 30 seconds, pausing to add 1 to 2 tablespoons of water as needed to create a smooth, creamy dressing. Add the avocado mixture to the cabbage. Toss well and set aside.

2 Sprinkle the fish with the seasoning. Heat the oil in a large cast-iron or heavy skillet over medium-high heat. Add the fish; cook until the fish is lightly browned and flakes easily with a fork, 2 minutes on each side. Serve the fish over or next to the slaw.

NUTRITION FACTS (SERVING SIZE: ¼ OF FISH AND SLAW): CALORIES 320; FAT 16 G (SAT 3 G); PROTEIN 36 G; CARB 9 G; FIBER 4 G; SUGARS 4 G (ADDED SUGARS 0 G); SODIUM 609 MG

TIP Blackened seasoning is typically made by combining several spices you may have on hand. If you prefer to make your own blackened seasoning instead of using store-bought, combine these spices in a small bowl: 2 tablespoons smoked or regular paprika; 2 teaspoons each of garlic powder and onion powder; 1½ teaspoons dried thyme; 1 teaspoon each of dried oregano, black pepper, and salt; and ¼ to ½ teaspoon cayenne pepper, depending on desired level of spice. This recipe makes 5 tablespoons; store any extra in an airtight container for up to six months.

NOTE Use 3 tablespoons of extra virgin olive oil in place of the mayonnaise for slightly less creamy slaw, if desired.

---

4 cups (280 g) finely shredded cabbage

¾ cup (112 g) cherry tomatoes, quartered

2 scallions, chopped

1 avocado, diced

¼ cup (60 ml) olive, canola, or avocado oil-based mayonnaise

3 tablespoons lime juice

1 teaspoon ground cumin

1 teaspoon garlic powder

½ teaspoon salt

1½ pounds (680 g) tilapia or other firm white fish

1 tablespoon blackened seasoning

1 tablespoon avocado oil

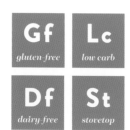

Gf *gluten-free*

Lc *low carb*

Df *dairy-free*

St *stovetop*

3 tablespoons hoisin sauce

2 tablespoons lime juice

¼ teaspoon garlic powder

2 tablespoons lower-sodium soy sauce or tamari

1½ tablespoons sesame oil

1 teaspoon grated ginger

1¼ pounds (505 g) salmon fillets

¼ teaspoon salt

One 12-ounce (340 g) bag fresh broccoli slaw

1½ cups (233 g) shelled edamame, thawed

2 scallions, chopped

Toasted sesame seeds (optional)

hoisin salmon with warm broccoli-edamame slaw

HANDS-ON: 15 MINUTES :: TOTAL: 15 MINUTES :: SERVES 4

This simple one-dish meal uses ingredients with bold flavors, like hoisin sauce, lime juice, and soy sauce. Only a little of each is needed, allowing the sodium to stay just under 600 mg per serving. With 5 grams of fiber and 41 grams of protein, it's a filling meal by itself, but you can also pair it with ready-to-heat brown rice or another whole grain, if desired.

1 In a small bowl, whisk together the hoisin sauce, 1 tablespoon of lime juice, and the garlic powder. In a separate small bowl, whisk together the soy sauce, 1 tablespoon lime juice, 1 tablespoon oil, and ginger. Set both aside.

2 Heat ½ tablespoon of the oil in a large skillet over medium heat. Sprinkle the fish with salt. Cook the salmon, skin side down, until the skin is lightly browned, 6 minutes. Flip the fish and brush with the hoisin mixture. Cook until the fish has reached desired degree of doneness, about 2 to 4 minutes. Transfer to a plate.

3 Wipe the skillet clean and increase the heat to medium-high. Add the broccoli slaw, edamame, and scallions; cook, stirring frequently, until the broccoli is crisp-tender, 2 minutes. Add the soy sauce mixture; sauté for 30 seconds. Remove the skillet from the heat. Serve the salmon over the warm broccoli slaw.

NUTRITION FACTS (SERVING SIZE: 1 FILLET WITH ¼ OF SLAW): CALORIES 390; FAT 18 G (SAT 2.5 G); PROTEIN 41 G; CARB 15 G; FIBER 5 G; SUGARS 4 G (ADDED SUGARS 2 G); SODIUM 593 MG

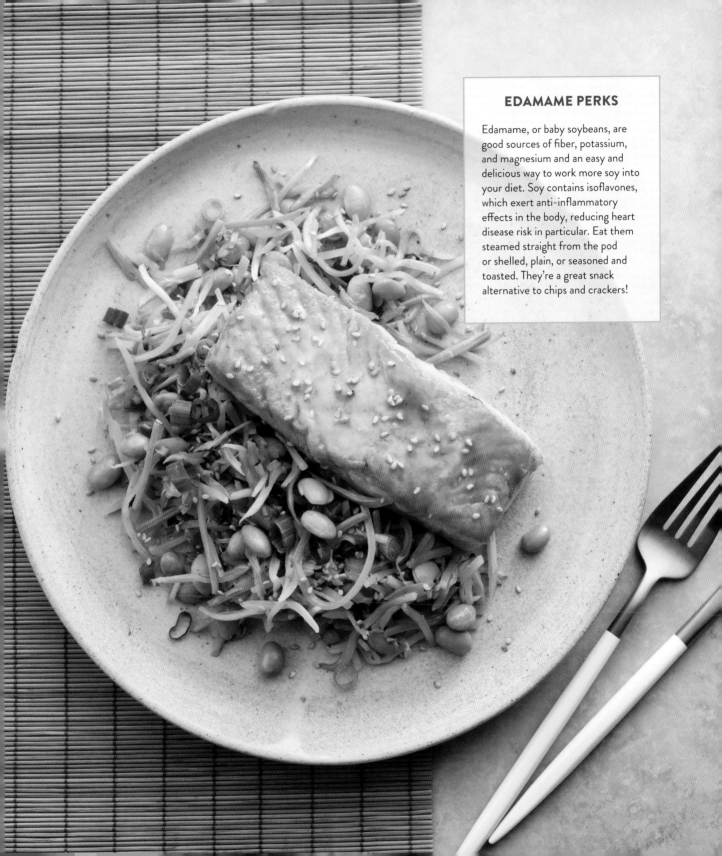

EDAMAME PERKS

Edamame, or baby soybeans, are good sources of fiber, potassium, and magnesium and an easy and delicious way to work more soy into your diet. Soy contains isoflavones, which exert anti-inflammatory effects in the body, reducing heart disease risk in particular. Eat them steamed straight from the pod or shelled, plain, or seasoned and toasted. They're a great snack alternative to chips and crackers!

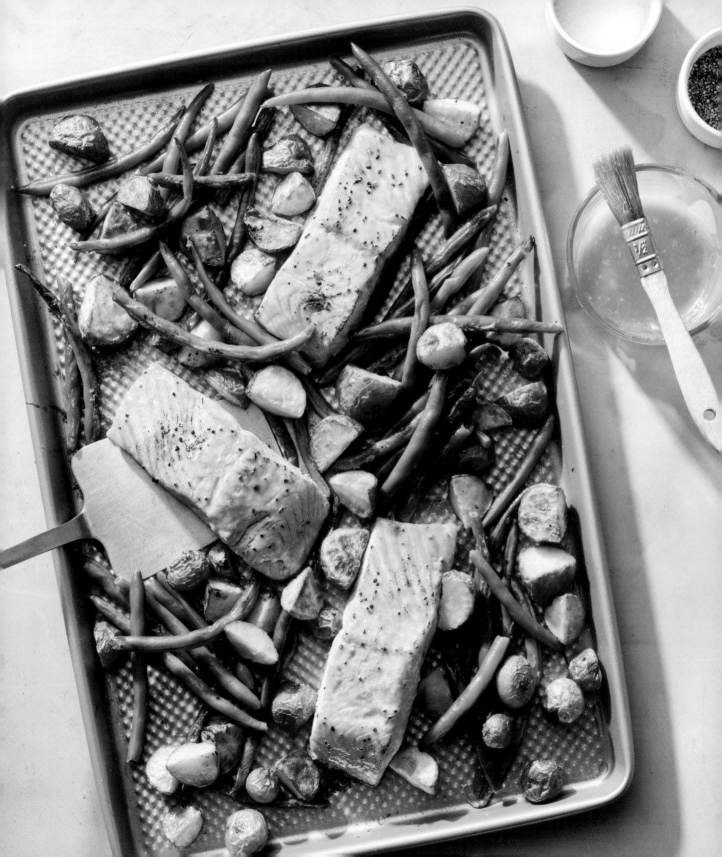

honey-dijon
sheet pan salmon

This sheet pan salmon dinner makes eating the recommended two to three servings of seafood a week so much easier! A tangy, sweet sauce made with honey, Dijon mustard, and butter is a delicious way to highlight the salmon's richness and pairs well with the crispy, roasted potatoes and green beans.

1 Preheat the oven to 450°F (220°C). Toss the potatoes with the oil, ½ teaspoon salt, and ½ teaspoon garlic powder on a rimmed baking sheet. Bake for 20 minutes.

2 While the potatoes cook, combine the honey, butter, and mustard in a small bowl; set aside. Coat the green beans with cooking spray, then toss with the remaining ½ teaspoon garlic powder and ¼ teaspoon salt.

3 Flip the potatoes, then add the salmon and green beans to the sheet pan in an even layer. Brush the honey mixture over the salmon and sprinkle with the remaining ¼ teaspoon salt and pepper. Return the sheet pan to the oven and bake for 8 minutes.

4 Turn the green beans. Bake for an additional 5 to 7 minutes, until the fish has reached your desired degree of doneness and the potatoes are tender.

NUTRITION FACTS (SERVING SIZE: ¼ OF SHEET PAN): CALORIES 420; FAT 18 G (SAT 3.5 G); PROTEIN 36 G; CARB 29 G; FIBER 4 G; SUGARS 9 G (ADDED SUGARS 4 G); SODIUM 652 MG

DAIRY-FREE OPTION Substitute a non-dairy buttery spread for the butter.

Ingredients

- 1 pound (454 g) small red potatoes, halved (quartered if large)
- 1½ tablespoons avocado oil
- 1 teaspoon salt
- 1 teaspoon garlic powder
- 1 tablespoon honey
- 2 teaspoons butter or ghee, melted
- 1 to 2 teaspoons Dijon mustard
- One 12-ounce (340 g) bag trimmed fresh green beans
- Cooking spray
- 1¼ pounds (505 g) salmon fillets
- ¼ teaspoon black pepper

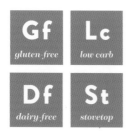

Gf gluten-free

Lc low carb

Df dairy-free

St stovetop

1¼ pounds (567 g) tuna steaks, cut into 4 pieces

¼ cup (60 ml) lower-sodium soy sauce or tamari

2 tablespoons rice vinegar

1 tablespoon sesame oil

2 teaspoons minced garlic

2 teaspoons minced ginger

1 tablespoon avocado oil

½ teaspoon salt

¼ teaspoon black pepper

5 cups (283 g) baby spinach

1 avocado, sliced or diced

½ cup (90 g) orange sections

⅓ cup (80 ml) Ginger-Soy Vinaigrette or bottled sesame-ginger dressing

GINGER-SOY VINAIGRETTE

3 tablespoons fresh orange juice

1 tablespoon rice vinegar

2 tablespoons lower-sodium soy sauce or tamari

2 teaspoons honey

1 tablespoon plus 1 teaspoon minced fresh ginger

½ teaspoon garlic salt

3 tablespoons avocado oil

1 tablespoon sesame oil

seared tuna over ginger-soy spinach and avocado

HANDS-ON: 15 MINUTES :: TOTAL: 35 MINUTES :: SERVES 4

Looking for a fish recipe that's a little different? Baby spinach and orange sections are tossed with a Ginger-Soy Vinaigrette, creating the perfect balance of flavor and texture to highlight seared tuna. This dish boasts 25 percent of the daily value for potassium, which is important for heart health since low-grade inflammation is a primary force behind the development and progression of hypertension.

1 Place the tuna steaks in a shallow dish or zip-top bag. Combine the soy sauce, vinegar, sesame oil, garlic, and ginger in a small bowl. Pour the mixture over the fish. Cover or seal the bag and marinate in the refrigerator for 20 minutes.

2 Heat the avocado oil in a large skillet over medium-high heat. Sprinkle the tuna with salt and pepper. Add the fish to the pan; cook until the fish is lightly browned on both sides and has reached your desired degree of doneness, 2 to 4 minutes on each side.

3 Combine the spinach, avocado, orange sections, and dressing in a large bowl. Toss well to combine. Evenly divide the spinach mixture among 4 plates and top with the tuna.

NUTRITION FACTS (SERVING SIZE: ¼ OF TUNA OVER TOSSED GREENS): CALORIES 354; FAT 18 G (SAT 2.5 G); PROTEIN 35 G; CARB 13 G; FIBER 5 G; SUGARS 5 G (ADDED SUGARS 1 G); SODIUM 626 MG

ginger-soy vinaigrette

MAKES ¾ CUP (180 ML)

Whisk together all ingredients in a small bowl. Refrigerate in a covered container for up to 5 days. Shake well before serving.

NUTRITION FACTS (SERVING SIZE: 1 TABLESPOON): CALORIES 51; FAT 4.5 G (SAT 1.5 G); PROTEIN 0 G; CARB 2 G; FIBER 0 G; SUGARS 1.5 G (ADDED SUGARS 1 G); SODIUM 92 MG

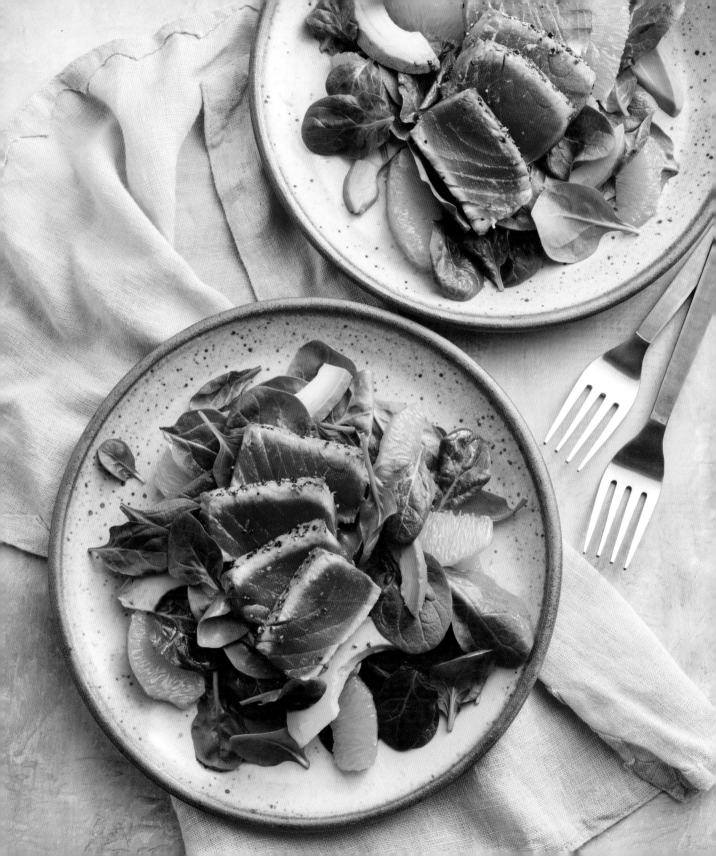

Gf
gluten-free

Df
dairy-free

St
stovetop

3 ears corn

Cooking spray

1 tablespoon avocado oil

1½ pounds (680 g) large sea
scallops, rinsed and patted dry

½ teaspoon ground cumin

¾ teaspoon salt

½ teaspoon black pepper

1½ cups (224 g) chopped tomato
or halved cherry tomatoes

1 avocado, diced

¼ cup (29 g) minced red onion

¼ cup (4 g) chopped fresh
cilantro or basil

2 tablespoons extra virgin olive
oil

1 tablespoon lime juice

½ teaspoon honey

¼ teaspoon garlic powder

NOTE If tomatoes and corn
aren't in season, you can still
enjoy this dish by using cherry
tomatoes and 2½ cups
(363 g) thawed, frozen corn
kernels that have been warmed
to room temperature in the
microwave.

seared scallops over summer corn salad

HANDS-ON: 10 MINUTES :: TOTAL: 15 MINUTES :: SERVES 4

This dish was inspired by an abundance of summer corn and tomatoes,
but this recipe is delicious year-round (see Note). Scallops are a great
source of selenium and zinc, two nutrients that can be challenging to
consume in adequate amounts but are crucial for the immune system to
work at 100 percent efficiency and reduce susceptibility to illness. One
serving of this recipe provides 42 percent of the daily value for selenium
and 20 percent of the daily value for zinc.

1 Remove the husks and silk from the corn. Cut the kernels off the cob
to yield 2½ cups (363 g).

2 Heat a large cast-iron or heavy skillet over medium-high heat.
Lightly coat the skillet with cooking spray. Add the corn kernels and
cook until lightly browned, stirring occasionally, 3 minutes. Sprinkle
the corn with ¼ teaspoon of salt and place in a large bowl. Return the
skillet to the heat.

3 Heat the avocado oil in the skillet. Sprinkle the scallops with cumin,
¼ teaspoon salt, and ¼ teaspoon pepper. Cook the scallops in the hot
oil, undisturbed, until the bottom of each scallop has browned edges
and is slightly opaque, for 1 minute. Turn the scallops over and cook
until firm and opaque, with browned edges, 1 to 2 minutes. Remove
from the skillet and let stand.

4 Add the tomatoes, avocado, onion, and cilantro to the corn. In
a small bowl, whisk together the olive oil, lime juice, honey, garlic
powder, and remaining ¼ teaspoon of salt and pepper. Pour over the
corn mixture and toss well to combine. Divide the corn mixture evenly
among 4 plates. Top with the scallops.

NUTRITION FACTS (SERVING SIZE: ¼ OF SCALLOPS AND CORN MIXTURE): CALORIES 361;
FAT 17.5 G (SAT 2.5 G); PROTEIN 25 G; CARB 29 G; FIBER 5 G; SUGARS 8 G (ADDED SUGARS
0.5 G); SODIUM 714 MG

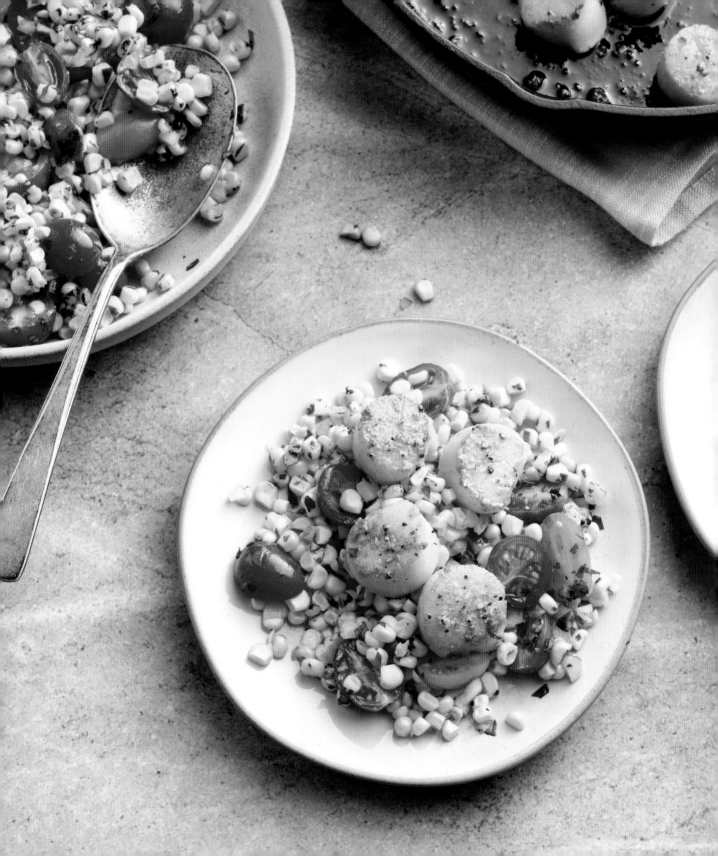

Gf *gluten-free*
 Df *dairy-free*
 V *vegan**
 St *stovetop*

spaghetti squash pad thai with shrimp

HANDS-ON: 15 MINUTES :: TOTAL: 15 MINUTES :: SERVES 4

This lower-carb riff on pad thai might be my all-time favorite way to eat spaghetti squash, and only minimal work is required at mealtime when you prep the spaghetti squash in advance. If I don't have shrimp, I'll use a rotisserie chicken or any other protein I happen to have on hand. Almost any protein would be delicious!

¾ cup (180 ml) lower-sodium chicken or vegetable broth

¼ cup (60 ml) creamy peanut butter

1½ tablespoons lower-sodium soy sauce or tamari

1 tablespoon rice vinegar

1 tablespoon oyster sauce

2 teaspoons grated ginger

1 teaspoon cornstarch

1 tablespoon plus 1 teaspoon sesame oil

1¼ pounds (567 g) large raw shrimp, peeled and deveined

3 cups (255 g) broccoli slaw

4 cups (620 g) cooked spaghetti squash strands

2 scallions, chopped

Coarsely chopped peanuts (optional)

1 Combine the broth, peanut butter, soy sauce, vinegar, oyster sauce, and ginger in a large skillet over medium heat. Cook, stirring frequently, until the mixture is fully combined and hot throughout, 2 minutes. Whisk in the cornstarch. Cook until thickened and reduced by one third, 2 minutes. Pour the peanut sauce into a small bowl; set aside. Rinse and wipe the skillet with a clean kitchen or paper towel. Return the skillet to the stovetop.

2 Heat 2 teaspoons of the oil in the skillet over medium-high heat. Add the shrimp; cook until pink, stirring frequently, 2 minutes. Remove the shrimp from the skillet; keep warm.

3 Heat the remaining 2 teaspoons oil in the skillet. Add the broccoli slaw; sauté until crisp-tender, 3 minutes. Add the squash strands and peanut sauce, gently stirring to combine all ingredients. Cook until hot throughout, 2 minutes. Stir in the shrimp and scallions. Top with coarsely chopped peanuts, if desired.

NUTRITION FACTS (SERVING SIZE: ¼ OF SKILLET): CALORIES 344; FAT 13.5 G (SAT 2 G); PROTEIN 35 G; CARB 20 G; FIBER 5 G; SUGARS 7 G (ADDED SUGARS 1 G); SODIUM 610 MG

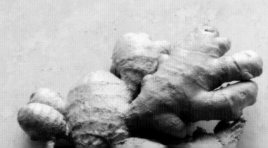

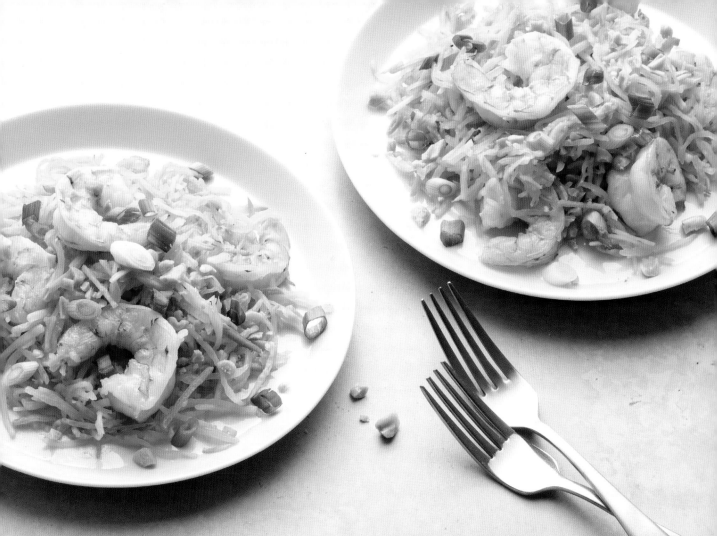

TIP I like to prep spaghetti squash at the start of the week because it keeps well in the refrigerator for 3 days, and my preferred cooking method is in the microwave. To do this, I carefully pierce a whole spaghetti squash (don't cut it in half) with a sharp knife in 5 to 6 places, making approximately 1-inch (26 mm) cuts. Place the squash in the microwave and cook on HIGH for 5 to 7 minutes. Turn the squash over and cook for an additional 2 to 3 minutes. Let stand for at least 15 minutes. Cut the top and bottom off, then cut the squash in half lengthwise. Discard the seeds and associated pulp. (Use a paring knife to loosen these strands for easy removal.) Then, use a fork to scrape out the strands. Season lightly with salt and pepper and refrigerate in an airtight container.

VEGAN OPTION Drain one 14-ounce (397 g) package of extra-firm tofu on clean kitchen or paper towels. Cut into ¾-inch (2 cm) pieces. Cook the tofu in 2 teaspoons of hot sesame oil in a large skillet over medium-high heat until lightly browned, stirring frequently, 3 minutes. Remove the tofu from the skillet, then return it to the skillet later in step 3 in place of the shrimp.

CALORIES 321; FAT 18 G (SAT 2.5 G); PROTEIN 17 G; CARB 22 G; FIBER 6 G; SUGARS 7 G (ADDED SUGARS 1 G); SODIUM 445

CHICKEN VARIATION Shred, chop, or slice cooked skinless chicken breasts to yield 2½ cups (350 g). Warm slightly in the microwave if the chicken is cold. Cook the broccoli slaw in 1 tablespoon plus 1 teaspoon sesame oil. Add the chicken to the skillet later in step 3 in place of the shrimp.

CALORIES 368; FAT 16 G (SAT 3 G); PROTEIN 34 G; CARB 20 G; FIBER 5 G; SUGARS 7 G (ADDED SUGARS 1 G); SODIUM 506

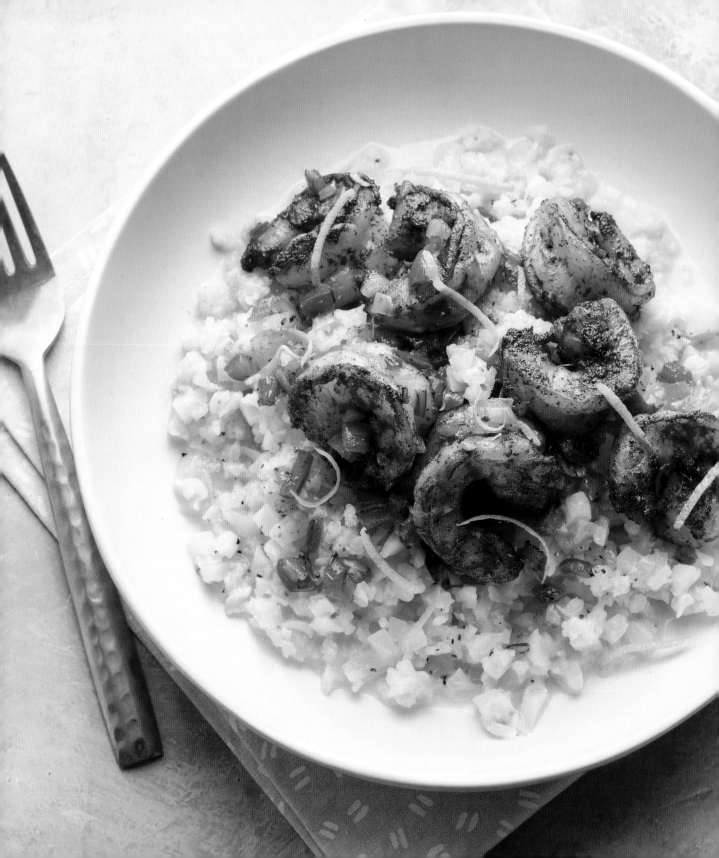

blackened shrimp over lemony cauliflower risotto

HANDS-ON: 15 MINUTES :: TOTAL: 15 MINUTES :: SERVES 4

Consider this a lightened-up take on shrimp and grits. As it cooks, the riced cauliflower creates a creamy risotto-like texture, which serves as a perfect base for blackened shrimp. The addition of lemon keeps the flavor light, not heavy.

1 Heat 2 teaspoons oil in a large skillet over medium-high heat. Sprinkle the shrimp with the blackening seasoning, tossing well to coat. Cook the shrimp in the hot oil until pink, stirring frequently, 1½ minutes per side. Transfer the shrimp to a bowl; keep warm.

2 Return the skillet to the stovetop and heat 1 teaspoon oil over medium-high heat. Set a ¼ cup (40 g) of the diced onion aside. Add the remaining onion, bell pepper, and 1 teaspoon garlic to the skillet. Sauté the vegetables until they are beginning to soften, 4 minutes. Transfer to the bowl with the shrimp. Sprinkle with ¼ teaspoon each of salt and pepper.

3 Wipe the skillet with a clean kitchen or paper towel and return it to the stovetop. Reduce the heat to medium and add 1 teaspoon oil. Sauté the reserved onion and 1 teaspoon garlic until the onion is just beginning to soften on the edges and the garlic is fragrant, 2 minutes. Add the cauliflower and broth and bring to a simmer. Cover and cook until the cauliflower is crisp-tender, 10 minutes.

4 Remove the lid and stir. Cook, uncovered, until the liquid has evaporated, 10 minutes. Add the Parmesan, butter, lemon zest, lemon juice, and ¼ teaspoon each of salt and pepper, stirring to melt the cheese and butter. Serve the shrimp and vegetables over the cauliflower risotto.

NUTRITION FACTS (SERVING SIZE: ¼ OF SHRIMP AND CAULIFLOWER): CALORIES 304; FAT 11 G (SAT 3 G); PROTEIN 44 G; CARB 8 G; FIBER 2 G; SUGARS 3 G (ADDED SUGARS 0 G); SODIUM 746 MG

Ingredients

- 1 tablespoon plus 1 teaspoon avocado oil
- 2 pounds (790 g) large shrimp, peeled and deveined
- 2 teaspoons blackening seasoning
- 1 small onion, diced
- 1 small bell pepper, diced
- 2 teaspoons minced garlic
- ½ teaspoon salt
- ½ teaspoon black pepper
- 4 cups (360 g) riced cauliflower
- 2 cups (480 ml) low-sodium chicken or vegetable broth
- ¼ cup (20 g) freshly grated Parmesan
- 1 tablespoon butter
- 1 teaspoon lemon zest
- 2 teaspoons lemon juice

Gf
gluten-free

Df
dairy-free

Sp
sheet pan

Cooking spray

One 12-ounce (340 g) package nitrate-free andouille chicken sausage links

½ onion, sliced

1 bell pepper, sliced

2 celery stalks, diced

3 garlic cloves, minced

1 tablespoon avocado oil

1 tablespoon plus 1 teaspoon salt-free Cajun or Creole seasoning

½ teaspoon salt

½ teaspoon black pepper

4 cups (567 g) fresh cauliflower crumbles

2 cups (480 ml) fresh refrigerated salsa or pico de gallo

2 scallions, chopped

1 pound (395 g) large raw shrimp, peeled and deveined

sheet pan jambalaya

HANDS-ON: 15 MINUTES :: TOTAL: 30 MINUTES :: SERVES 4

It's not unusual for a traditional jambalaya to contain anywhere from 2500 to 5000 mg of sodium per serving, thanks to the andouille sausage, stock, and salt-heavy spice blends. Although a little higher in sodium compared to other recipes in this book, this Sheet Pan Jambalaya cuts down the sodium significantly yet keeps the classic flavors by using a little less sausage (nitrate-free), a salt-free seasoning, and fresh salsa. Since keeping tabs on sodium intake is important, balance your daily intake with lower-sodium foods when you make this.

1 Preheat the oven to 425°F (220°C). Line a large baking sheet with foil, then lightly coat with cooking spray.

2 Cut the sausage links into ½-inch (13 mm) thick slices. Place the sausage, onion, bell pepper, celery, and garlic onto the baking sheet. Drizzle with the oil and toss well to coat. Sprinkle with 2 teaspoons of the seasoning, ¼ teaspoon salt, and ¼ teaspoon pepper. Gently toss to combine and spread the ingredients evenly across the pan. Bake for 10 minutes.

3 In a large bowl, combine the cauliflower crumbles, salsa, scallions, and ¼ teaspoon each of salt and pepper. Add the cauliflower mixture to the sheet pan, gently stirring to incorporate, then spread them evenly across the pan. Bake for 5 minutes.

4 Toss the shrimp with 2 teaspoons of the seasoning. Add the shrimp to the pan, then return to the oven. Bake for an additional 5 to 7 minutes, until the shrimp is pink and the cauliflower is crisp-tender.

NUTRITION FACTS (SERVING SIZE: ¼ OF SHEET PAN):
CALORIES 329; FAT 10 G (SAT 2 G); PROTEIN 40 G;
CARB 18 G; FIBER 5 G; SUGARS 5 G (ADDED
SUGARS 0 G); SODIUM 980 MG

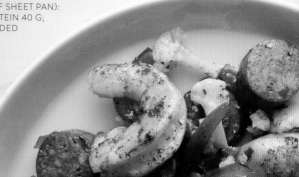

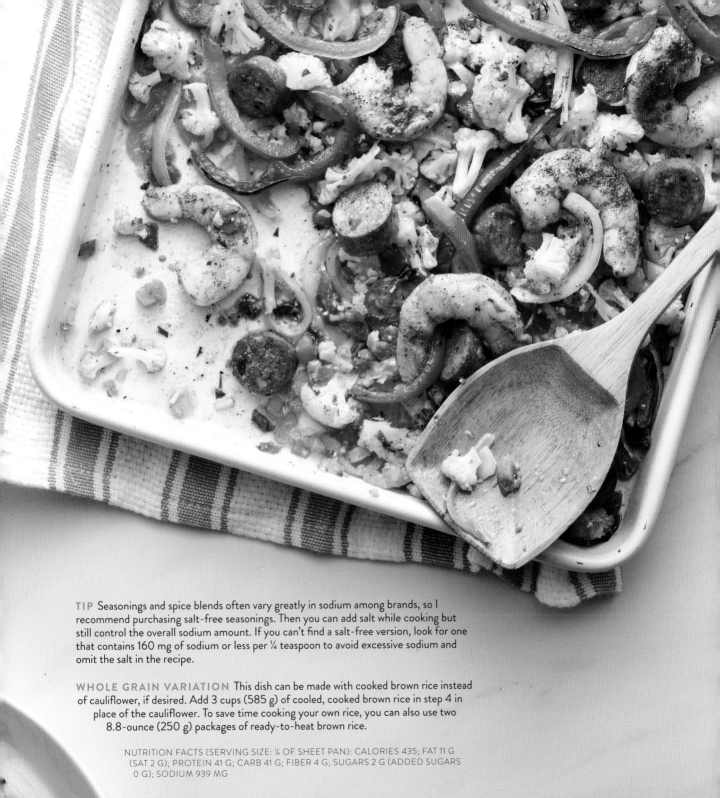

TIP Seasonings and spice blends often vary greatly in sodium among brands, so I recommend purchasing salt-free seasonings. Then you can add salt while cooking but still control the overall sodium amount. If you can't find a salt-free version, look for one that contains 160 mg of sodium or less per ¼ teaspoon to avoid excessive sodium and omit the salt in the recipe.

WHOLE GRAIN VARIATION This dish can be made with cooked brown rice instead of cauliflower, if desired. Add 3 cups (585 g) of cooled, cooked brown rice in step 4 in place of the cauliflower. To save time cooking your own rice, you can also use two 8.8-ounce (250 g) packages of ready-to-heat brown rice.

NUTRITION FACTS (SERVING SIZE: ¼ OF SHEET PAN): CALORIES 435; FAT 11 G (SAT 2 G); PROTEIN 41 G; CARB 41 G; FIBER 4 G; SUGARS 2 G (ADDED SUGARS 0 G); SODIUM 939 MG

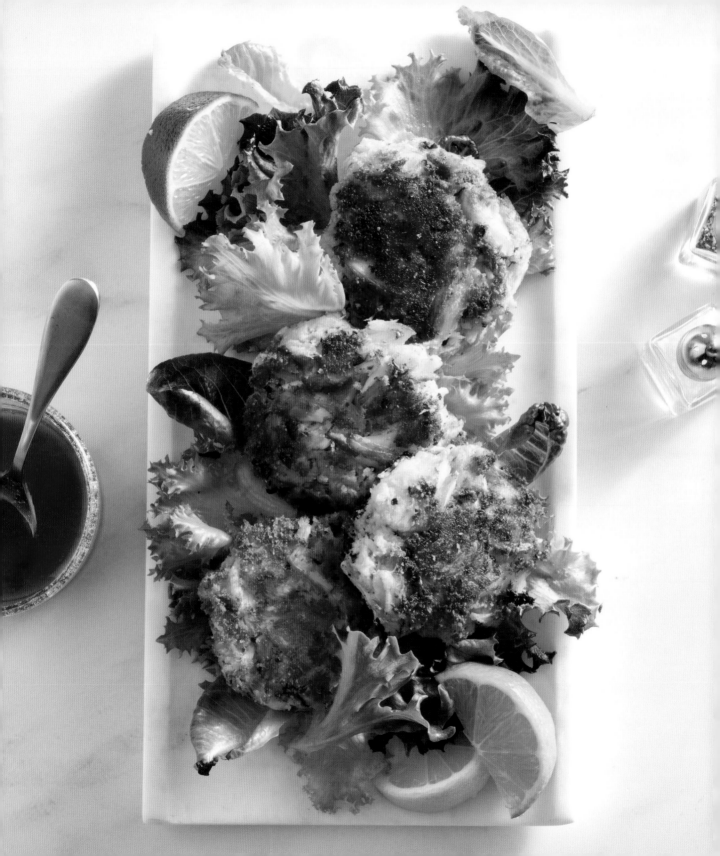

chile-lime crab cakes

HANDS-ON: 15 MINUTES :: TOTAL: 15 MINUTES :: SERVES 4

Thai cuisine is one of my favorites because of the bold flavors in traditional ingredients like chili paste, lime juice, fish sauce, soy sauce, lemongrass, and curry paste. While this dish is far from authentic, those flavors inspired me to try infusing ordinary crab cakes with basil, chili sauce, and lime. I serve them over greens dressed with a light soy sauce–based vinaigrette.

1 Drain the crabmeat on a clean kitchen towel or several layers of paper towels and pick out any remaining pieces of shell.

2 Combine the mayonnaise, scallion, basil, chili-garlic sauce, lime zest, lime juice, and garlic in a mixing bowl, stirring well. Stir in the almond flour. Add the crabmeat; stir gently to combine. Cover and chill until ready to cook.

3 Divide the crab mixture into 8 equal portions; gently shape each portion into a ¾-inch (2 cm) thick cake.

4 Heat 1 tablespoon oil in a large nonstick or cast-iron skillet over medium-high heat; swirl to coat. Add 4 crab cakes to the pan; cook until golden, 3 minutes on each side. Remove the cakes from the pan; keep warm. Repeat with the remaining 1 tablespoon oil and 4 crab cakes.

5 Toss the spring mix with the vinaigrette and divide among 4 plates. Top with the crab cakes.

1 pound (454 g) lump crabmeat

¼ cup (60 ml) olive oil mayonnaise

1 scallion, chopped

3 tablespoons chopped basil or cilantro

2 tablespoons chili-garlic sauce

1 teaspoon lime zest

2 teaspoons lime juice

1 teaspoon minced garlic

⅔ cup (75 g) almond flour

2 tablespoons avocado oil

4 cups (170 g) spring mix or baby greens

¼ cup (60 ml) Ginger-Soy Vinaigrette (page 170) or bottled sesame-ginger dressing

NUTRITION FACTS (SERVING SIZE: 2 CRAB CAKES OVER TOSSED GREENS): CALORIES 342; FAT 23 G (SAT 2 G); PROTEIN 22 G; CARB 11 G; FIBER 3 G; SUGARS 5 G (ADDED SUGARS 1 G); SODIUM 649 MG

TIP Chill the cakes for 20 minutes before cooking to make them less likely to stick or fall apart. If prepping ahead, the uncooked cakes can be covered and refrigerated for up to 24 hours.

Gf
gluten-free

Df
dairy-free

Nc
no-cook

3 cups (505 g) cooked brown rice

3 tablespoons rice vinegar

3 tablespoons lower-sodium soy sauce or tamari

¾ pound (303 g) cooked salmon, flaked into bite-size pieces

1 cup (104 g) chopped cucumber

½ cup (55 g) grated or shredded carrot

¼ cup (25 g) chopped scallion

1 tablespoon sesame oil

¼ cup (60 ml) olive oil mayonnaise

2 teaspoons sriracha

1 avocado, diced

Sesame seeds (optional)

quick poke bowls

HANDS-ON: 15 MINUTES ∷ TOTAL: 15 MINUTES. ∷ SERVES 4

Don't want the hassle and prevision of rolling your own sushi? These poke bowls are a quick solution where brown rice serves as a base for lightly seasoned salmon and vegetables.

1 Warm the brown rice in the microwave or heat according to package directions. Stir 2 tablespoons each of vinegar and soy sauce into the rice.

2 Place the salmon, cucumber, carrot, and scallion in a bowl. Add 1 tablespoon each of vinegar, soy sauce, and sesame oil. Toss gently to combine. In a separate small bowl, combine the mayonnaise and sriracha.

3 To assemble, divide the rice among 4 bowls and top each evenly with the salmon mixture and avocado. Add a dollop of the sriracha mixture to each bowl. Sprinkle with sesame seeds, if desired.

NUTRITION FACTS (SERVING SIZE: 1 BOWL): CALORIES 464; FAT 22 G (SAT 3 G); PROTEIN 24 G; CARB 41 G; FIBER 6 G; SUGARS 2 G (ADDED SUGARS 0 G); SODIUM 677 MG

TIP Cook and refrigerate two salmon fillets (approximately 1 pound/454 g raw salmon) at the start of the week to use in this recipe for quick meal prep. If you don't have time to do this at the start of the week? No problem! Cooking salmon in the oven requires minimal effort. Here's how:

Preheat the oven to 400°F (200°C). Place the salmon on a roasting pan or in a baking dish. Brush lightly with oil to prevent the outside from drying out, and season with salt and pepper, if desired. A common rule of thumb is to cook salmon for 4 to 5 minutes per ½-inch (13 mm), based on the fillet's thickest part. For example, you'd cook a 1-inch (2.5 cm) fillet for 8 to 10 minutes.

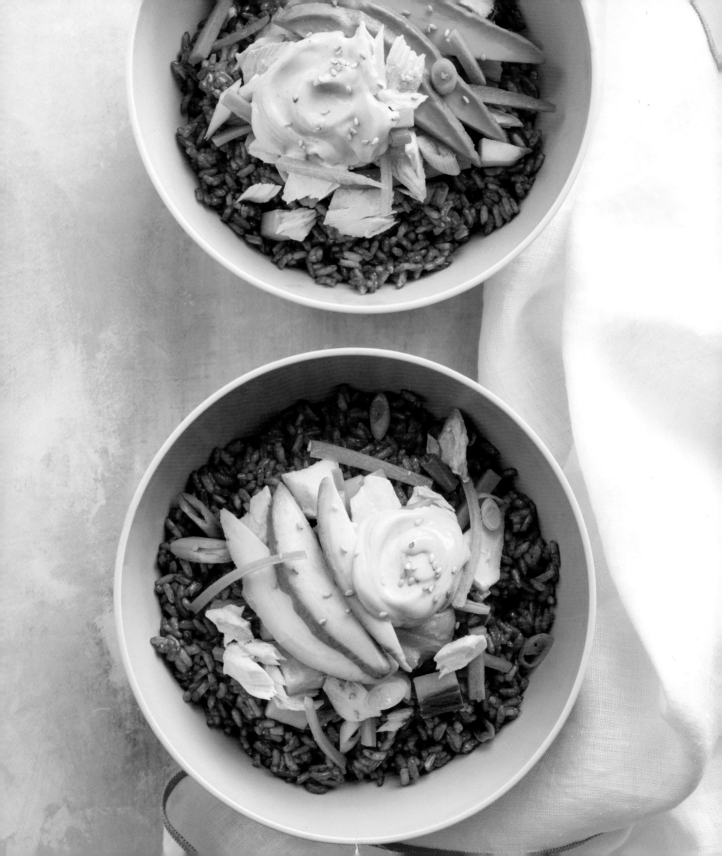

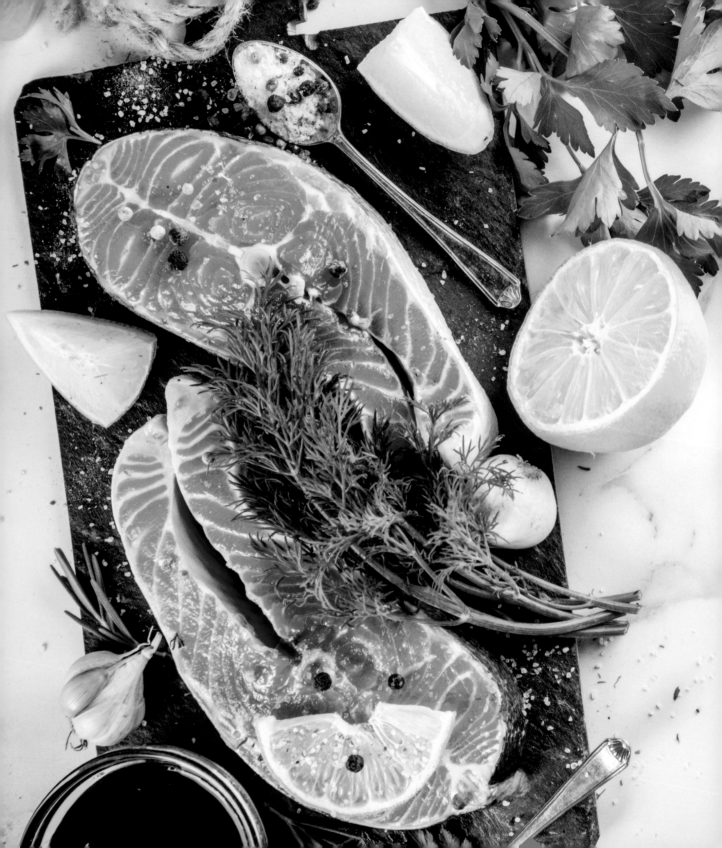

fish and seafood lowest in mercury

Aside from being an excellent source of nutrient-dense protein, fish and seafood also contain varying amounts of some key anti-inflammatory nutrients like omega-3 fatty acids, vitamin D, selenium, zinc, and B vitamins. However, they also can be a source of toxins, such as the heavy metal mercury. It's safe to say all fish and seafood contain at least trace amounts of mercury (and likely POPs, see page 25), but this isn't a reason to avoid them. In fact, incorporating fish and seafood regularly is part of an anti-inflammatory diet, but the key is choosing ones that are lowest in mercury. The following list specifies "Best" and "Good" fish and seafood choices, as well as ones to avoid, based on mercury levels. It was issued jointly by the EPA and FDA and includes the following recommendations:

- Consume 8 to 12 ounces (225 to 340 g) of fish and seafood (about 2 to 3 servings) a week from the "Best" list.

- Or consume 4 ounces (about 1 serving) a week from the "Good" list.

- Fish and seafood contain nutrients important for development, so pregnant people and children shouldn't avoid them but rather choose a variety of sources on the "Best" list.

- Children starting at 2 years can consume 1 to 2 servings (approximately 1 ounce/28 g each) from the "Best" list and slowly increase the serving size to 4 ounces (115 g) by 11 years, slowly increasing the amount with age.

BEST

Anchovy	Cod	Lobster (American and spiny)	Perch (freshwater and ocean)	Shad	Trout, freshwater
Atlantic mackerel	Crab	Mullet	Pollock	Shrimp	Canned light tuna (includes skipjack)
Black sea bass	Crawfish	Oyster	Salmon	Skate	Whitefish
Butterfish	Flounder	Pacific chub mackerel	Sardine	Smelt	Whiting
Catfish	Haddock		Scallop	Sole	
Clam	Hake			Squid	
	Herring			Tilapia	

GOOD

Bluefish	Halibut	Snapper	Tilefish (Atlantic Ocean)	Tuna (albacore or white tuna; canned, fresh, or frozen)	Weakfish/ seatrout
Carp	Mahi-mahi	Spanish mackerel			White croaker/ Pacific croaker
Chilean sea bass	Monkfish	Striped bass (ocean)		Tuna (yellowfin)	
Grouper	Rockfish				
	Sablefish				

AVOID

King mackerel	Orange roughy	Swordfish	Tilefish (Gulf of Mexico)	Tuna (bigeye)
Marlin	Shark			

These recommendations are from the Fish Advice published by the EPA and the FDA.

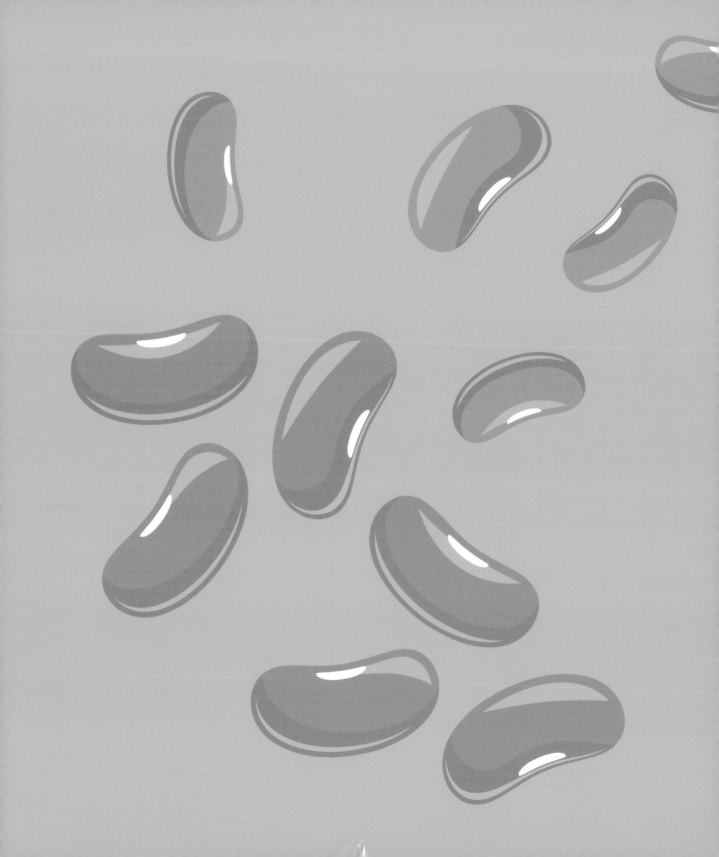

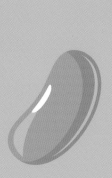

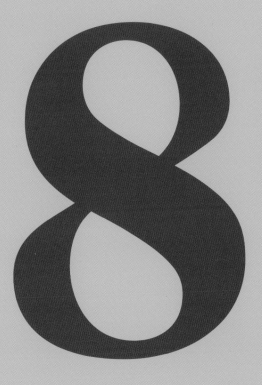

8

· · · · · · · · · · · ·

MEATLESS MAINS

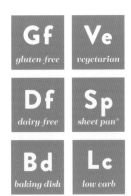

Gf — *gluten-free*
Ve — *vegetarian*
Df — *dairy-free*
Sp — *sheet pan*
Bd — *baking dish*
Lc — *low carb*

Cooking spray

One 12-ounce (340 g) package broccoli florets

1 cup (149 g) cherry tomatoes, halved

1 small red onion, cut into wedges

1 tablespoon avocado oil

1 teaspoon garlic powder

¾ teaspoon salt

8 large eggs

2 large egg whites

¼ cup (60 ml) low-fat milk or nondairy milk alternative

¼ teaspoon black pepper

roasted vegetable frittata

HANDS-ON: 10 MINUTES :: TOTAL: 40 MINUTES :: SERVES 4

Always in the fridge but easy to overlook, eggs are a quick, high-quality protein source. They're also one of the best sources of two anti-inflammatory nutrients: selenium and choline. In fact, two eggs provide 50 percent of your daily needs for both nutrients. For extra flavor, I'll incorporate ½ cup (56 g) of crumbled feta by stirring half into the whisked egg mixture and then sprinkling the other half over the top before baking.

1 Heat the oven to 375°F (190°C). Generously coat a 9 x 13-inch (23 x 33 cm) metal or ceramic baking dish with cooking spray.

2 Place the broccoli, tomatoes, and onion in the baking dish. Drizzle with oil and toss to coat the vegetables. Sprinkle with garlic powder and ½ teaspoon salt. Spread the vegetables in a single layer.

3 Bake for 12 to 15 minutes, until the broccoli is crisp-tender, stirring the vegetables after 8 minutes.

4 While the vegetables roast, whisk together the eggs, egg whites, milk, ¼ teaspoon salt, and pepper in a large bowl.

5 Pour the egg mixture over the vegetables. Bake for 18 to 20 minutes, until the frittata is set in the center and starting to turn golden and puff around the edges.

NUTRITION FACTS (SERVING SIZE: ¼ OF FRITTATA): CALORIES 231; FAT 13 G (SAT 2.5 G); PROTEIN 18 G; CARB 9 G; FIBER 3 G; SUGARS 4 G (ADDED SUGARS 0 G); SODIUM 541 MG

SHEET PAN VARIATION To prepare the frittata on a sheet pan, follow the directions above using a 13 x 18-inch (33 x 46 cm) sheet pan instead of a baking dish. Then, in step 5, bake for 15 to 18 minutes, until the frittata is set in the center.

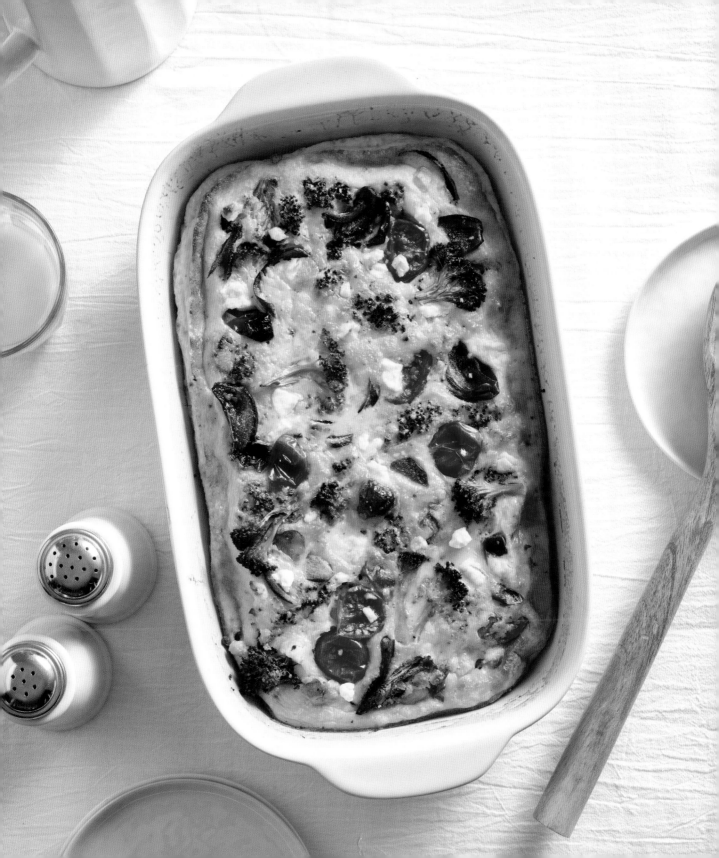

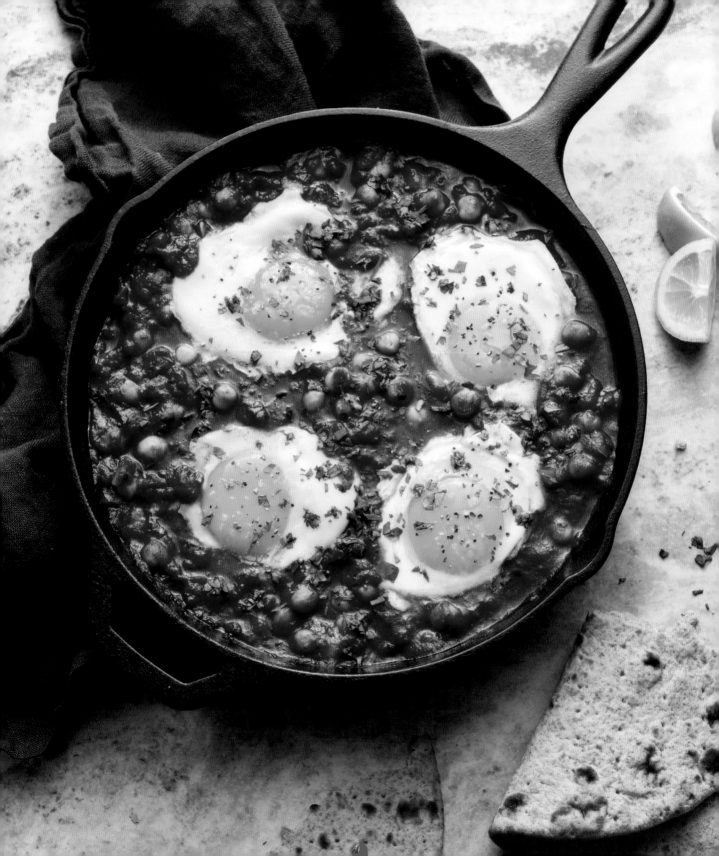

skillet shakshuka

HANDS-ON: 10 MINUTES :: TOTAL: 20 MINUTES :: SERVES 4

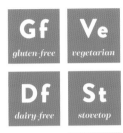

Shakshuka, eggs poached in a fragrant tomato-based sauce, is a dish that originated in North Africa and the Middle East. This version comes together quickly on the stovetop, but it can also be made in the Instant Pot. The pressure cooker variation requires the addition of broth or water to prevent scorching, which creates a slightly saucier dish—but I think it's just as good as the original.

1 Heat the oil in a large skillet over medium heat. Add the shallots and garlic; cook, stirring frequently, until fragrant, 2 minutes.

2 Add the tomatoes, tomato paste, paprika, chili powder, honey, cumin, salt, cinnamon, and cayenne, if desired. Stir well to combine. Reduce the heat to medium-low. Add the chickpeas and simmer until slightly thickened and hot throughout, 5 minutes.

3 Using the back of a spoon, make four wells in the sauce. Crack one egg into each well. Cover, and cook until the egg whites are set, 6 to 8 minutes.

NUTRITION FACTS (SERVING SIZE: ¼ OF SKILLET): CALORIES 320; FAT 9 G (SAT 1.5 G); PROTEIN 16 G; CARB 42 G; FIBER 11 G; SUGARS 14 G (ADDED SUGARS 3 G); SODIUM 561 MG

INSTANT POT VARIATION Set the pressure cooker to the SAUTÉ function. Add the oil to the pot and heat for 2 minutes. Sauté the shallots and garlic as directed in step 1. Add 2 cups (480 ml) of low-sodium vegetable broth or water, along with all of the remaining ingredients, except the eggs. Cover the pressure cooker and fasten the lid. Lock and seal the steam valve. Set to HIGH pressure for 5 minutes. Manually release the pressure. Uncover and turn off. Using the back of a spoon, make four wells in the sauce. Crack one egg into each well. Cover the pressure cooker and fasten the lid. Lock and seal the steam valve. Set to HIGH pressure for 1 minute. Manually release the pressure, then uncover. To cook eggs longer, press SAUTÉ and cook for 1 to 2 minutes or until desired degree of doneness.

1 tablespoon avocado oil

2 shallots, chopped

5 garlic cloves, minced

One 28-ounce (740 g) can no-salt-added crushed tomatoes

2 tablespoons tomato paste

1½ tablespoons smoked paprika

2 teaspoons chili powder

2 teaspoons honey

1 teaspoon ground cumin

1 teaspoon salt

¼ teaspoon ground cinnamon

⅛ teaspoon cayenne pepper (optional)

One 15-ounce (425 g) can no-salt-added chickpeas, rinsed and drained

4 large eggs

Chopped fresh cilantro and lemon wedges (optional)

Gf *gluten-free*

Ve *vegetarian*

Sp *sheet pan*

Cooking spray

Two 12-ounce (340 g) packages cauliflower florets

1 tablespoon olive oil

1 tablespoon lower-sodium taco seasoning

10 ultra-thin slices sharp cheddar

1 cup (260 g) no-salt-added black beans, drained and rinsed

2 Roma tomatoes, chopped

2 scallions, chopped

Diced avocado, chopped fresh cilantro, and sliced jalapeños (optional)

fork-and-knife cauliflower nachos

HANDS-ON: 10 MINUTES :: TOTAL: 20 MINUTES :: SERVES 4

Roasted cauliflower creates a sturdy base for all your favorite toppings, and using slices of cheese, rather than shredded, helps to secure the cauliflower and create a layer for holding the other toppings. These aren't easy to eat with your hands, so plan to eat them with a fork and knife.

1 Preheat the oven to 425°F (220°C). Line a baking sheet with foil; lightly coat with cooking spray.

2 Place the cauliflower florets on the baking sheet. Add the oil and toss to combine. Then, lightly spray with cooking spray so that cauliflower is well coated. Sprinkle with the taco seasoning and toss again to combine. Arrange the cauliflower in a single layer.

3 Bake for 12 to 14 minutes, until the cauliflower is crisp-tender and the edges are starting to brown.

4 Push the cauliflower together and toward the center of the pan in a single layer. Top with the cheese slices. Bake for 4 minutes, or until the cheese is melted. Top the nachos with the black beans. Cook for 2 minutes or until the nachos are hot throughout and the cheese is beginning to brown.

5 Top with tomato, scallions, and, if desired, avocado, cilantro, sliced jalapenos, and any other desired toppings.

NUTRITION FACTS (SERVING SIZE: ¼ OF NACHOS): CALORIES 255; FAT 13 G (SAT 5.5 G); PROTEIN 15 G; CARB 20 G; FIBER 7 G; SUGARS 4 G (ADDED SUGARS 0 G); SODIUM 319 MG

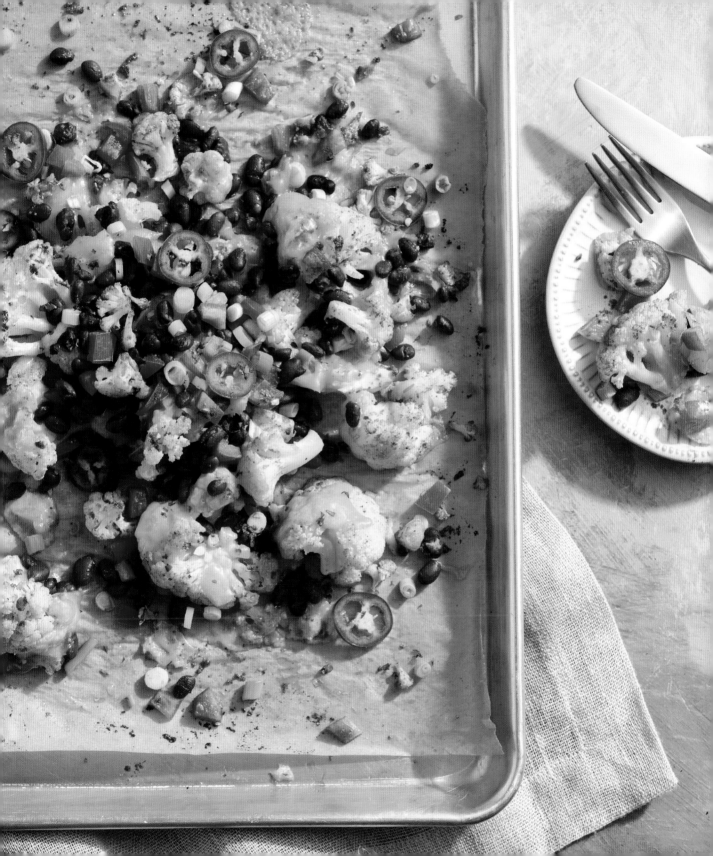

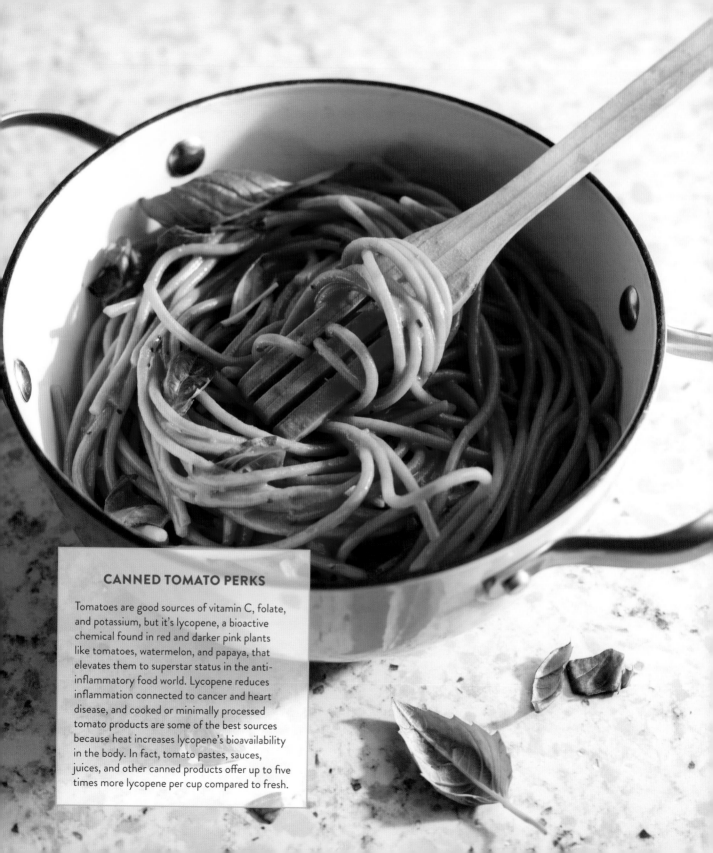

CANNED TOMATO PERKS

Tomatoes are good sources of vitamin C, folate, and potassium, but it's lycopene, a bioactive chemical found in red and darker pink plants like tomatoes, watermelon, and papaya, that elevates them to superstar status in the anti-inflammatory food world. Lycopene reduces inflammation connected to cancer and heart disease, and cooked or minimally processed tomato products are some of the best sources because heat increases lycopene's bioavailability in the body. In fact, tomato pastes, sauces, juices, and other canned products offer up to five times more lycopene per cup compared to fresh.

spaghetti alla vodka

HANDS-ON: 12 MINUTES :: TOTAL: 20 MINUTES :: SERVES 7

Creamy and comforting, this one-pot pasta is one of my family's favorites. I like to use a multigrain pasta that offers 5 grams or more of protein per ounce and is fortified with plant-based protein flours made from legumes like chickpeas or lentils. The extra protein provides a little more satiety, and it has a sturdier texture for the sauce to cling to.

1 Heat the oil in a 2½ to 3-quart (2.4 to 2.8 L) saucepan or Dutch oven over medium heat. Sauté the garlic in the hot oil until golden and fragrant, 2 minutes.

2 Add the tomato paste and seasoning. Cook, stirring frequently, until the tomato paste has a looser consistency and has slightly darkened in color, 3 minutes. Add the vodka and cook, stirring constantly, until the liquid has evaporated, 30 seconds.

3 Add 2⅔ cups (640 ml) of water to the tomato paste mixture, stirring to mix well. Break the spaghetti into thirds and add to the tomato paste mixture. Bring to a simmer, stirring occasionally, making sure that the liquid fully covers the spaghetti.

4 Simmer until the sauce is reduced and the pasta is not quite al dente, 10 to 12 minutes.

5 Add the coconut milk, salt, and pepper, stirring to fully combine. Simmer until the pasta is al dente, 3 minutes. Gently fold in the basil.

NUTRITION FACTS (SERVING SIZE: 1 CUP/143 G): CALORIES 279; FAT 10 G (SAT 5 G); PROTEIN 9 G; CARB 39 G; FIBER 4 G; SUGARS 8 G (ADDED SUGARS 0 G); SODIUM 393 MG

1½ tablespoons avocado oil

2 teaspoons minced garlic

One 12-ounce can (309 g) tomato paste

1 teaspoon Italian herb seasoning

⅓ cup (80 ml) vodka

8 ounces (227 g) dry gluten-free or multigrain protein-enriched spaghetti

1 cup (240 ml) canned coconut milk

1 teaspoon salt

¼ teaspoon black pepper

⅓ cup (3 g) chopped fresh basil

Gf
gluten-free

Ve
vegetarian

St
stovetop

Two 8-ounce (227 g) boxes legume-based shell pasta

2 teaspoons butter

1 tablespoon gluten-free all-purpose flour or arrowroot flour

2 cups (480 ml) low-fat milk

One 15-ounce (425 g) can pumpkin puree

¾ teaspoon salt

½ teaspoon garlic powder

½ teaspoon dry mustard

½ teaspoon black pepper

One 8-ounce (226 g) block reduced-fat sharp white cheddar, grated

¾ cup (60 g) freshly grated Parmesan

white cheddar–pumpkin mac and cheese

HANDS-ON: 15 MINUTES :: TOTAL: 25 MINUTES :: SERVES 9

Pumpkin is the secret ingredient that adds creaminess and a healthy dose of carotenoids to the cheese sauce, but I promise picky eaters will never know it's in there! Responsible for giving many deep orange and green fruits and vegetables their rich colors, carotenoids are a phytochemical family that includes beta-carotene, lycopene, lutein, and zeaxanthin. They act as antioxidants to prevent free radicals from creating new inflammation in the body.

1 Cook the pasta in a large saucepan or Dutch oven to the lower end of the time range specified on the package. Drain, set aside, and keep warm.

2 Melt the butter in the saucepan over medium heat. Add the flour and cook, stirring constantly, until slightly golden, 1 minute. Slowly whisk in the milk. Continue to stir constantly until slightly thickened, 3 minutes.

3 Add the pumpkin, salt, garlic powder, dry mustard, and pepper; stir well to combine. Stir in the cheeses and cook 2 minutes, or until the cheeses are completely melted. Gently fold in the pasta. Cook until hot throughout, 1 minute.

NUTRITION FACTS (SERVING SIZE: 1 CUP/186 G): CALORIES 323; FAT 11 G (SAT 5 G); PROTEIN 23 G; CARB 37 G; FIBER 8 G; SUGARS 9 G (ADDED SUGARS 0 G); SODIUM 514 MG

TIP Make sure to watch the time carefully when cooking legume-based pastas. I've found they can quickly go from al dente to overdone and mushy. If you're not a fan of legume-based pasta, substitute two 8-ounce (227 g) boxes of a whole-grain pasta.

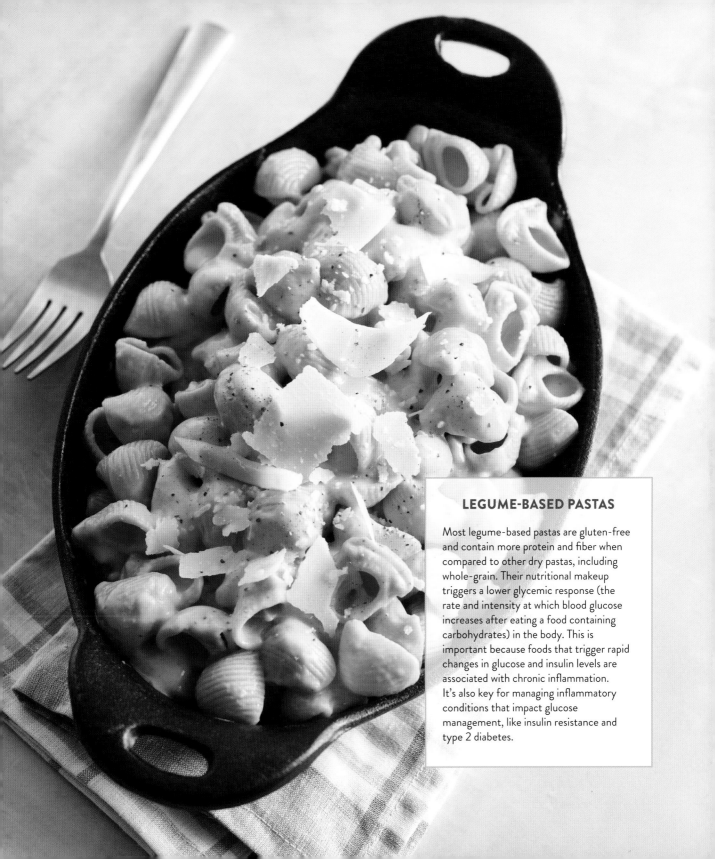

LEGUME-BASED PASTAS

Most legume-based pastas are gluten-free and contain more protein and fiber when compared to other dry pastas, including whole-grain. Their nutritional makeup triggers a lower glycemic response (the rate and intensity at which blood glucose increases after eating a food containing carbohydrates) in the body. This is important because foods that trigger rapid changes in glucose and insulin levels are associated with chronic inflammation. It's also key for managing inflammatory conditions that impact glucose management, like insulin resistance and type 2 diabetes.

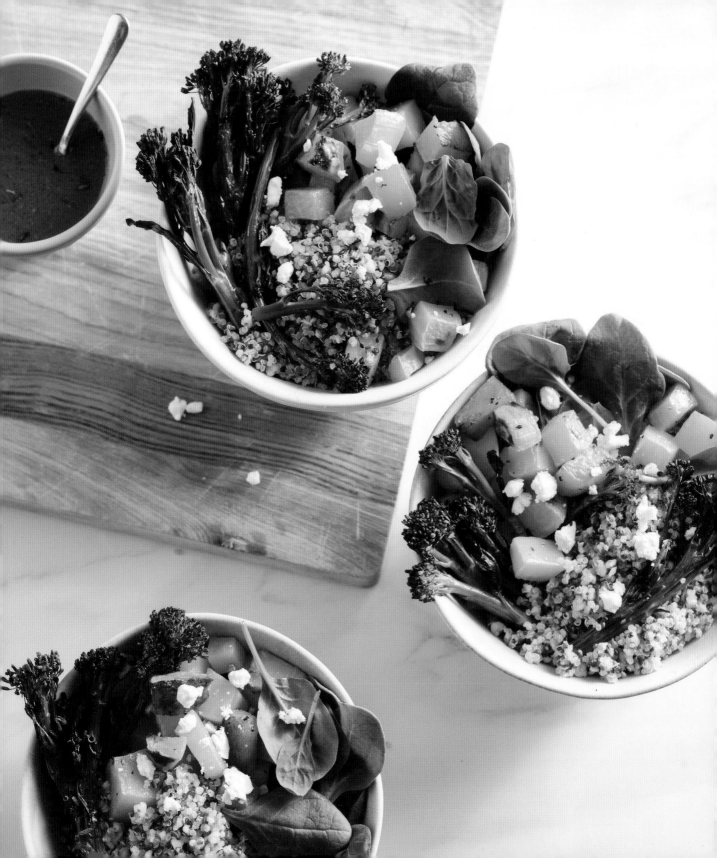

roasted fall vegetable grain bowl

HANDS-ON: 12 MINUTES :: TOTAL: 30 MINUTES :: SERVES 4

Craving healthy comfort food? A filling, one-dish meal like this autumn-inspired grain bowl is your answer! Assembly is easy: Simply top baby spinach with warm quinoa and roasted vegetables. Then, drizzle with a balsamic vinaigrette. For an extra touch of flavor and protein, sprinkle a little crumbled feta or goat cheese over the top, if desired.

1 Preheat the oven to 425°F (220°C).

2 Toss the squash with 1 tablespoon oil, ½ teaspoon garlic powder, and ¼ teaspoon salt in a medium bowl. Toss the Broccolini and onion with 1 tablespoon oil, ½ teaspoon garlic powder, and ¼ teaspoon salt in a separate bowl.

3 Spread the squash evenly across a baking sheet. Bake for 12 minutes, or until the edges are just beginning to brown. Remove from the oven and stir.

4 Add the Broccolini to the baking sheet. Bake for 8 to 10 minutes, until the vegetables are crisp-tender and the edges are browned.

5 Divide the spinach evenly among 4 bowls. Top each with the quinoa and vegetables. Drizzle each with 1½ tablespoons of the vinaigrette.

NUTRITION FACTS (SERVING SIZE: 1 BOWL): CALORIES 358; FAT 16 G (SAT 2 G); PROTEIN 9 G; CARB 46 G; FIBER 8 G; SUGARS 5 G (ADDED SUGARS 0 G); SODIUM 549 MG

NOTE Prefer a homemade dressing? In a small bowl, whisk together 3 tablespoons of extra virgin olive oil, 1 tablespoon each of balsamic vinegar and maple syrup, 2 teaspoons of Dijon mustard, and a dash each of salt and pepper. Use in place of the bottled dressing in step 5.

2 cups (280 g) cubed (1 inch/2.5 cm) butternut squash

2 tablespoons olive oil

1 teaspoon garlic powder

½ teaspoon salt

1 bunch Broccolini (about ½ pound/227 g)

1 small red onion, sliced

2 cups (113 g) baby spinach or arugula

3 cups (555 g) cooked quinoa, warmed

¼ cup plus 2 tablespoons (90 ml) bottled balsamic vinaigrette

greek fried quinoa

HANDS-ON: 10 MINUTES :: TOTAL: 10 MINUTES :: SERVES 4

Proof that vegan food can be both hearty and satisfying, this skillet packs it all—whole grains, legumes, and vegetables—in one dish. No time to prep quinoa? Use two 8-ounce (227 g) ready-to-heat pouches of quinoa or brown rice instead. Don't heat the packages; just add them directly to the skillet.

1 tablespoon olive oil

½ cup (80 g) chopped red onion

1 garlic clove, minced

3 cups (555 g) cooked quinoa, chilled

¾ teaspoon salt

3 cups (170 g) baby spinach

1 cup (260 g) no-salt-added canned chickpeas, rinsed and drained

½ teaspoon lemon zest

1 cup (149 g) cherry tomatoes, halved or quartered

¾ cup (100 g) chopped cucumber

2 teaspoons lemon juice

Crumbled feta (optional)

1 Heat the oil in a large skillet over medium-high heat. Cook the onion and garlic in the hot oil until the onion is just beginning to soften, 3 minutes. Stir in the quinoa and salt. Cook, stirring frequently, until the quinoa is hot throughout, 3 minutes.

2 Add the spinach, chickpeas, and lemon zest; cook until the spinach begins to wilt, 1 to 2 minutes.

3 Remove the skillet from the heat. Add the tomatoes, cucumber, and lemon juice, stirring to combine. Sprinkle with cheese, if desired.

NUTRITION FACTS (SERVING SIZE: 1½ CUPS/336 G): CALORIES 291; FAT 7 G (SAT 1 G); PROTEIN 11 G; CARB 45 G; FIBER 8 G; SUGARS 4 G (ADDED SUGARS 0 G); SODIUM 421 MG

CHICKEN VARIATION Add 1½ cups (170 g) shredded rotisserie chicken breast with the other ingredients in step 2.

NUTRITION FACTS (SERVING SIZE: APPROXIMATELY 1¾ CUPS/379 G): CALORIES 349; FAT 8 G (SAT 1 G); PROTEIN 23 G; CARB 45 G; FIBER 8 G; SUGARS 4 G (ADDED SUGARS 0 G); SODIUM 554 MG

LAMB VARIATION Brown ½ pound (227 g) of lean ground lamb in a skillet lightly coated with cooking spray before starting step 1. Remove the cooked lamb from the skillet and set aside. Wipe out the skillet; then proceed to step 1. Add ½ teaspoon of ground cumin along with the quinoa and salt in step 1. Then, add the cooked lamb with the other ingredients in step 2.

NUTRITION FACTS (SERVING SIZE: APPROXIMATELY 1¾ CUPS/393 G): CALORIES 372; FAT 10 G (SAT 2 G); PROTEIN 22 G; CARB 45 G; FIBER 8 G; SUGARS 4 G (ADDED SUGARS 0 G); SODIUM 460 MG

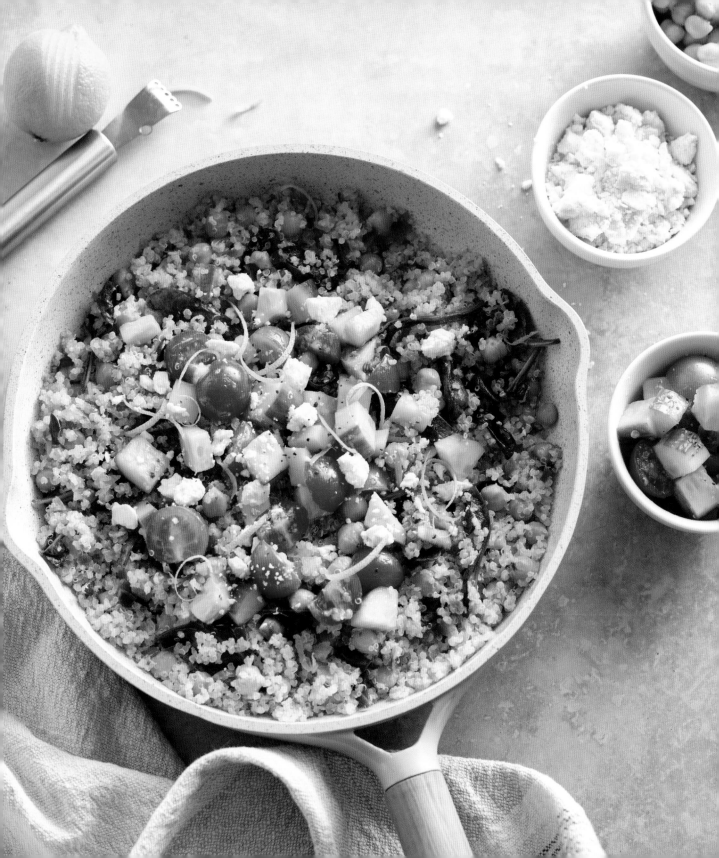

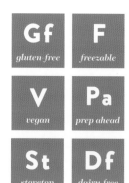

1 tablespoon plus 1 teaspoon avocado oil

1 cup (70 g) finely chopped mushrooms

½ cup (80 g) finely chopped onion

1 teaspoon minced garlic

One 15-ounce (425 g) can no-salt-added black beans, rinsed and drained

1 cup (218 g) cooked brown rice, cooled to room temperature

2 tablespoons gluten-free panko or bread crumbs

¾ teaspoon salt

½ teaspoon ground cumin

⅛ teaspoon chili powder

½ cup (120 g) refrigerated salsa or pico de gallo

1 avocado, diced

Romaine lettuce leaves

open-faced black bean burgers

HANDS-ON: 15 MINUTES :: TOTAL: 45 MINUTES :: SERVES 4

Topped with melted cheese, eaten over a bed of greens, or served on a bun, these burgers are good any way you serve them. But my favorite way to eat them is on a crisp lettuce leaf topped with fresh salsa and avocado. I like to use a fresh or refrigerated salsa since they tend to be substantially lower in sodium than jarred varieties. Look for them in the refrigerated produce case.

1 Heat 2 teaspoons of the oil in a skillet over medium heat. Add the mushrooms, onion, and garlic. Cook, stirring frequently, until very tender, 8 minutes. Remove from the heat and let cool.

2 Place the beans in a large bowl and mash them with clean hands or a fork. (Note: The mixture won't be smooth, and a few whole beans may remain.)

3 Drain any excess liquid from the cooled mushroom mixture, then add it to the beans along with the rice, panko, salt, cumin, and chili powder. Mix well with clean hands, then let chill for at least 30 minutes in the refrigerator.

4 Shape the chilled bean mixture into 4 patties (about ⅓ cup/208 g each). Flatten each patty slightly with the palm of your hand so that they are 1-inch (2.5 cm) thick.

5 Heat the remaining 2 teaspoons oil in a large skillet over medium-high heat. Add the patties and cook until browned and warm throughout, 4 to 5 minutes on each side.

6 Combine the salsa and avocado in a small bowl. Serve the burgers on top of the lettuce leaves, then top evenly with the avocado mixture.

NUTRITION FACTS (SERVING SIZE: 1 BURGER AND ¼ OF AVOCADO MIXTURE): CALORIES 276; FAT 11 G (SAT 1 G); PROTEIN 9 G; CARB 36 G; FIBER 9 G; SUGARS 2 G (ADDED SUGARS 0 G); SODIUM 394 MG

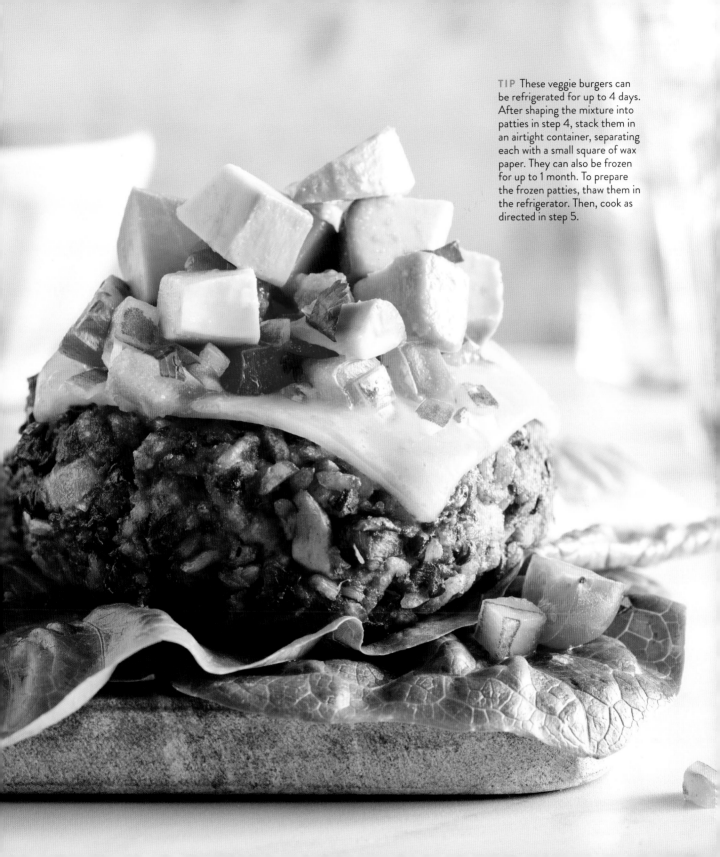

TIP These veggie burgers can be refrigerated for up to 4 days. After shaping the mixture into patties in step 4, stack them in an airtight container, separating each with a small square of wax paper. They can also be frozen for up to 1 month. To prepare the frozen patties, thaw them in the refrigerator. Then, cook as directed in step 5.

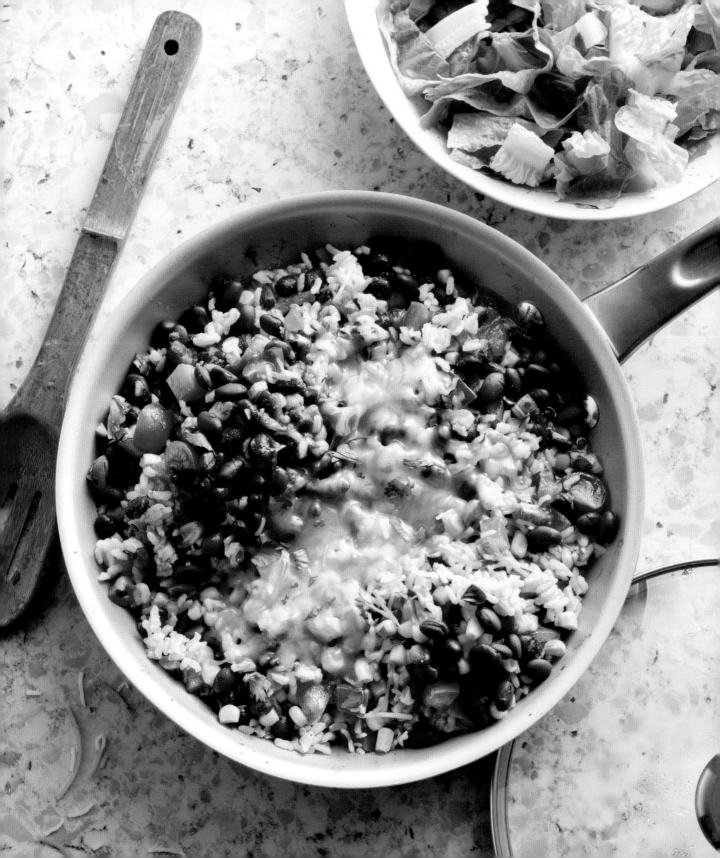

skillet mexican rice casserole

HANDS-ON: 15 MINUTES :: TOTAL: 25 MINUTES :: SERVES 5

Thanks to instant brown rice, this family-friendly dinner comes together in less time than it takes to cook a pot of regular brown rice. Sometimes labeled as 10-minute rice, these instant varieties contain rice grains that are partially cooked and then dehydrated before packaging so that they require less time to prepare later. Yet, they still retain the fiber and many of the B vitamins in the rice grain.

1 Heat the oil in a large skillet over medium-high heat. Add the onion and sauté until the onion is just beginning to soften, 4 minutes.

2 Add the beans, salsa, rice, corn, and taco seasoning, along with 1½ cups (360 ml) of water, stirring well to combine. Bring to a boil. Cover, and reduce the heat to medium-low. Cook until the rice is tender, 10 minutes.

3 Stir the cilantro into the rice mixture. Sprinkle the cheese over the top. Cover the skillet and remove from the heat. Let stand, covered, until the cheese is melted, 1 to 2 minutes. Serve the casserole over the lettuce.

NUTRITION FACTS (SERVING SIZE: ⅕ OF CASSEROLE): CALORIES 373; FAT 11 G (SAT 4.5 G); PROTEIN 15 G; CARB 53 G; FIBER 9 G; SUGARS 3 G (ADDED SUGARS 0 G); SODIUM 232 MG

NOTE For an extra kick of spice, add a seeded and diced jalapeño with the other ingredients in step 3.

1 tablespoon avocado oil

1 small red onion, chopped

One 15-ounce (425 g) can no-salt-added black beans, rinsed and drained

One 12-ounce (340 g) carton refrigerated salsa or pico de gallo

1½ cups (150 g) quick-cooking brown rice

1 cup (145 g) fresh or thawed frozen corn kernels

2 tablespoons lower-sodium taco seasoning

¼ cup (4 g) chopped fresh cilantro

1 cup (90 g) shredded Mexican-blend cheese

5 cups (235 g) chopped romaine lettuce

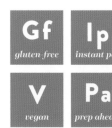

Gf *gluten-free*

Ip *instant pot*

V *vegan*

Pa *prep ahead*

Df *dairy-free*

instant pot hoppin' john

HANDS-ON: 10 MINUTES :: TOTAL: 45 MINUTES :: SERVES 6

Hoppin' John is a Southern dish that features black-eyed peas and rice. Traditionally, the peas are seasoned by cooking them with a small amount of pork to give the dish a meaty flavor. However, I've found that there are a few plant-based ingredients that can yield a similar hearty umami flavor, and soy sauce is one of them. I also like to add a little balsamic vinegar for extra flavor when cooking and again at the table.

1 tablespoon olive oil

2 cups (320 g) chopped yellow onion

4 garlic cloves, minced

3 cups (720 ml) low-sodium vegetable broth

One 14.5-ounce (411 g) can no-salt-added fire-roasted diced tomatoes

1½ cups (210 g) dried black-eyed peas

2 tablespoons lower-sodium soy sauce or tamari

1 tablespoon balsamic vinegar (plus more for serving)

1 teaspoon smoked paprika

¼ teaspoon salt

½ teaspoon black pepper

4 cups (780 g) hot cooked brown rice

1 Set the pressure cooker to the SAUTÉ function. Add the oil to the pot and heat for 2 minutes. Sauté the onion and garlic in the hot oil until fragrant, 2 minutes.

2 Add the broth, tomatoes, peas, soy sauce, vinegar, paprika, salt, and pepper, stirring to combine. Cover the pressure cooker and fasten the lid. Lock and seal the steam valve. Set to HIGH pressure for 17 minutes.

3 Manually release the pressure. Uncover and turn off the pressure cooker.

4 To serve, divide the rice among 6 bowls. Top evenly with the black-eyed peas. Serve with extra balsamic vinegar, if desired.

NUTRITION FACTS (SERVING SIZE: APPROXIMATELY 1 CUP/291 G PEAS AND ⅔ CUP/130 G RICE): CALORIES 355; FAT 1 G (SAT 1 G); PROTEIN 14 G; CARB 65 G; FIBER 12 G; SUGARS 9 G (ADDED SUGARS 0 G); SODIUM 519 MG

NOTE To give the dish a little heat, add a small seeded and diced jalapeño with the other ingredients in step 2. To keep things simple, heat two 8.8-ounce (250 g) pouches of ready-to-heat brown rice in place of the cooked brown rice.

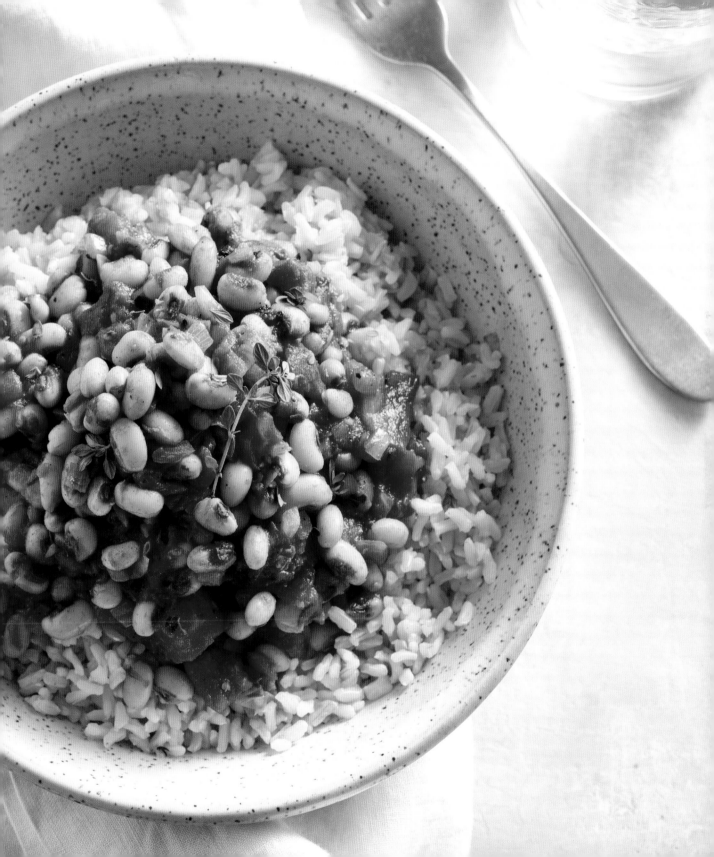

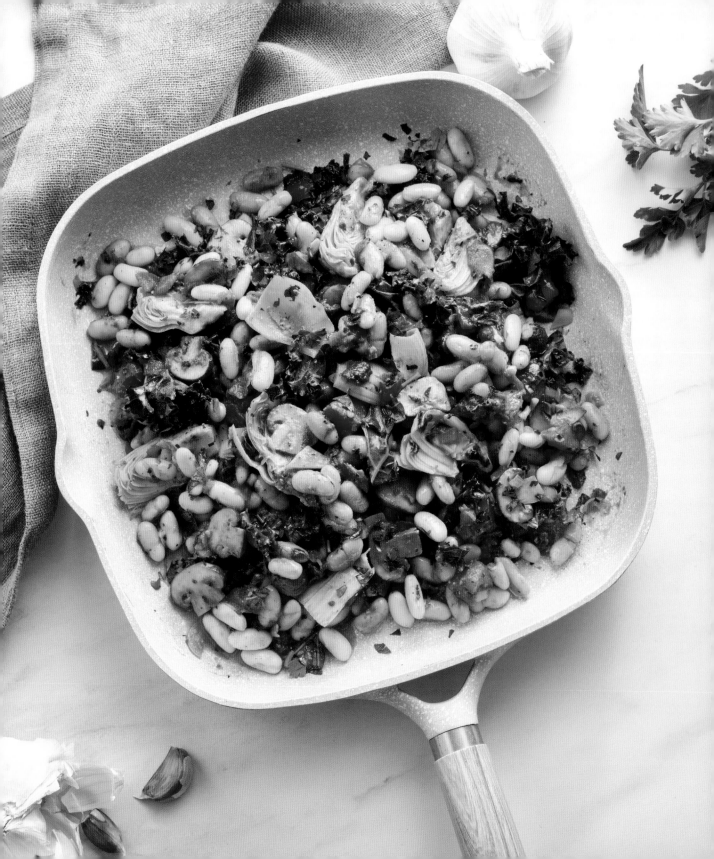

tuscan white bean skillet

HANDS-ON: 15 MINUTES :: TOTAL: 20 MINUTES :: SERVES 5

Perfect when you need a quick dinner on a cold night, this dish packs in 30 percent of the daily value for iron and 25 percent of the daily value for potassium. It also provides one third of your daily fiber needs. While it's hearty enough to be a stand-alone meal, I like to pair it with Lemony Arugula Salad with Parmesan (page 215).

1 Heat the oil in a large skillet over medium-high heat. Sauté the onion in the hot oil until just tender, 5 minutes. Add the mushrooms, sun-dried tomatoes, and garlic. Cook until the garlic is fragrant and the edges of the mushrooms are beginning to soften, 2 minutes.

2 Reduce the heat to medium. Add the beans, tomatoes, artichoke hearts, kale, Italian seasoning, salt, and pepper, stirring to combine. Cover and cook until bubbly and hot throughout, 8 to 10 minutes. Sprinkle with parsley, if desired.

NUTRITION FACTS (SERVING SIZE: 1½ CUPS/515 G): CALORIES 274; FAT 6 G (SAT 0.5 G); PROTEIN 14 G; CARB 42 G; FIBER 10 G; SUGARS 8 G (ADDED SUGARS 0 G); SODIUM 517 MG

1 tablespoon olive oil

1 cup (160 g) diced yellow onion

One 8-ounce (227 g) package sliced mushrooms

½ cup (55 g) drained, chopped oil-packed sun-dried tomatoes

3 garlic cloves, minced

Two 14.5-ounce (411 g) cans no-salt-added cannellini beans, rinsed and drained

Two 14.5-ounce (411 g) cans no-salt-added fire-roasted diced tomatoes

One 14.5-ounce (411 g) can artichoke hearts in water, drained and chopped

3 cups (48 g) chopped kale

1 teaspoon Italian seasoning

½ teaspoon salt

¼ teaspoon black pepper

Chopped fresh parsley (optional)

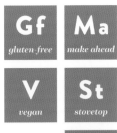

Gf gluten-free

Ma make ahead

V vegan

St stovetop

Df dairy-free

1 tablespoon avocado oil

1 large onion, finely chopped

8 garlic cloves, minced

2 tablespoons fresh minced ginger

1 tablespoon plus 1 teaspoon garam masala

1 tablespoon ground coriander

1 tablespoon ground cumin

1 tablespoon ground turmeric

1 tablespoon paprika

2 teaspoons chili powder

One 28-ounce (794 g) can no-salt-added tomato sauce

One 15-ounce (425 g) can no-salt added chickpeas, rinsed and drained

One 13.5-ounce (383 g) can coconut milk

1 tablespoon tomato paste

2 cups (32 g) chopped kale

chana masala

HANDS-ON: 15 MINUTES :: TOTAL: 15 MINUTES :: SERVES 6

This vegan dish is a hit for everyone, even nonvegetarians. Chickpeas give the dish a meat-like texture and fiber to make this dish hearty and filling. Traditional Indian masala dishes are usually served over hot white basmati rice. White rice isn't considered whole grain, which means it doesn't have the bran, the outer fibrous covering that contains most of the grain's fiber. This dish can be served over brown rice or another whole grain, like quinoa or farro, but I prefer to serve over a little bit of white rice, as originally intended, to appreciate the complex mixture of spices in the coconut sauce.

1 Heat the oil in a large pot over medium heat. Sauté the onion, garlic, and ginger until the onion is beginning to soften, 4 minutes.

2 Add the garam masala, coriander, cumin, turmeric, paprika, and chili powder. Sauté until fragrant, 30 seconds, stirring constantly.

3 Add the tomato sauce, chickpeas, coconut milk, and tomato paste, along with ½ cup (120 ml) of water, stirring to combine. Bring to a simmer. Stir in the kale; cook until just wilted, 5 minutes.

NUTRITION FACTS (SERVING SIZE: 1 CUP/315 G): CALORIES 286; FAT 13 G (SAT 9 G); PROTEIN 8 G; CARB 31 G; FIBER 7 G; SUGARS 10 G (ADDED SUGARS 0 G); SODIUM 436 MG

NOTE An equivalent amount of ginger paste can be used in place of the fresh minced ginger. Look for tubes of ginger paste in the refrigerated produce section.

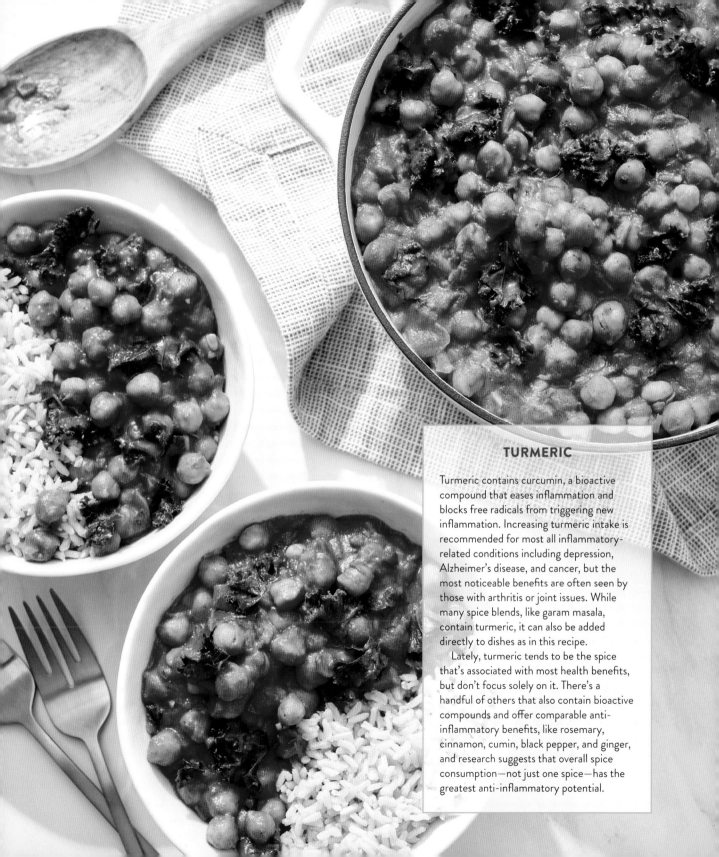

TURMERIC

Turmeric contains curcumin, a bioactive compound that eases inflammation and blocks free radicals from triggering new inflammation. Increasing turmeric intake is recommended for most all inflammatory-related conditions including depression, Alzheimer's disease, and cancer, but the most noticeable benefits are often seen by those with arthritis or joint issues. While many spice blends, like garam masala, contain turmeric, it can also be added directly to dishes as in this recipe.

Lately, turmeric tends to be the spice that's associated with most health benefits, but don't focus solely on it. There's a handful of others that also contain bioactive compounds and offer comparable anti-inflammatory benefits, like rosemary, cinnamon, cumin, black pepper, and ginger, and research suggests that overall spice consumption—not just one spice—has the greatest anti-inflammatory potential.

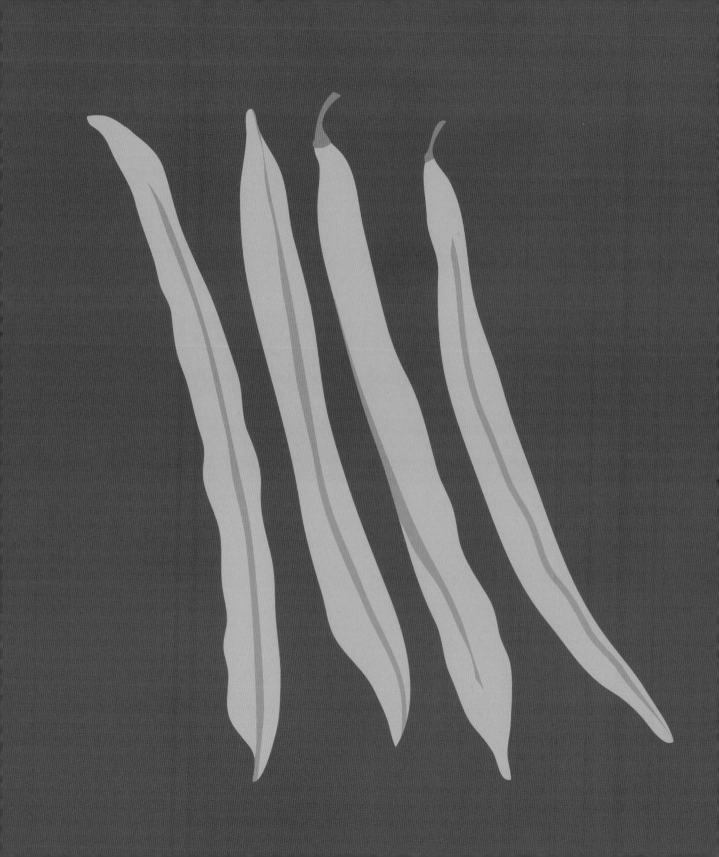

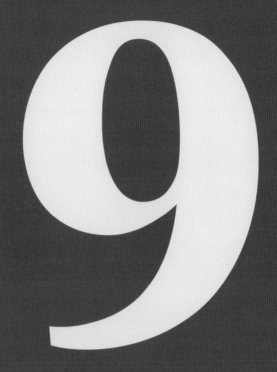

9

·················

SIDES & SALADS

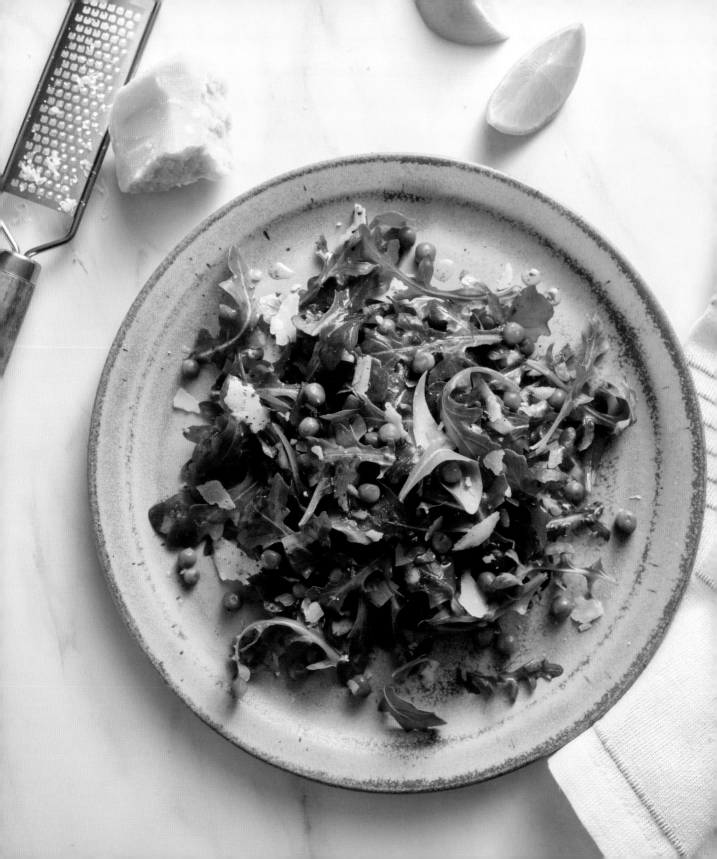

lemony arugula
salad with parmesan

HANDS-ON: 5 MINUTES :: TOTAL: 5 MINUTES :: SERVES 6

One of my favorite tricks for perking up a bottled salad dressing is to add a squeeze of lemon or lime juice. The fresh juice brightens and enhances the dressing's flavors, and this tangy lemon version is a perfect complement to peppery greens, green peas, and Parmesan.

Combine the arugula and peas in a large bowl. Whisk together the vinaigrette and lemon juice and pour over the greens. Add the cheese and toss well.

NUTRITION FACTS (SERVING SIZE: ⅙ OF SALAD): CALORIES 120; FAT 9 G (SAT 2 G); PROTEIN 6 G; CARB 4 G; FIBER 2 G; SUGARS 2 G (ADDED SUGARS 0 G); SODIUM 233 MG

DAIRY-FREE/VEGAN OPTION Replace the Parmesan with ⅓ cup (34 g) coarsely chopped roasted salted cashews or other nut.

NOTE Dress the salad up by adding 1 cup (180 g) of trimmed, slightly blanched fresh asparagus pieces before tossing with the dressing.

One 5-ounce (142 g) container baby arugula

1 cup (145 g) fresh peas or thawed frozen peas

¼ cup (60 ml) bottled olive oil vinaigrette

1 to 2 teaspoons lemon juice

2 ounces (57 g) freshly shaved Parmesan

ARUGULA

Arugula is a leafy green akin to spinach, kale, and lettuces like romaine, red leaf, and radicchio, but it has a lighter, leafier texture and a slight peppery flavor that makes it perfect to toss with a citrus dressing or vinaigrette and top with ripe berries. Its anti-inflammatory perks come from antioxidants, like beta-carotene and vitamin C. This leafy green is also a member of the cruciferous vegetable family, which contains powerful anti-inflammatory compounds. (See page 15 for more information on cruciferous vegetables).

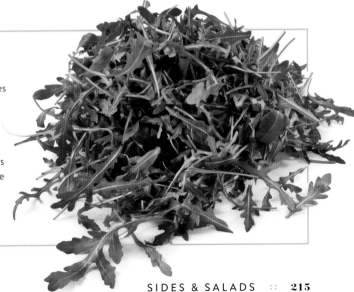

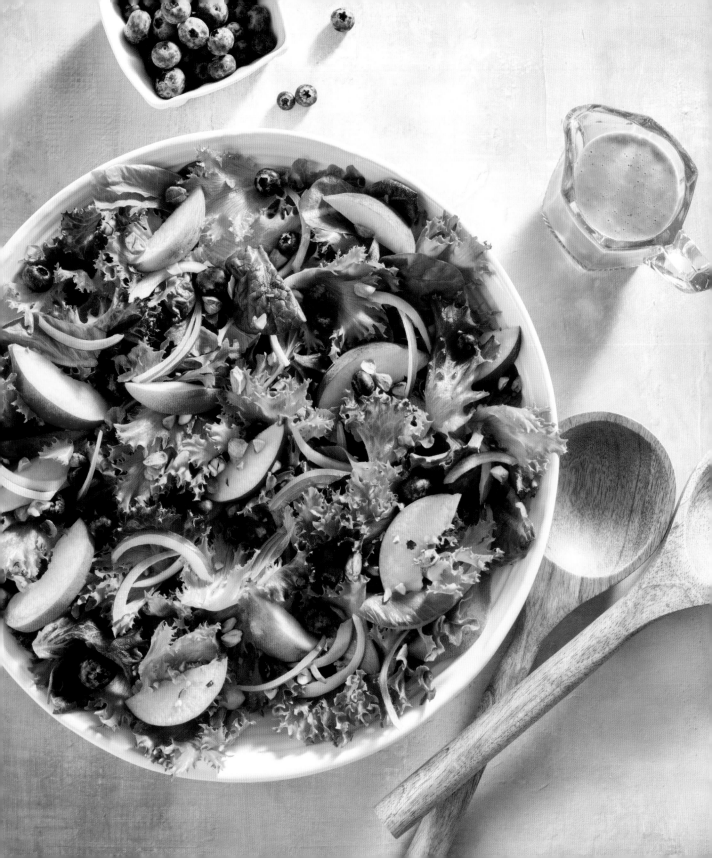

summer salad with lime-basil vinaigrette

HANDS-ON: 7 MINUTES :: TOTAL: 10 MINUTES :: SERVES 6

Summer peaches and berries are hard to beat, and this quick salad is one of my favorite ways to feature their sweet, juicy flavors. The crunchy tang from the pistachios and onion and the citrus-herb dressing are perfect complements to highlight the summer fruits.

Combine the greens, pistachios, onion, peach slices, and blueberries in a large salad bowl. Drizzle with the vinaigrette. Toss well to combine and serve immediately.

NUTRITION FACTS (SERVING SIZE: ⅙ OF SALAD): CALORIES 139; FAT 11 G (SAT 1.5 G); PROTEIN 2 G; CARB 9 G; FIBER 2 G; SUGARS 5 G (ADDED SUGARS 1 G); SODIUM 112 MG

lime-basil vinaigrette

MAKES ABOUT 1 CUP (240 ML)

Combine all of the ingredients in the bowl of a food processor. Cover and process until smooth, 30 seconds, pausing to scrape down the sides with a spatula as needed. Refrigerate in a sealed container for up to 4 days. Shake well before using. Use extra dressing to toss with other leafy greens or drizzle over sliced tomatoes.

NUTRITION FACTS (SERVING SIZE: 1 TABLESPOON): CALORIES 64; FAT 7 G (SAT 1 G); PROTEIN 0 G; CARB 1 G; FIBER 0 G; SUGARS 1 G (ADDED SUGARS 0.5 G); SODIUM 60 MG

A TRICK FOR EATING RAW RED ONIONS

Love the flavor that a little uncooked red onion adds to a salad but not the lingering taste? If so, try soaking red onion slices in a bowl of cold water for 10 to 15 minutes. Then, drain and use. The onion slices will have a less pungent flavor that won't stay with you for the next few hours.

---

5 cups (213 g) mixed greens

¼ cup (30 g) coarsely chopped pistachios

¼ cup (29 g) thinly sliced red onion

1 ripe peach, sliced

½ cup (74 g) blueberries

½ cup (120 ml) Lime-Basil Vinaigrette or bottled olive oil vinaigrette

LIME-BASIL VINAIGRETTE

½ cup (21 g) packed fresh basil leaves

½ cup (120 ml) extra virgin olive oil

¼ cup (60 ml) lime juice

2 tablespoons water

2 teaspoons honey

2 garlic cloves

½ teaspoon salt

¼ teaspoon black pepper

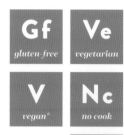

Gf *gluten-free* **Ve** *vegetarian*

V *vegan+* **Nc** *no cook*

Lc *low carb*

winter greens with maple-cider vinaigrette

HANDS-ON: 10 MINUTES :: TOTAL: 10 MINUTES :: SERVES 6

Tossed with a quick homemade vinaigrette, this salad adds the perfect pop of color to a fall or holiday table. I love the way the toasted pecans pair with the citrus sections and cherries, but you can substitute another toasted nut like walnuts, almonds, or cashews, if desired.

One 5-ounce (142 g) package baby spinach and arugula salad mix

1 orange, peeled and sectioned

⅓ cup (36 g) toasted pecan pieces

¼ cup (38 g) crumbled feta or blue cheese

¼ cup (30 g) dried cherries or cranberries

⅓ cup (80 ml) Maple-Cider Vinaigrette

MAPLE-CIDER VINAIGRETTE

2 tablespoons apple cider vinegar

1 tablespoon orange juice

2 teaspoons maple syrup or honey

½ teaspoon Dijon mustard

½ teaspoon garlic salt

¼ teaspoon black pepper

2½ tablespoons extra virgin olive oil

Place the salad greens in a large mixing bowl. Add the orange sections, pecans, cheese, cherries, and vinaigrette to the salad greens. Toss well and serve immediately.

NUTRITION FACTS (SERVING SIZE: ⅙ OF SALAD): CALORIES 147; FAT 12 G (SAT 2 G); PROTEIN 2 G; CARB 10 G; FIBER 2 G; SUGARS 8 G (ADDED SUGARS 3 G); SODIUM 244 MG

DAIRY-FREE/VEGAN OPTION Omit the cheese. Increase to ⅓ cup (36 g) of cranberries and ½ cup (55 g) of pecans.

NUTRITION FACTS (SERVING SIZE: ⅙ OF SALAD): CALORIES 155; FAT 12 G (SAT 1.5 G); PROTEIN 2 G; CARB 11 G; FIBER 2 G; SUGARS 9 G (ADDED SUGARS 4 G); SODIUM 186 MG

TIP Substitute approximately 5 cups (150 g) of any dark leafy green for the 5-ounce package. Need to skip the homemade dressing to save time? Use ⅓ cup (80 ml) of any olive oil-based bottled vinaigrette instead.

maple-cider vinaigrette

MAKES ABOUT ⅓ CUP (80 ML)

Combine the vinegar, juice, syrup, mustard, garlic salt, and pepper in a small mixing bowl, stirring to combine. Slowly whisk in the oil. Refrigerate in a sealed container for up to 4 days. Shake well before using. Toss the remaining vinaigrette with spinach, arugula, or lettuces (like Bibb or romaine) for a quick salad at a later meal.

NUTRITION FACTS (SERVING SIZE: 1 TABLESPOON): CALORIES 57; FAT 6 G (SAT 1 G); PROTEIN 0 G; CARB 2 G; FIBER 0 G; SUGARS 2 G (ADDED SUGARS 1 G); SODIUM 174 MG

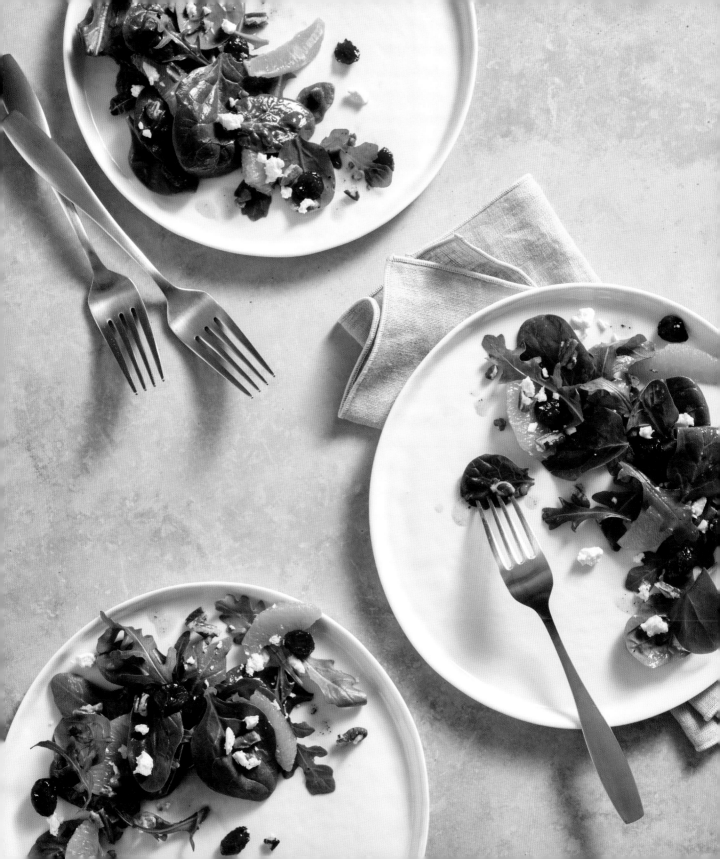

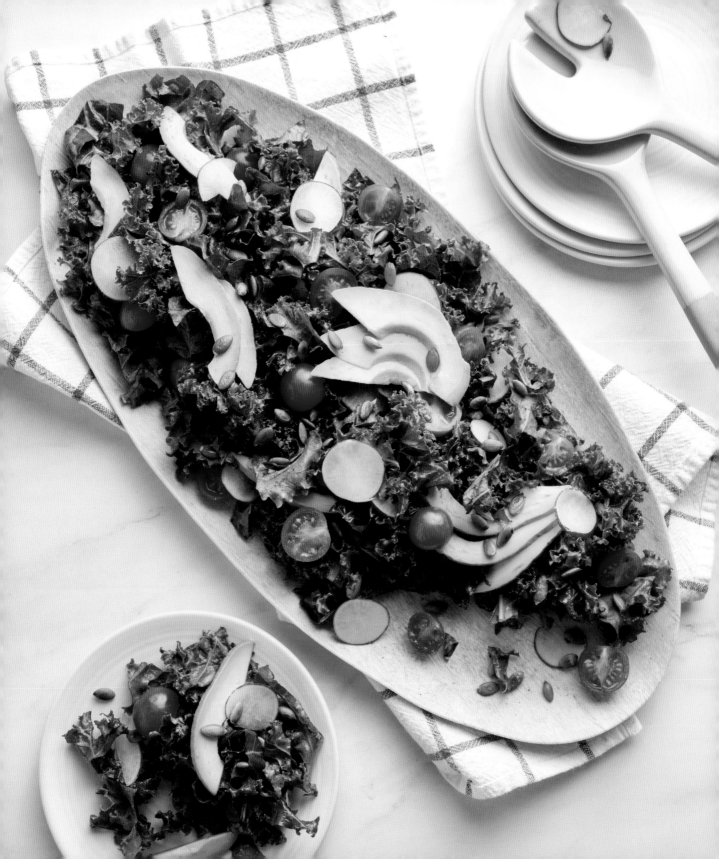

southwestern kale salad

HANDS-ON: 7 MINUTES :: TOTAL: 17 MINUTES :: SERVES 6

A bright, slightly nutty dressing made with olive oil, lime juice, cilantro, and tahini makes this kale salad anything but ordinary. The dressing's creamy texture is also a perfect thickness for coating the kale, which minimizes the massage time that kale usually requires to soften. Since kale is a heartier green, leftovers of the tossed salad generally hold well when covered in the refrigerator for 1 to 2 days.

1   Combine the oil, lime zest, lime juice, cilantro, jalapeño, tahini, garlic, honey, cumin, and salt in the bowl of a food processor. Cover and process until smooth, 30 seconds, pausing to scrape down the sides with a spatula as needed.

2   Place the kale in a large bowl. Pour the dressing over the kale. Using clean hands, massage the dressing into the kale for 1 to 2 minutes. Let the kale stand until the leaves are beginning to soften, 10 minutes.

3   Add the tomatoes, avocado, radishes, and pepitas and toss well.

NUTRITION FACTS (SERVING SIZE: ⅙ OF SALAD): CALORIES 198; FAT 17 G (SAT 2 G); PROTEIN 4 G; CARB 11 G; FIBER 4 G; SUGARS 3 G (ADDED SUGARS 1 G); SODIUM 110 MG

MEATLESS MAIN VARIATION Rinse and drain one 15-ounce (425 g) can of no-salt-added black beans. Add the beans and 2 cups (370 g) of cooked quinoa in step 3. Toss well before serving.

NUTRITION FACTS (SERVING SIZE: ⅙ OF SALAD): CALORIES 332; FAT 19 G (SAT 2.5 G); PROTEIN 11 G; CARB 34 G; FIBER 9 G; SUGARS 4 G (ADDED SUGARS 1 G); SODIUM 123 MG

¼ cup (60 ml) olive oil

1 teaspoon lime zest

¼ cup (60 ml) lime juice

¼ cup (4 g) chopped fresh cilantro

1 small jalapeño, seeded and roughly chopped

2 tablespoons tahini

2 garlic cloves

1 teaspoon honey

½ teaspoon ground cumin

¼ teaspoon fine sea salt

One 10-ounce (284 g) package trimmed chopped kale

1 cup (149 g) cherry tomatoes, halved

1 avocado, sliced

3 radishes, thinly sliced

2 tablespoons toasted pepitas (pumpkin seeds)

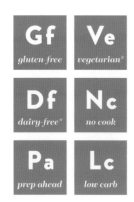

shaved brussels slaw

HANDS-ON: 5 MINUTES :: TOTAL: 25 MINUTES :: SERVES 8

Shredded brussels sprouts can be stir-fried in a skillet or used raw in a slaw like this one. Both methods create a delicious way to eat this cruciferous vegetable—they taste very different from the boiled sprouts you may be remembering from your childhood! One serving of this slaw provides 60 percent of the daily value for vitamin C, and you can quickly turn it into a main dish by topping it with grilled shrimp or chicken.

Two 9-ounce (255 g) packages shaved or shredded brussels sprouts

⅓ cup (80 ml) balsamic vinaigrette

½ cup (87 g) pomegranate arils

¼ cup (28 g) uncured bacon crumbles

¼ cup (27 g) chopped toasted pecans

¼ cup (20 g) freshly grated Manchego or Parmesan

½ teaspoon black pepper

Combine the brussels sprouts and vinaigrette in a large bowl, tossing well to combine. Gently fold in the pomegranate, bacon, pecans, cheese, and pepper. Cover and refrigerate for at least 20 minutes before serving.

NUTRITION FACTS (SERVING SIZE: ABOUT ⅔ CUP/95 G): CALORIES 120; FAT 8 G (SAT 1.5 G); PROTEIN 5 G; CARB 10 G; FIBER 3 G; SUGARS 3 G (ADDED SUGARS 0 G); SODIUM 173 MG

TIP Shave or shred brussels sprouts yourself using a box grater. To do this, purchase 1½ pounds (612 g) of whole brussels sprouts to yield approximately 6 cups (528 g) of shaved brussels sprouts.

DAIRY-FREE OPTION Omit the cheese and increase the pecans to ½ cup (54 g). Add ¼ teaspoon salt with the pepper.

NUTRITION FACTS (SERVING SIZE: ABOUT ⅔ CUP/95 G): CALORIES 134; FAT 10 G (SAT 1.5 G); PROTEIN 4 G; CARB 10 G; FIBER 4 G; SUGARS 4 G (ADDED SUGARS 0 G); SODIUM 188 MG

VEGETARIAN OPTION Omit the bacon crumbles and increase the pecans to ½ cup (54 g).

NUTRITION FACTS (SERVING SIZE: ABOUT ⅔ CUP/95 G): CALORIES 132; FAT 10 G (SAT 1.5 G); PROTEIN 4 G; CARB 10 G; FIBER 4 G; SUGARS 4 G (ADDED SUGARS 0 G); SODIUM 108 MG

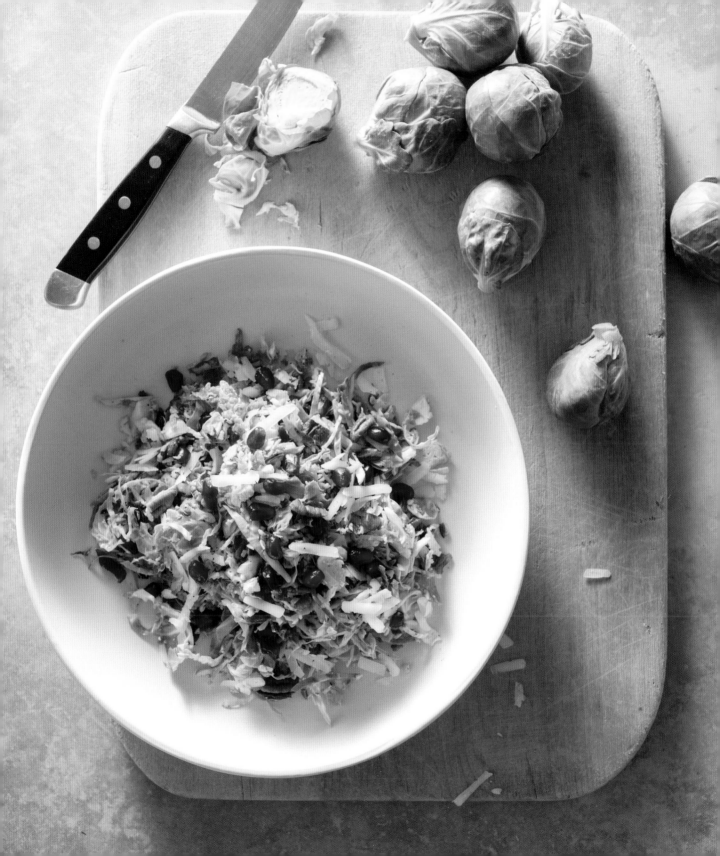

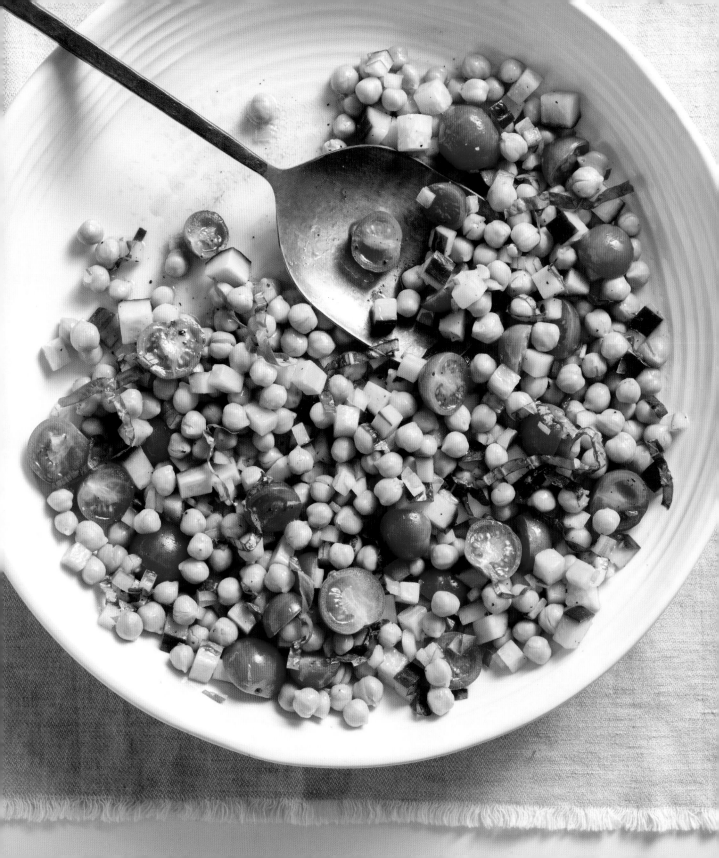

tomato, cucumber, and chickpea salad

HANDS-ON: 10 MINUTES :: TOTAL: 40 MINUTES :: SERVES 8

This recipe is a perfect example of how you can quickly create a fresh, flavorful side dish with simple produce and pantry staples. It's hard to beat the combination of fresh basil and tomato, but you can substitute other fresh herbs like oregano, thyme, or dill, if desired.

1 Combine the chickpeas, tomatoes, cucumber, and onion in a large bowl. In a small bowl, whisk together the oil, vinegar, basil, salt, and pepper. Pour over the chickpea mixture, stirring to coat all ingredients.

2 Cover and chill for at least 30 minutes or until ready to serve.

NUTRITION FACTS (SERVING SIZE: ABOUT ¾ CUP/149 G): CALORIES 114; FAT 6 G (SAT 0.5 G); PROTEIN 4 G; CARB 12 G; FIBER 3 G; SUGARS 2 G (ADDED SUGARS 0 G); SODIUM 195 MG

NOTE This salad can be made up to 24 hours in advance. Cover and refrigerate leftovers to use within 3 days for best taste and quality.

One 15-ounce (425 g) can no-salt-added chickpeas, rinsed and drained

2 cups (298 g) cherry tomatoes, halved

1 English cucumber, diced

½ cup (80 g) finely chopped red onion

3 tablespoons extra virgin olive oil

2 tablespoons red wine vinegar

¼ cup (11 g) fresh sliced basil

¾ teaspoon salt

½ teaspoon black pepper

Gf
gluten-free

Ve
vegetarian

St
stovetop

street corn salad

HANDS-ON: 15 MINUTES :: TOTAL: 15 MINUTES :: SERVES 8

Always a hit at summer cookouts, this fresh corn salad comes together in just a few minutes with minimal work. Serve it at room temperature or chilled as a side dish or a dip. You can't go wrong! For a little heat, add a chopped, seeded jalapeño pepper in step 3.

6 ears corn

Cooking spray

½ teaspoon salt

½ cup (113 g) nonfat plain Greek yogurt

⅓ cup (80 ml) lime juice

¼ cup (60 g) olive oil mayonnaise

2 teaspoons honey

1 teaspoon chili powder

1 teaspoon smoked paprika

½ teaspoon ground cumin

½ cup (8 g) chopped fresh cilantro

½ cup (60 g) crumbled cotija

Chopped fresh cilantro or lime wedges (optional)

1 Remove the husks and silk from the corn. Cut the kernels off the cob to yield 5 cups (770 g).

2 Coat a large skillet with cooking spray, then heat over medium-high heat. Add the corn and cook, stirring occasionally, until lightly browned, 3 minutes. Remove the skillet from the heat. Sprinkle the corn with salt.

3 In a large bowl, whisk together the yogurt, lime juice, mayonnaise, honey, chili powder, paprika, and cumin. Gently fold in the corn, cilantro, and cotija.

NUTRITION FACTS (SERVING SIZE: ABOUT ¾ CUP/139 G): CALORIES 156; FAT 6.5 G (SAT 2 G); PROTEIN 6 G; CARB 22 G; FIBER 3 G; SUGARS 5 G (ADDED SUGARS 1 G); SODIUM 315 MG

TIP Substitute 5 cups (770 g) of thawed frozen roasted corn kernels in place of the fresh corn, if desired. In place of step 2, warm the corn in the microwave or over low heat in the skillet. Then, incorporate the corn in step 3.

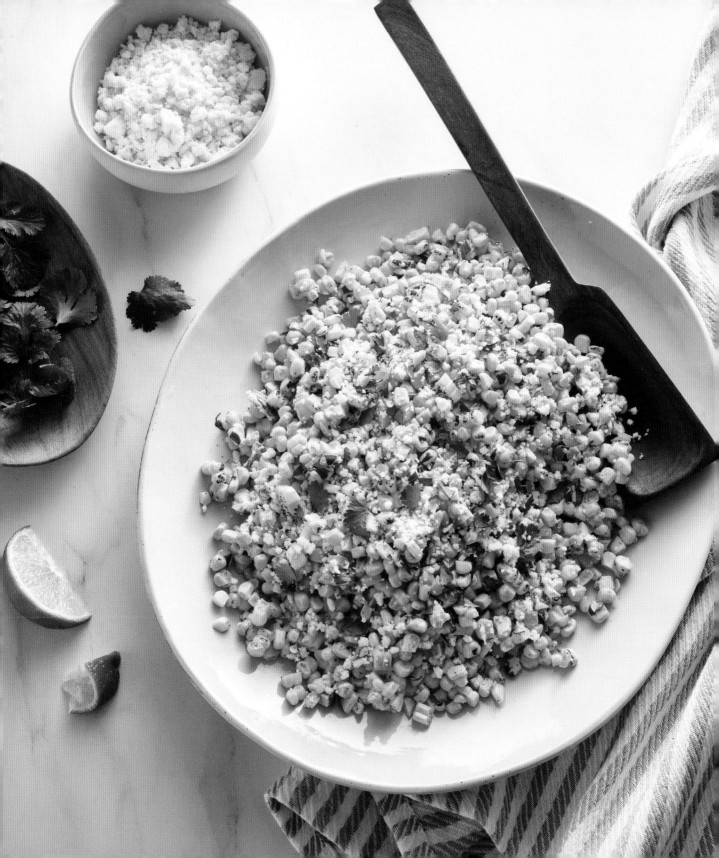

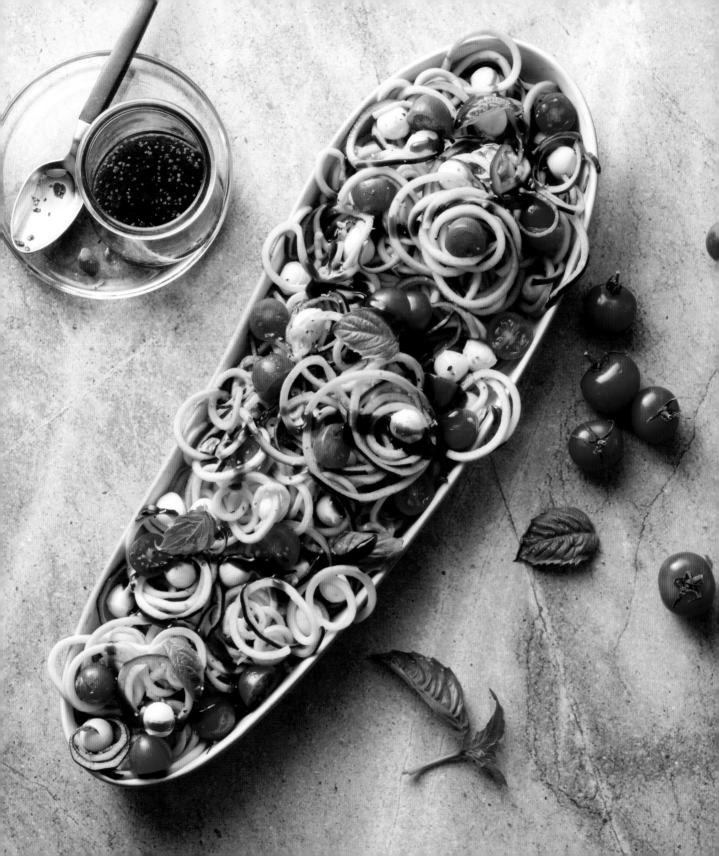

caprese zoodles

HANDS-ON: 5 MINUTES :: TOTAL: 20 MINUTES :: SERVES 6

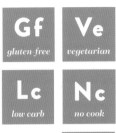

"Fresh and summery" is how one taste tester described this dish. Even better, preparing this recipe is easy and quick so you can get back outside and enjoy your summer. Speaking of summer: If you have a bumper crop of zucchini, you can try making your own zucchini spirals instead of buying them. Keep this recipe on hand in the cooler months, too—it's a fresh pick-me-up and calls for produce that is readily available at most markets, no matter the season.

1 In a large bowl, combine the zucchini spirals, vinegar, oil, salt, and pepper. Toss well and let stand 15 minutes.

2 Add the tomatoes, mozzarella, and basil to the zucchini spirals. Gently toss to combine all ingredients. Drizzle with the balsamic glaze, if desired.

NUTRITION FACTS (SERVING SIZE: ABOUT ¾ CUP/99 G): CALORIES 83; FAT 6 G (SAT 2 G); PROTEIN 4 G; CARB 4 G; FIBER 1 G; SUGARS 2 G (ADDED SUGARS 0 G); SODIUM 223 MG

TIP Purchase fresh zucchini spirals from the produce section or use 1 to 2 whole zucchini to create your own fresh spirals. I've found that ¾ pound (340 g) of zucchini will yield the amount of spirals needed for this recipe (approximately 2½ to 3 cups).

One 10-ounce (284 g) package fresh zucchini spirals

1½ tablespoons balsamic vinegar

1 tablespoon extra virgin olive oil

½ teaspoon salt

¼ teaspoon black pepper

1 cup (149 g) cherry tomatoes, halved

4 ounces (113 g) mozzarella pearls, halved

¼ cup (10 g) chopped fresh basil leaves

Balsamic glaze (optional)

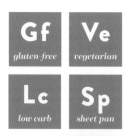

Gf *gluten-free* **Ve** *vegetarian*

Lc *low carb* **Sp** *sheet pan*

Af *air fryer**

Cooking spray

½ cup (40 g) freshly grated Parmesan

1 teaspoon garlic powder

½ teaspoon dried thyme

¼ teaspoon salt

¼ teaspoon black pepper

2 large zucchini, cut into ¼-inch (6 mm) thick slices

roasted parmesan zucchini

HANDS-ON: 10 MINUTES :: TOTAL: 22 MINUTES :: SERVES 5

One of my kids' favorite ways to eat zucchini is sliced, lightly breaded, and baked until crisp, but this is pretty labor-intensive for a weeknight since it involves an egg wash and breading. I decided to simplify the process by skipping the egg wash and breading and using a little Parmesan and seasonings instead. The result is crisp, lightly "breaded" zucchini slices that are much quicker to make and gives the original version a run for its money when it comes to taste.

1 Preheat the oven to 400°F (200°C). Line a sheet pan with foil. Place a metal cooling rack on top of the pan. Lightly coat the rack with cooking spray.

2 Combine the Parmesan, garlic powder, thyme, salt, and pepper in a shallow bowl. Working in batches, lightly coat the zucchini slices with cooking spray on both sides and toss with the cheese mixture. Place the coated zucchini slices on the rack. Repeat with the remaining zucchini slices.

3 Sprinkle any remaining cheese mixture over the zucchini on the rack and lightly coat the zucchini slices with cooking spray. Bake for 10 minutes, or until the zucchini is crisp-tender. Turn the oven to broil and cook for 2 minutes, or until the zucchini slices are beginning to crisp and turn golden brown.

NUTRITION FACTS (SERVING SIZE: ⅕ OF ZUCCHINI SLICES): CALORIES 55; FAT 2.5 G (SAT 1.5 G); PROTEIN 4 G; CARB 5 G; FIBER 1 G; SUGARS 2 G (ADDED SUGARS 0 G); SODIUM 249 MG

AIR FRYER OPTION Preheat the air fryer to 400°F (200°C). Lightly coat the air fryer pan with cooking spray. Combine the Parmesan, garlic powder, thyme, salt, and pepper as directed in step 2. Working in batches, lightly coat the zucchini slices with cooking spray on both sides and toss with the cheese mixture. Place the zucchini slices on the air fryer pan and lightly coat with cooking spray. Bake for 10 to 12 minutes, until the zucchini slices are beginning to crisp and turn golden brown, turning the slices halfway through the cooking process. Let the zucchini cool slightly before removing from the pan. Repeat with the remaining zucchini slices.

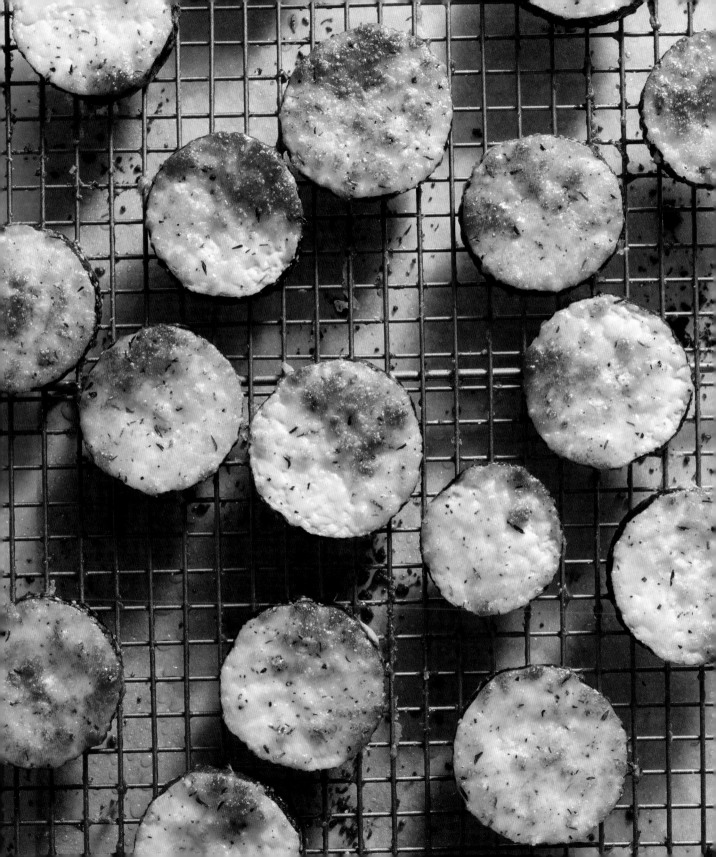

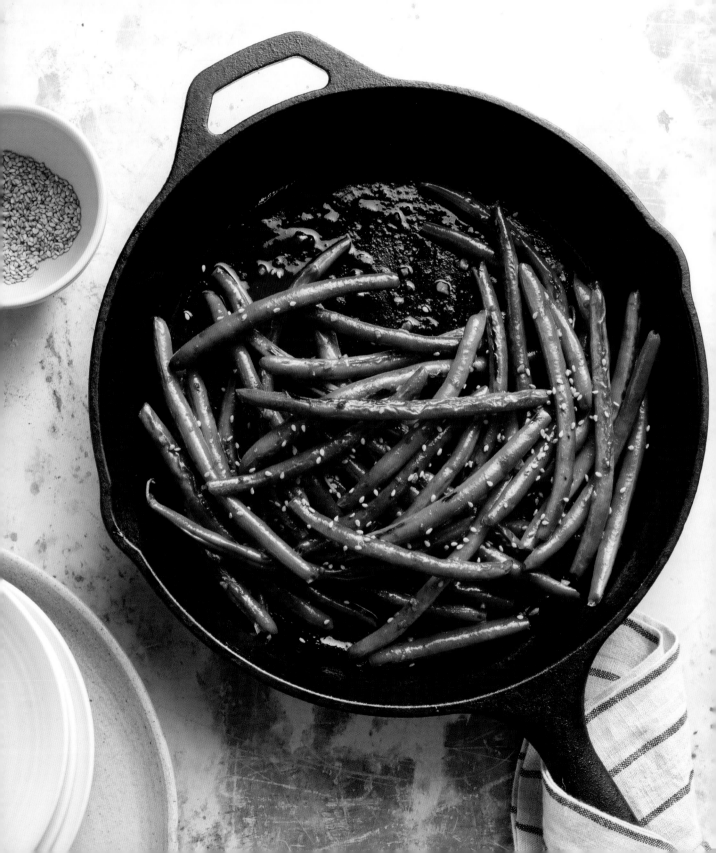

charred sriracha green beans

HANDS-ON: 10 MINUTES :: TOTAL: 12 MINUTES :: SERVES 4

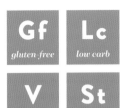

Every time I make these, at least half of the pan is completely gone by the time we sit down to eat. While I don't usually allow eating straight from the pan, I make an exception any time my kids get excited about green vegetables. Sriracha adds a small amount of heat to this amazing green bean recipe, but it's more subtle and a little milder than vinegar-heavy hot sauces like Tabasco. Feel free to decrease or omit, if desired.

1 Heat a large cast-iron pan over medium-high heat. Add the oil and beans and cook, without stirring, until seared or lightly charred, 5 to 7 minutes.

2 Push the green beans to one side of the skillet. Add the garlic to the other side and sauté until fragrant, 1 minute. Combine the garlic and green beans in the skillet. Add the soy sauce and sriracha, tossing to coat the beans. Sprinkle with sesame seeds, if desired.

NUTRITION FACTS (SERVING SIZE: ¼ OF GREEN BEANS): CALORIES 66; FAT 4 G (SAT 0.5 G); PROTEIN 2 G; CARB 7 G; FIBER 2 G; SUGARS 3 G (ADDED SUGARS 0 G); SODIUM 189 MG

1 tablespoon avocado oil

One 12-ounce (340 g) package trimmed green beans

1 teaspoon minced garlic

1 tablespoon lower-sodium soy sauce or tamari

2 teaspoons sriracha

2 teaspoons toasted sesame seeds (optional)

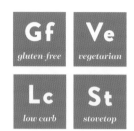

Gf *gluten-free*

Ve *vegetarian*

Lc *low carb*

St *stovetop*

wild mushroom "risotto"

HANDS-ON: 15 MINUTES :: TOTAL: 30 MINUTES :: SERVES 6

Risotto is typically made by slowly adding hot broth to short-grain rice, but this recipe uses riced cauliflower instead. The result is a creamy, risotto-like texture that's significantly lower in carbs and has a lower glycemic impact on blood glucose (see page 48 for more on glycemic index). Mushrooms, thyme, and Parmesan give the dish a rich, hearty flavor. The mushrooms also serve as a source of vitamin D, a nutrient that's hard to find in food.

1½ tablespoons olive oil

1½ tablespoons butter

8 ounces (226 g) fresh wild mushrooms (any mix of cremini, shiitake, baby portobello, oyster, or button), sliced

½ teaspoon salt

½ teaspoon black pepper

1 yellow onion, finely chopped

2 teaspoons minced garlic

Two 12-ounce (340 g) packages fresh cauliflower crumbles

1½ cups (360 ml) low-sodium vegetable or chicken broth

2 fresh thyme sprigs

⅓ cup (27 g) freshly grated Parmesan

1 Heat ½ tablespoon oil and ½ tablespoon butter in a large skillet over medium-high heat. Add the mushrooms and cook until lightly browned and beginning to soften, 5 minutes. Season with ¼ teaspoon salt and ¼ teaspoon pepper. Remove the mushroom mixture from the skillet and wipe clean.

2 Heat the remaining 1 tablespoon oil in the skillet over medium heat. Add the onion and garlic; cook until the onion begins to soften, 5 minutes. Add the cauliflower, broth, and thyme, and bring to a simmer. Cover and cook until the cauliflower is crisp-tender, 10 minutes.

3 Remove the lid and stir. Cook, uncovered, until almost all of the liquid has evaporated, 10 to 12 minutes. Gently stir in the mushrooms, remaining 1 tablespoon of butter, Parmesan, and remaining ¼ teaspoon each of salt and pepper.

NUTRITION FACTS (SERVING SIZE: ABOUT ¾ CUP/182 G): CALORIES 82; FAT 4 G (SAT 1.5 G); PROTEIN 4 G; CARB 8 G; FIBER 3 G; SUGARS 3 G (ADDED SUGARS 0 G); SODIUM 227 MG

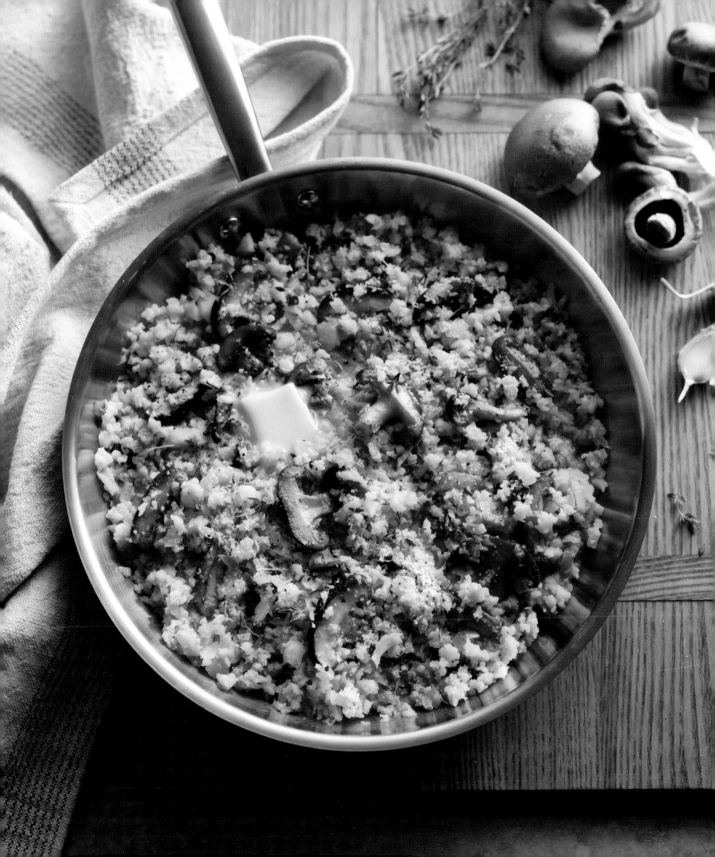

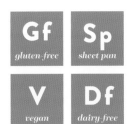

Gf
gluten-free

Sp
sheet pan

V
vegan

Df
dairy free

Cooking spray

One 2½ to 3-pound (1134 to 1361 g) butternut squash

1½ tablespoons avocado oil

1 tablespoon maple syrup

2 tablespoons chopped fresh rosemary

2 teaspoons garlic powder

¾ teaspoon salt

¼ teaspoon black pepper

roasted rosemary butternut squash

HANDS-ON: 15 MINUTES :: TOTAL: 35 MINUTES :: SERVES 5

Struggling to get your family to eat more vegetables? Give butternut squash a try! Roasting emphasizes butternut squash's sweet flavor by caramelizing the squash's natural sugars, and one serving boasts almost 99 percent of the daily value of vitamin A and 40 percent of vitamin C.

1 Preheat the oven to 425°F (215°C). Line a baking sheet with foil and lightly coat with cooking spray.

2 Peel the outside of the squash with a vegetable peeler or paring knife. Cut the squash in half and use a knife to loosen the seeds and stringy pulp. Scoop out the seeds and discard. Cut the squash into ¾ to 1-inch (2 to 2.5 cm) cubes to yield approximately 6 cups (840 g) of cubes.

3 Place the squash on the baking sheet. In a small bowl, whisk together the oil, syrup, and rosemary. Pour the mixture over the squash and toss well to coat. Spread the cubes evenly across the baking sheet. Sprinkle with the garlic powder, salt, and pepper.

4 Bake for 23 to 28 minutes, until the squash is tender.

NUTRITION FACTS (SERVING SIZE: ⅕ OF SQUASH): CALORIES 129; FAT 4 G (SAT 0.5 G); PROTEIN 2 G; CARB 23 G; FIBER 4 G; SUGARS 6 G (ADDED SUGARS 2 G); SODIUM 296 MG

HOW TO CUT BUTTERNUT SQUASH

I've always loved the flavors in roasted butternut squash, but I was intimidated to purchase a whole squash to prepare for years. Then, I got a hands-on lesson from a chef and learned how simple prepping it can be.

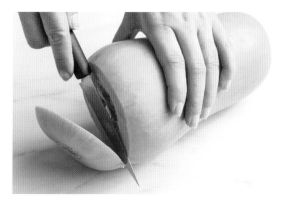

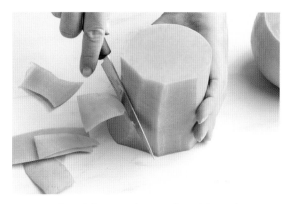

STEP 1: Lay the squash on its side on a cutting board. Cut off and discard the top and bottom ½-inch (13 mm) of the squash. This gets rid of the stem and creates a flat, stable base for peeling.

STEP 2: Stand the squash up and peel the sides using a vegetable peeler or paring knife. Discard the peel. If your squash is really hard and tough to peel, see below.

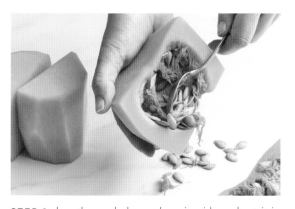

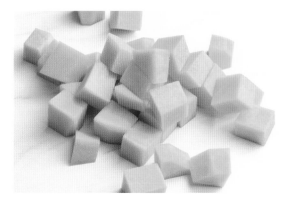

STEP 3: Lay the peeled squash on its side and cut it in half vertically (from top to bottom). Use a paring knife to loosen the seeds and stringy pulp. Scoop out with a spoon or fork and discard.

STEP 4: Now you're ready to cut into cubes! Make sure your cube size is uniform so they will roast evenly.

Got a really tough squash? Soften it in the microwave before peeling and cutting. First, pierce the squash with a sharp knife 5 to 6 times. Then, microwave for 1½ to 2 minutes. Let stand for 5 minutes.

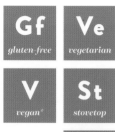

Gf *gluten-free*

Ve *vegetarian*

V *vegan**

St *stovetop*

Lc *low carb*

lower-carb
mashed potatoes

HANDS-ON: 15 MINUTES :: TOTAL: 40 MINUTES :: SERVES 6

If you're a potato fan, you'll love this lightened version that slashes carbs by using cauliflower along with the potatoes. Greek yogurt, broth, and a little butter also deliver a lower-fat but still creamy end product. If doubling the recipe, use a Dutch oven or large saucepan to boil the vegetables and garlic.

One 12-ounce (340 g) package cauliflower florets

¾ pound (340 g) small red potatoes, cubed

2 garlic cloves, peeled

½ cup (120 ml) low-sodium vegetable or chicken broth

2 tablespoons butter

¼ cup (56 g) plain low-fat Greek yogurt

¾ teaspoon salt

½ teaspoon black pepper

1 Combine the cauliflower, potato cubes, and garlic cloves in a Dutch oven or large saucepan. Add cold water to cover by about 1 inch (2.5 cm). Place over medium-high heat and bring to a boil. Reduce the heat, and simmer until the potatoes and cauliflower are very tender, 16 minutes. Drain well; return to the saucepan.

2 Using a slotted spoon, carefully remove the cauliflower florets and garlic cloves and place them in the bowl of a food processor, leaving the potato in the saucepan. Set the potatoes in the saucepan aside.

3 Add ¼ cup (60 ml) broth to the food processor. Cover and process until coarsely pureed, stopping to scrape down sides of the bowl during processing as needed, 1 to 2 minutes.

4 Add the remaining ¼ cup (60 ml) broth and the butter to the potatoes. Coarsely mash the potatoes with a potato masher or large spatula. Add the cauliflower mixture, yogurt, salt, and pepper to the potatoes, stirring to combine well.

NUTRITION FACTS (SERVING SIZE: ABOUT ⅔ CUP/128 G): CALORIES 84; FAT 4 G (SAT 2 G); PROTEIN 3 G; CARB 11 G; FIBER 2 G; SUGARS 2 G (ADDED SUGARS 0 G); SODIUM 263 MG

DAIRY-FREE/VEGAN OPTION Substitute 2 tablespoons of nondairy butter spread for the butter and use 3 tablespoons of extra-creamy plain oat milk in place of the yogurt. Add additional oat milk as needed, 1 tablespoon at a time, to reach desired consistency.

NUTRITION FACTS (SERVING SIZE: ABOUT ⅔ CUP/124 G): CALORIES 84; FAT 4 G (SAT 2 G); PROTEIN 2 G; CARB 11 G; FIBER 2 G; SUGARS 2 G (ADDED SUGARS 0 G); SODIUM 301 MG

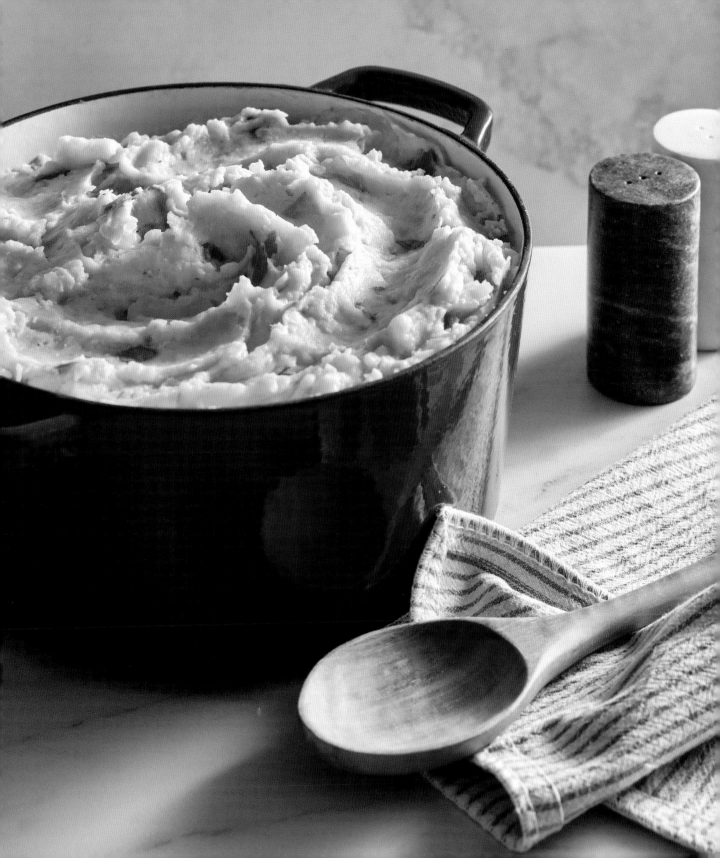

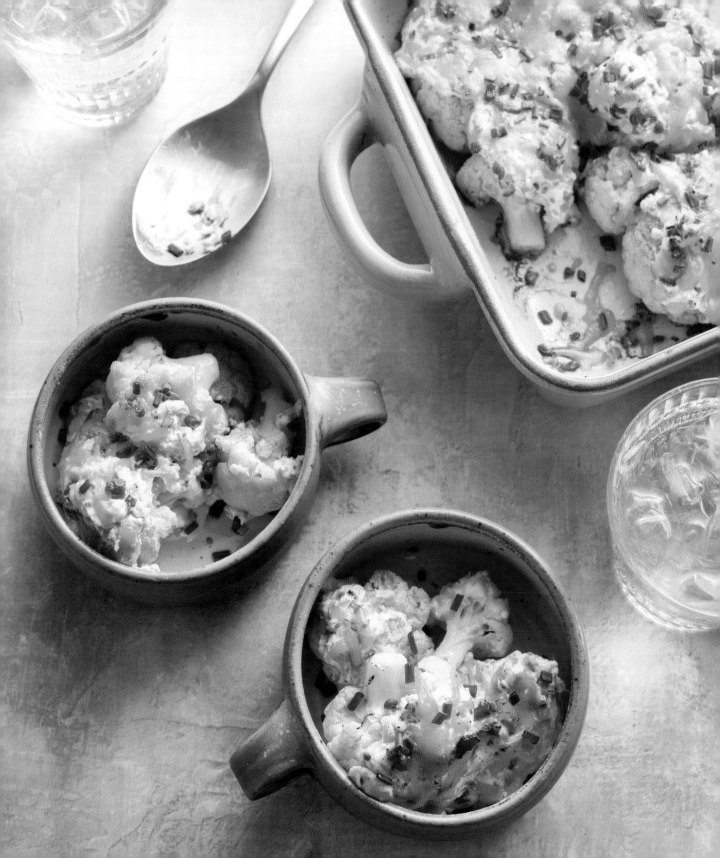

twice-baked cauliflower casserole

HANDS-ON: 10 MINUTES :: TOTAL: 45 MINUTES :: SERVES 10

This casserole is a healthier riff on traditional twice-baked potatoes, which tend to be carbohydrate dense and high in saturated fat and sodium. Roasted cauliflower serves as a base for a lightened cheesy filling that would typically be scooped into potato skins and baked.

1 Preheat the oven to 425°F (215°C). Coat a 9 x 13-inch (23 x 33 cm) metal or ceramic baking dish with cooking spray.

2 Toss the cauliflower with the oil, garlic powder, and ½ teaspoon salt in the baking dish. Spread the cauliflower out evenly in the baking dish. Bake for 30 minutes, or until the florets are tender and golden, stirring after 15 minutes.

3 In a medium bowl, mix the cream cheese and yogurt until smooth. Stir in ½ cup (56 g) cheddar, bacon, onion powder, and ¼ teaspoon salt. Carefully spoon the mixture over the cauliflower. Sprinkle the remaining ½ cup (56 g) cheddar over the top.

4 Bake for 7 to 9 minutes, until the cheese is melted and golden brown. Top with chives, if desired.

NUTRITION FACTS (SERVING SIZE: ABOUT ½ CUP/109 G): CALORIES 125; FAT 8 G (SAT 3 G); PROTEIN 8 G; CARB 6 G; FIBER 2 G; SUGARS 3 G (ADDED SUGARS 0 G); SODIUM 353 MG

VEGETARIAN OPTION Omit the bacon crumbles.

NUTRITION FACTS (SERVING SIZE: ABOUT ½ CUP/106 G): CALORIES 112; FAT 7 G (SAT 3 G); PROTEIN 7 G; CARB 6 G; FIBER 2 G; SUGARS 3 G (ADDED SUGARS 0 G); SODIUM 284 MG

Cooking spray

- Cooking spray
- 6 cups (642 g) cauliflower florets
- 2 tablespoons avocado oil
- 1 teaspoon garlic powder
- ¾ teaspoon salt
- 4 ounces (113 g) reduced-fat cream cheese
- ⅔ cup (150 g) nonfat plain Greek yogurt
- 1 cup (113 g) shredded reduced-fat cheddar
- ⅓ cup (37 g) uncured bacon crumbles
- 1 teaspoon onion powder
- Chopped fresh chives (optional)

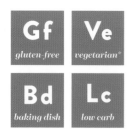

Gf — gluten-free
Ve — vegetarian*
Bd — baking dish
Lc — low carb

Cooking spray

5 zucchini, halved lengthwise

½ teaspoon salt

¼ teaspoon black pepper

6 ounces (170 g) ⅓-less-fat cream cheese, softened

½ teaspoon garlic powder

½ teaspoon onion powder

1 cup (113 g) shredded reduced-fat cheddar

⅓ cup (34 g) uncured bacon crumbles

2 jalapeños, seeded and minced

jalapeño popper zucchini boats

HANDS-ON: 15 MINUTES :: TOTAL: 40 MINUTES :: SERVES 10

This riff on jalapeño poppers maintains all the flavor of this game-day favorite but fits into an anti-inflammatory lifestyle. It's an excellent example of making smarter choices while not giving up favorite foods. Zucchini "boats" are great vehicles to load up with ingredients commonly used to make jalapeño poppers, especially because they taste mild enough to not detract from the spicy, cheesy filling.

1 Preheat the oven to 375°F (190°C). Coat a baking dish with cooking spray.

2 Scoop out the pulp in the center of each zucchini, using a spoon to create approximately ¾-inch (2 cm) thick shells. Reserve and finely chop the zucchini pulp; place the chopped pulp on a clean kitchen or paper towel to drain.

3 Place the hollowed zucchini halves, cut sides up, into the prepared baking dish. Lightly coat with cooking spray and sprinkle with salt and pepper.

4 Combine the cream cheese, garlic powder, onion powder, zucchini pulp, ½ cup (56 g) cheddar, bacon, and jalapeños in a large bowl. Using an electric hand mixer, beat on medium-high speed until soft and fluffy.

5 Spoon the cream cheese mixture into the zucchini boats. Sprinkle with the remaining ½ cup (56 g) cheddar. Bake for 15 minutes, or until the cheese is melted and the zucchini is crisp-tender.

NUTRITION FACTS (SERVING SIZE: 1 ZUCCHINI BOAT): CALORIES 84; FAT 5 G (SAT 3 G); PROTEIN 6 G; CARB 3 G; FIBER 0 G; SUGARS 1 G (ADDED SUGARS 0 G); SODIUM 288 MG

VEGETARIAN OPTION Omit the bacon and increase the cheddar to 1¼ cups (142 g).

NUTRITION FACTS (SERVING SIZE: 1 ZUCCHINI BOAT): CALORIES 81; FAT 5 G (SAT 3 G); PROTEIN 5 G; CARB 3 G; FIBER 0 G; SUGARS 1 G (ADDED SUGARS 0 G); SODIUM 244 MG

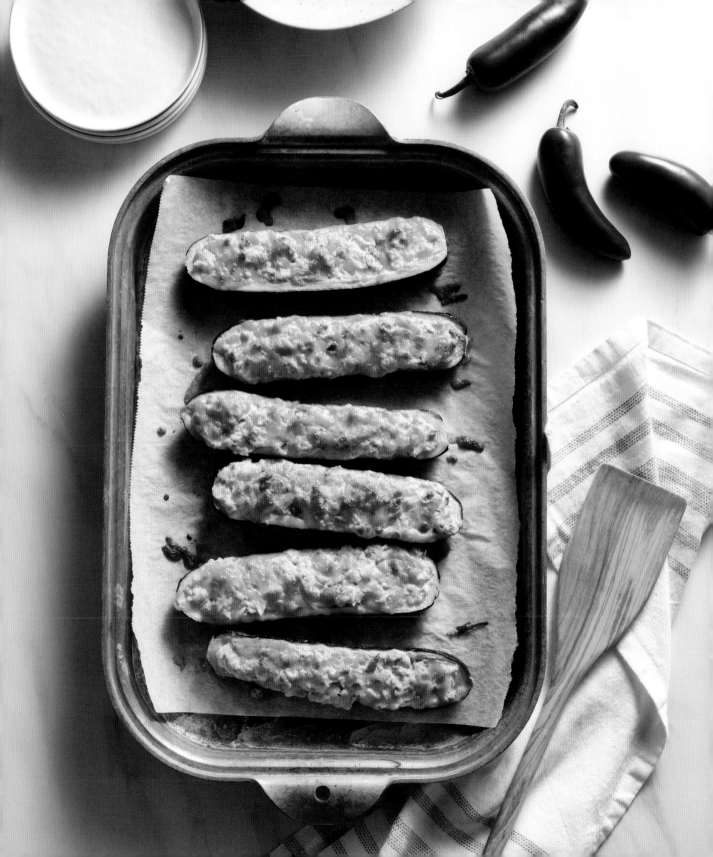

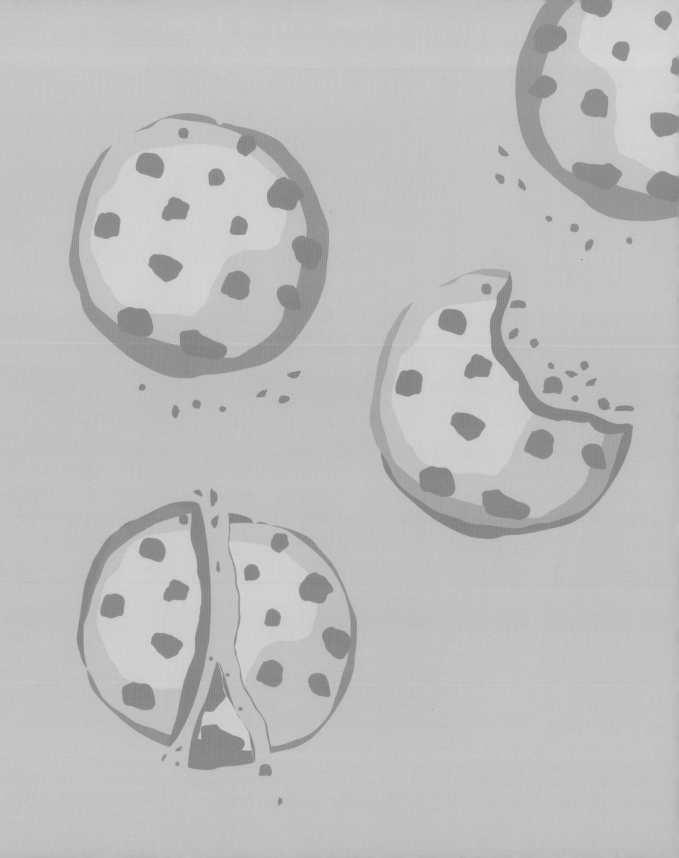

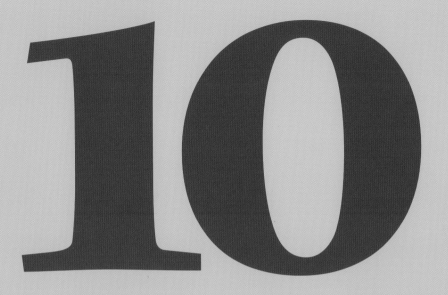

10

SNACKS, TREATS & DRINKS

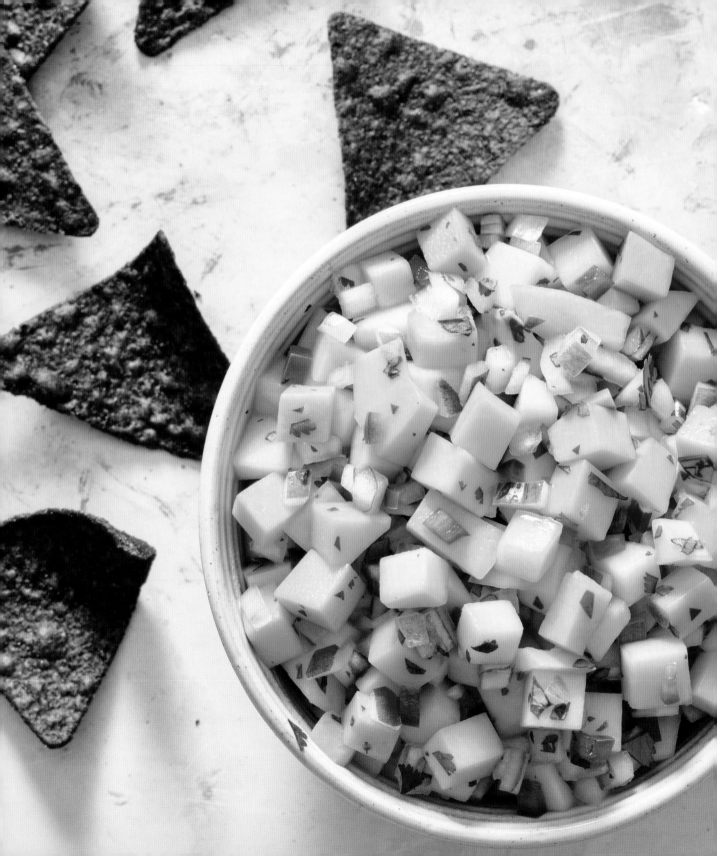

mango salsa

HANDS-ON: 10 MINUTES :: TOTAL: 10 MINUTES :: SERVES 6

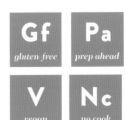

This six-ingredient salsa takes only a few minutes to prepare and is a delicious alternative to store-bought savory tomato salsas. Serve with tortilla chips, as a topping for fish tacos, or as a side for grilled chicken or pork. This salsa can be made in advance but is best served within 36 hours of preparation.

Combine all of the ingredients in a large bowl; toss well. Cover and refrigerate until serving.

NUTRITION FACTS (SERVING SIZE: ⅓ CUP/69 G): CALORIES 54; FAT 0 G (SAT 0 G); PROTEIN 1 G; CARB 13 G; FIBER 2 G; SUGARS 11 G (ADDED SUGARS 0 G); SODIUM 83 MG

TIP Two mangos yield approximately 2 ½ cups (413 g) of diced fruit. Substitute another sweet tropical or summer fruit such as pineapple, watermelon, or strawberries, if desired.

2 mangoes, diced

1 cup (160 g) diced red onion

1 jalapeño, diced and seeded

½ cup (8 g) chopped fresh cilantro

1 to 2 tablespoons lime juice

¼ teaspoon salt

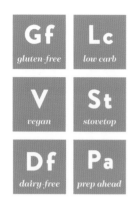

Gf *gluten-free* **Lc** *low carb* **V** *vegan* **St** *stovetop* **Df** *dairy-free* **Pa** *prep ahead*

lima bean hummus

HANDS-ON: 12 MINUTES :: TOTAL: 35 MINUTES :: SERVES 16

Lima beans in hummus may sound odd, but trust me on this one: Pureeing the lima beans creates a decadent texture that's creamier than hummus made with the traditional chickpeas. Adding lemon juice and thyme gives the hummus a fresh flavor, and soy sauce adds the perfect amount of umami. Serve it as a dip for veggies and pitas or use it as a spread on wraps.

One 15-ounce (425 g) bag frozen baby lima beans

3 to 4 tablespoons lemon juice

2 tablespoons tahini

2 tablespoons extra virgin olive oil

2 teaspoons lower-sodium soy sauce or tamari

½ teaspoon ground cumin

½ teaspoon minced garlic

½ teaspoon salt

2 tablespoons chopped fresh thyme or cilantro (optional)

1 Bring 2 cups (480 ml) of salted water to a boil in a small saucepan. Add the lima beans. Return to a boil, cover, reduce the heat to low, and cook until the beans are very tender, 20 minutes. (Note: The beans will cook slightly longer than what is suggested on the packaging and should be very soft.) Remove from the heat. Drain the beans, reserving ¼ cup (60 ml) of the cooking liquid.

2 Place the beans in the bowl of a food processor. Add 3 tablespoons lemon juice, tahini, oil, soy sauce, cumin, garlic, salt, and 2 tablespoons of the reserved cooking water. Process until almost smooth, 1 minute, stopping to scrape down sides with a spatula as needed. Adding the remaining cooking liquid, 1 tablespoon at a time, as needed to reach desired consistency. If desired, add the remaining 1 tablespoon lemon juice and the thyme. Process until smooth.

3 Refrigerate in an airtight container for up to 5 days.

NUTRITION FACTS (SERVING SIZE: 2 TABLESPOONS): CALORIES 63; FAT 3 G (SAT 0.5 G); PROTEIN 2 G; CARB 7 G; FIBER 2 G; SUGARS 0 G (ADDED SUGARS 0 G); SODIUM 99 MG

TIP Use 2½ cups (410 g) of frozen lima beans if you can't find a 15-ounce (425 g) package.

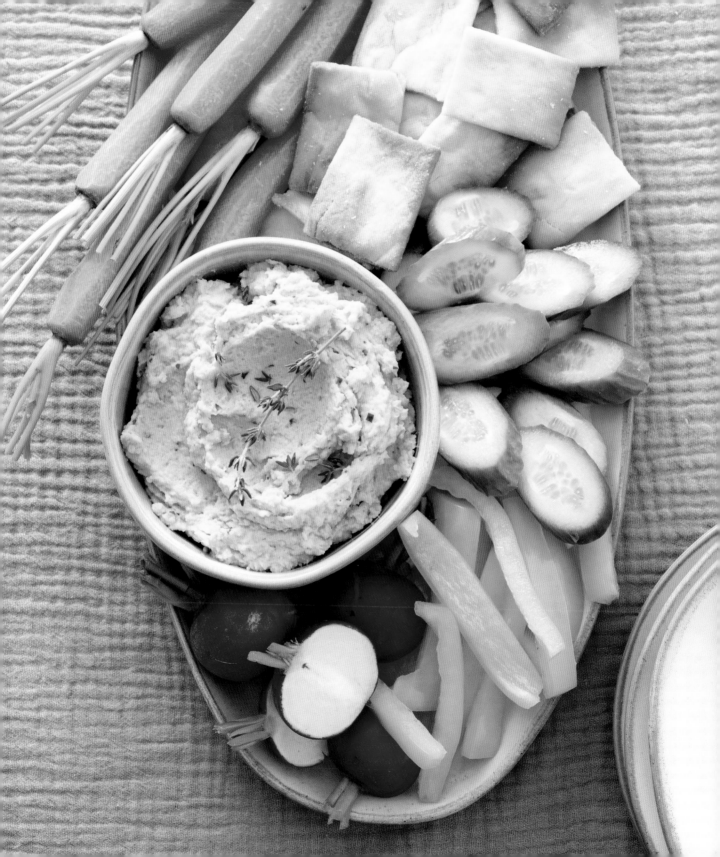

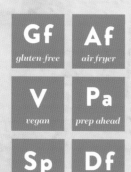

Gf *gluten-free* **Af** *air fryer*

V *vegan* **Pa** *prep ahead*

Sp *sheet pan** **Df** *dairy free*

crispy ranch chickpeas

HANDS-ON: 10 MINUTES :: TOTAL: 30 MINUTES :: SERVES 5

These toasted chickpeas are a tasty, nutritious snack that people of all ages—including kids—will love. I like to make a big batch at the start of the week, so I have a healthy snack option ready to go. Rinsing the chickpeas is a key step because it washes away some of the sodium in the beans.

One 15-ounce (425 g) can unsalted chickpeas, rinsed and drained

1 tablespoon avocado oil

½ teaspoon salt

1½ teaspoons dried dill

1½ teaspoons garlic powder

1 teaspoon onion powder

1 teaspoon dried parsley

Cooking spray

1 Preheat the air fryer to 390°F (199°C).

2 Spread the chickpeas over a layer of clean kitchen or paper towels. Using another towel, gently rub the chickpeas to remove any moisture and remove the thin membrane covering. Place the chickpeas, oil, and ¼ teaspoon salt in a small bowl; toss gently to combine. In a separate small bowl, combine the remaining ¼ teaspoon of salt, dill, garlic powder, onion powder, and parsley; set aside.

3 Spread the chickpeas across the air fryer tray or within the basket. Cook for 18 minutes, shaking the basket every 6 minutes. Remove the tray or basket from the air fryer and lightly coat the chickpeas with cooking spray. Add the dill mixture, tossing to combine. Cook for 4 to 5 minutes, until the chickpeas are golden brown and crispy. Let cool completely before storing in an airtight container for up to 5 days.

NUTRITION FACTS (SERVING SIZE: ¼ CUP/88 G): CALORIES 116; FAT 3 G (SAT 0.5 G); PROTEIN 5 G; CARB 15 G; FIBER 4 G; SUGARS 1 G (ADDED SUGARS 0 G); SODIUM 214 MG

SHEET PAN OPTION Preheat the oven to 325°F (165°C). Follow the directions as written in step 2. Lightly coat a rimmed sheet pan with cooking spray. Spread the chickpeas evenly across the pan. Bake for 40 minutes, shaking the pan to rotate the chickpeas at the 15 and 30-minute marks. Remove from the oven and lightly coat the chickpeas with cooking spray. Add the dill mixture and toss to combine. Bake for 10 minutes, or until the chickpeas are golden brown and crispy. Let cool completely before storing in an airtight container for up to 5 days.

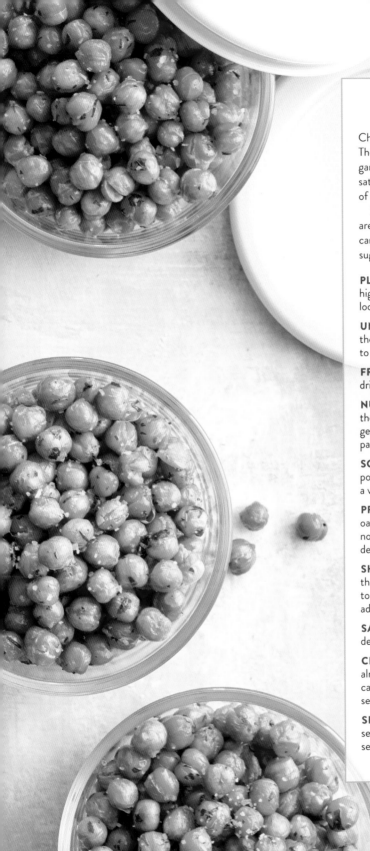

HOW TO PICK A HEALTHY SNACK

Chickpeas are high in protein and fiber (as are other legumes)! These two nutrients are what make chickpeas (also called garbanzo beans) such a great snack for keeping you fueled and satisfied throughout the day. A little healthy fat (in the form of avocado oil here) adds staying power to this snack.

Shopping for healthy snacks (and weeding out which ones are healthy and which ones just look like they're healthy) can feel like a daunting task. Here, I've listed some snack suggestions and snack-picking guidelines to help you out.

PLAIN OR LIGHTLY SALTED POPCORN. This low-cal, high-fiber snack is also a whole grain. Season a plain variety or look for one that's not too sodium heavy.

UNSALTED MIXED NUTS. Nuts are a great snack because they contain protein, fiber, and healthy fat. Look for unsalted to keep your sodium in check.

FREEZE-DRIED FRUIT. Sugar isn't typically added to freeze-dried varieties, but it is often added to dried fruit.

NUT BUTTER PACKS. Easy to find in single-serve containers, these (and their seed butter counterparts) are a great way to get protein, fiber, and healthy fats. Eat them straight up or pair them with fruit or whole-grain crackers.

SOUS-VIDE EGG BITES. Easy to find in stores, these are portion-controlled and high in protein. For a little fiber, select a variety that includes vegetables instead of meat.

PREMADE OVERNIGHT OATS. Usually made with milk and oats, these are even easier than oatmeal cups because there's no prep required. Look for one that's lower in sugar and delivers a few grams of protein.

SHRIMP COCKTAIL. Packed with protein and low in calories, these are great to keep on hand. Eat them plain, add them to a salad, or pair them with freshly sliced veggies (for some added fiber).

SALMON JERKY. This is another high-protein snack that also delivers good-for-you omega-3s.

CHICKEN (OR TUNA) POUCHES. You can find these already seasoned and in single-serve bags alongside the canned versions of these proteins. Pump up your snack by serving the chicken or tuna atop a whole-grain cracker.

SINGLE-SERVE DIPS. In the deli or refrigerated produce section of your grocery store is where you'll usually find single servings of hummus and guacamole, among others.

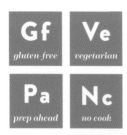

Gf
gluten-free

Ve
vegetarian

Pa
prep ahead

Nc
no cook

Lc
low carb

One 8-ounce (227 g) block firm Greek feta

¾ cup (180 ml) extra virgin olive oil, plus more for drizzling

1 tablespoon lemon zest

1 tablespoon chopped dill

2 teaspoons chopped parsley

½ teaspoon pepper

½ teaspoon red pepper flakes (optional)

1 English cucumber

24 cherry tomatoes

Twenty-four 5-inch (12.5 cm) wooden skewers

marinated feta-veggie skewers

HANDS-ON: 15 MINUTES :: TOTAL: 24 HOURS 45 MINUTES :: MAKES 24 SKEWERS

My favorite thing about this recipe is that the final product looks like you put in much more effort than you really did. Cute toothpicks go a long way, too! When assembling, skewer the feta cube last: It's a nice base for the veggies, and it's less likely to crumble if you don't skewer it all the way through. If you need a dairy-free version, consider using kalamata olives in place of the feta—both add a salty punch. If you don't have fresh herbs on hand, use 1 tablespoon of Greek seasoning instead.

1 Drain the feta and cut into ½-inch (13 mm) cubes.

2 In a medium bowl, combine the oil, lemon zest, dill, parsley, black pepper, and pepper flakes, if desired. Add the feta, stirring to fully coat. If needed, add additional oil to the bowl to cover the top of the cheese cubes. Cover and refrigerate for at least 24 hours.

3 When ready to assemble and serve, remove the bowl from the refrigerator. Let sit for 30 minutes, or until the oil returns to room temperature consistency. Trim the cucumber and cut into ½-inch (13 mm) cubes to yield approximately 1 cup (240 ml), reserving extra cucumber for another use. Add the cucumber and tomatoes to the cheese, stirring gently to fully coat with oil.

4 Drain the feta and vegetables, reserving the oil for another use (see Note). Assemble by placing a tomato and a cucumber cube on each skewer followed by a feta cube. Place on a serving platter or in a shallow serving dish. If desired, drizzle with additional extra virgin olive oil or some of the reserved oil. Cover and refrigerate until ready to serve.

NUTRITION FACTS (SERVING SIZE: 1 SKEWER): CALORIES 84; FAT 8 G (SAT 2 G); PROTEIN 2 G; CARB 1 G; FIBER 0 G; SUGARS 1 G (ADDED SUGARS 0 G); SODIUM 126 MG

NOTE The discarded oil can be used to make a great salad dressing! Refrigerate the oil if not using immediately.

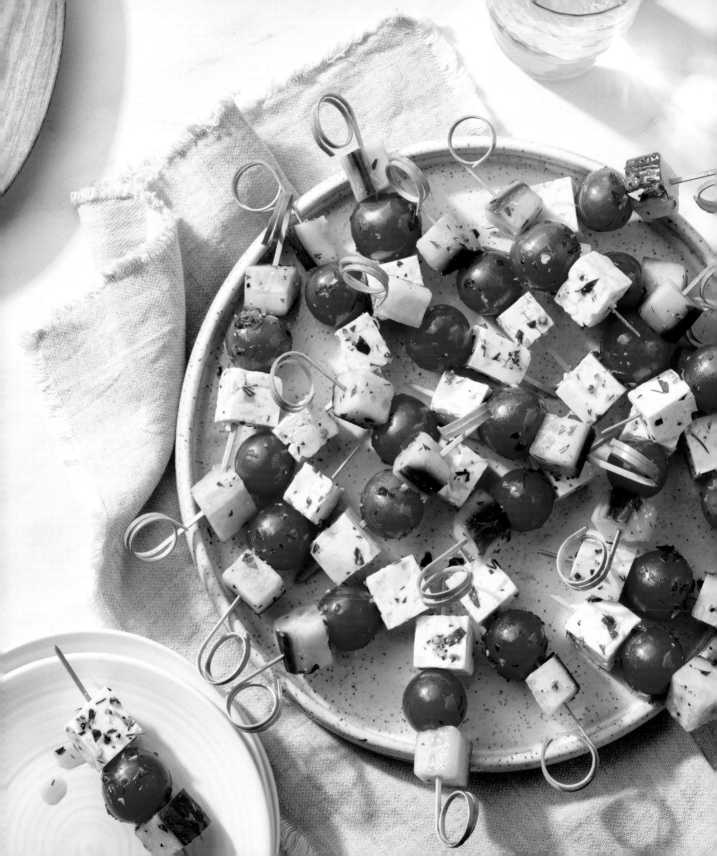

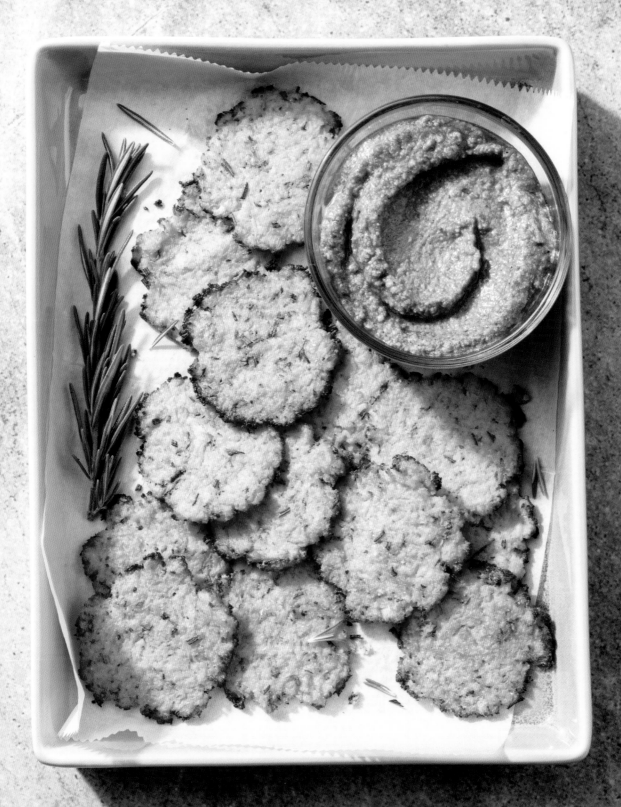

rosemary-parmesan cauliflower crisps

HANDS-ON: 10 MINUTES :: TOTAL: 25 MINUTES :: MAKES 20 CRISPS

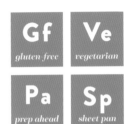

Cheesy and crispy, these low-carb "crackers" are delicious eaten plain! You could also serve them on a tray with a favorite pesto, roasted and sliced red peppers, or even smoked salmon. Or eat them as a crispy topper for soup. This recipe calls for freshly grated Parmesan, and the extra step of doing it yourself is worth it—it holds the crisp together better, and the results are crunchier than with pre-shredded Parmesan.

One 10-ounce (283 g) package frozen riced cauliflower

¾ cup (60 g) freshly grated Parmesan

2 teaspoons fresh chopped rosemary

½ teaspoon garlic powder

Pinch of salt

1 Preheat the oven to 425°F (215°C). Line a baking sheet with parchment paper.

2 Cook the cauliflower in the microwave according to package directions. Place on a clean kitchen or paper towel and squeeze to remove excess moisture.

3 Combine the cauliflower, Parmesan, rosemary, garlic powder, and salt in the bowl of a food processor. Cover and process by pulsing for 30 to 60 seconds, until the mixture has a smooth, doughlike consistency.

4 Scoop the cauliflower mixture by tablespoons and place 1-inch (2.5 cm) apart evenly across the baking sheet. Flatten each with the bottom of a glass or the back of a fork to a 1-inch (13 mm) thickness.

5 Bake for 15 to 20 minutes, until golden brown. Cool on the baking sheet for 5 minutes. Use a spatula to gently transfer the crisps to a cooling rack. Let cool completely before storing in an airtight container for 2 days.

NUTRITION FACTS (SERVING SIZE: 2 CRISPS): CALORIES 35; FAT 2 G (SAT 1 G); PROTEIN 2 G; CARB 2 G; FIBER 1 G; SUGARS 1 G (ADDED SUGARS 0 G); SODIUM 181 MG

NOTE These crisps are best when eaten immediately, so if prepared in advance, I recommend popping them in the oven to reheat them quickly. To do this, preheat the oven to 425°F (215°C), place the crisps on a baking sheet, and bake for 2 to 3 minutes, until hot.

Gf *gluten-free* :: Ve *vegetarian*

V *vegan** :: Nc *no cook*

½ cup (75 g) frozen strawberries

½ cup (83 g) frozen mango pieces

1 cup (16 g) trimmed kale

⅓ cup (80 ml) vanilla low-fat Greek yogurt

¾ cup (180 ml) unsweetened vanilla almond milk

Protein powder, flaxseed, chia seed, walnuts (optional)

strawberry-mango green smoothie

HANDS-ON: 3 MINUTES :: TOTAL: 5 MINUTES :: SERVES 1 :: MAKES APPROX. 1¾ CUPS (420 ML)

You've heard the phrase "don't judge a book by its cover." It applies here: The tangy, fruity, refreshing flavor of this creamy smoothie more than makes up for its muted green color. If you prefer a sweeter smoothie, add half of a frozen banana or a scoop of vanilla protein powder to dial back the tanginess.

Place all of the ingredients in a blender. Cover and blend until smooth. Serve immediately.

NUTRITION FACTS (SERVING SIZE: 1 SMOOTHIE): CALORIES 197; FAT 5 G (SAT 1 G); PROTEIN 10 G; CARB 30 G; FIBER 4 G; SUGARS 23 G (ADDED SUGARS 2 G); SODIUM 182 MG

DAIRY-FREE/VEGAN OPTION Substitute an equivalent amount of any vanilla plant-based yogurt in place of the Greek yogurt.

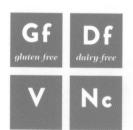

Gf *gluten-free* :: Df *dairy-free*

V :: Nc *no cook*

1 ripe banana, sliced and frozen

½ cup (120 ml) cold brew coffee

½ cup (120 ml) unsweetened nondairy milk

¼ cup (20 g) rolled oats

1 tablespoon chopped pecans

1 tablespoon chocolate-flavored plant-based protein powder

cold brew breakfast smoothie

HANDS-ON: 3 MINUTES :: TOTAL: 5 MINUTES :: SERVES 1 :: MAKES ABOUT 1¾ CUPS (420 ML)

Oats plus pecans plus protein powder make this an ultra-filling smoothie. It's a great on-the-go, drinkable breakfast that also caffeinates you so you can skip your usual coffee run. Nutrition-wise, this smoothie wins awards, too: It delivers 30 percent of your daily protein value and a quarter of your daily fiber goal.

Place all of the ingredients in a blender. Cover and blend until smooth. Serve immediately.

NUTRITION FACTS (SERVING SIZE: 1 SMOOTHIE): CALORIES 306; FAT 9 G (SAT 1 G); PROTEIN 15 G; CARB 46 G; FIBER 7 G; SUGARS 16 G (ADDED SUGARS 0 G); SODIUM 169 MG

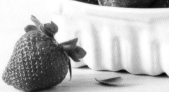

peanut butter–banana smoothie

HANDS-ON: 3 MINUTES :: TOTAL: 5 MINUTES :: SERVES 2 :: MAKES APPROX. 1 ½ CUPS (360 ML)

This creamy, thick, peanut buttery smoothie tastes more like a milkshake than a nondairy smoothie. You can easily turn it into ice cream by cutting back on the almond milk—use a ½ cup (120 ml) instead of ¾ cup (180 ml). To keep added sugars in check, look for unsweetened almond milk. Some almond milks labeled as "original" may have sugar added, so check the ingredient list.

1 large ripe banana, sliced and frozen

¾ cup (180 ml) unsweetened almond milk

3 tablespoons (48 g) creamy peanut butter

Protein powder, flaxseed, chia seed, walnuts (optional)

Place all of the ingredients in a blender. Cover and blend until smooth. Serve immediately.

NUTRITION FACTS (SERVING SIZE: ¾ CUP/180 ML): CALORIES 217; FAT 13 G (SAT 2.5 G); PROTEIN 7 G; CARB 21 G; FIBER 3 G; SUGARS 11 G (ADDED SUGARS 1 G); SODIUM 171 MG

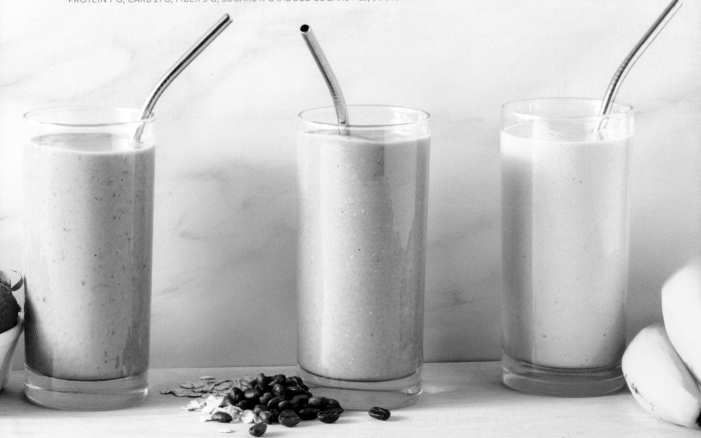

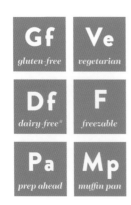

Gf *gluten-free* **Ve** *vegetarian*

Df *dairy-free** **F** *freezable*

Pa *prep ahead* **Mp** *muffin pan*

1¾ cups (210 g) all-purpose gluten-free flour

⅓ cup (60 g) granulated sugar

⅓ cup (66 g) packed brown sugar

3 teaspoons pumpkin pie spice

1 teaspoon baking soda

½ teaspoon salt

2 eggs

One 15-ounce (425g) can pumpkin puree

¼ cup (120 ml) avocado oil

1 teaspoon vanilla extract

½ cup (120 g) dark chocolate chips

pumpkin chocolate chip mini-muffins

HANDS-ON: 15 MINUTES :: TOTAL: 45 MINUTES :: MAKES 45 MUFFINS

When my kids were little, they loved a pumpkin muffin recipe that called for three things: a can of pumpkin puree, a box of spice cake mix, and water. While I loved the recipe's simplicity, I wasn't crazy about the sugar, additives, and gluten in the mix, so I created this homemade alternative. We tend to eat muffins as a snack, so I added dark chocolate chips, which complement the flavors in the pumpkin and spice blend. Make sure you purchase canned pumpkin puree and not pumpkin pie filling to avoid additional added sugars.

1 Preheat the oven to 350°F (180°C). Line a mini-muffin pan with paper liners or lightly coat with cooking spray; set aside.

2 Whisk together the flour, sugars, pumpkin pie spice, baking soda, and salt and in a large bowl. Add the eggs, pumpkin puree, oil, and vanilla, mixing until blended. Gently fold in the chocolate chips. Spoon 1 heaping tablespoon of the batter into the muffin cups so that they are approximately ¾ of the way full.

3 Bake for 12 to 15 minutes, until a toothpick inserted into the center of a muffin comes out clean. Cool completely before serving. Store in an airtight container at room temperature or in the refrigerator for up to 4 days. Store in an airtight container in the freezer for up to one month. Allow muffins to thaw at room temperature or warm in the microwave for 10 to 15 seconds.

NUTRITION FACTS (SERVING SIZE: 3 MINI-MUFFINS): CALORIES 163; FAT 7 G (SAT 2.3 G); PROTEIN 1 G; CARB 26 G; FIBER 2 G; SUGARS 12 G (ADDED SUGARS 11 G); SODIUM 155 MG

TIP You can make your own pumpkin pie spice by combining a few spices you already have on hand. Combine 1¼ teaspoon ground cinnamon, ½ teaspoon ground ginger, and ¼ teaspoon each of allspice, ground cloves, and ground nutmeg. Use in place of the pumpkin pie spice.

DAIRY-FREE OPTION Use ⅔ cup (107 g) vegan dark chocolate baking morsels in place of the chocolate chips.

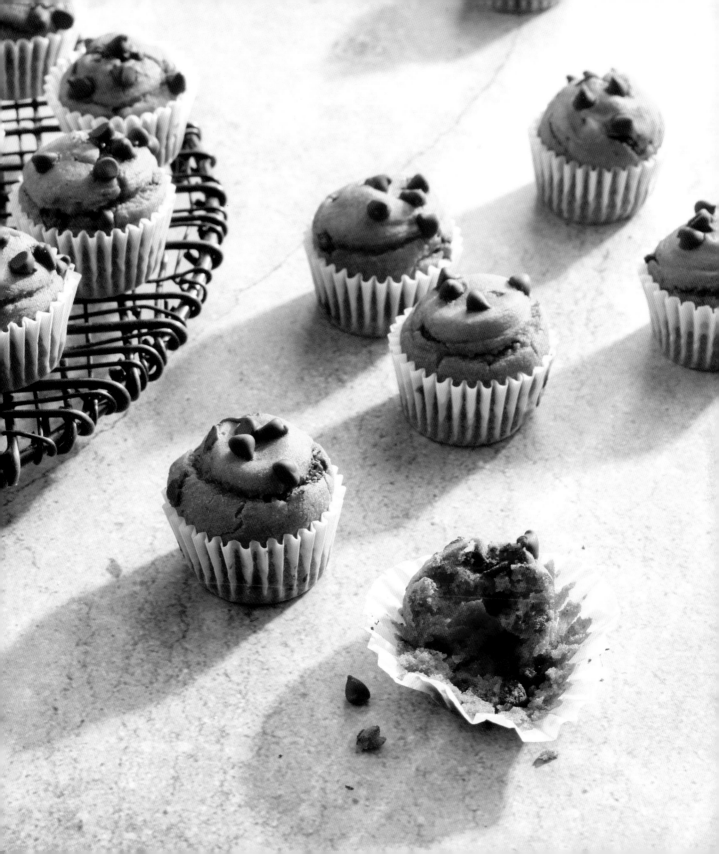

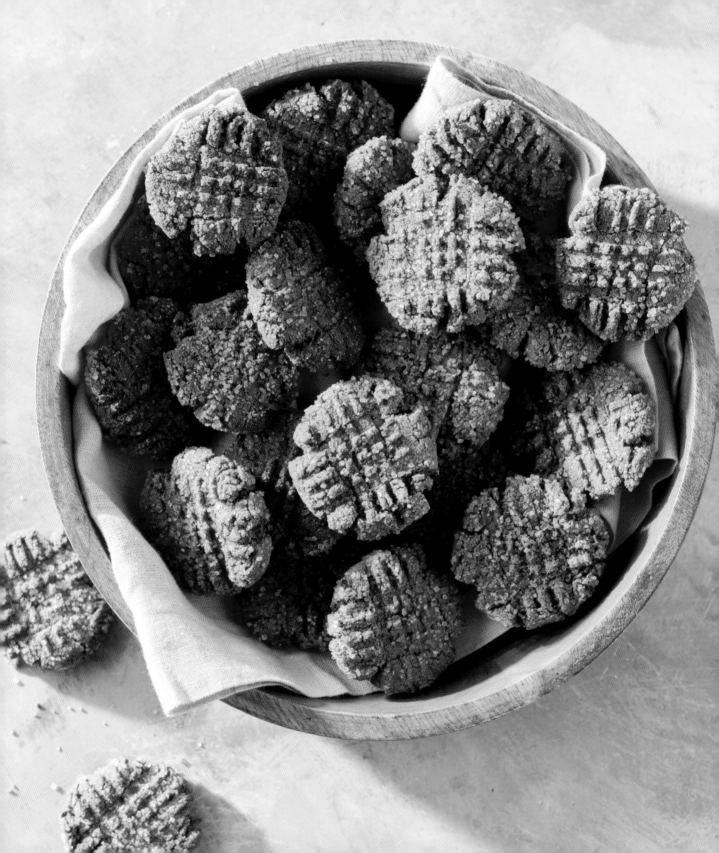

lemony ginger cookies

HANDS-ON: 10 MINUTES :: TOTAL: 20 MINUTES :: MAKES 15 COOKIES

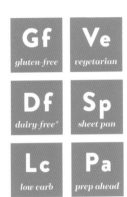

These cookies are soft, chewy, and full of sweet lemony ginger flavor. It took testing several batches with different amounts of gluten-free flours until we found a winning combination, and I'm betting you won't be able to tell they're gluten-free.

1 Preheat the oven to 350°F (180°C).

2 Whisk together the butter, sugar, molasses, egg, lemon zest, and vanilla in a large bowl. Stir in the flours, baking soda, spices, and salt until combined.

3 Scoop about 1 tablespoon of dough, roll into a ball, and lightly roll in sugar, if desired. Place on a baking sheet. Repeat with the remaining dough to form about 15 cookies. Use a fork to flatten each slightly in a cross-like shape. Sprinkle the tops lightly with the turbinado sugar, if desired.

4 Bake for 8 to 10 minutes, until the cookies are beginning to turn golden brown on the edges. Let the cookies cool on the sheet pan for 10 minutes before transferring to a wire rack. Let cool completely before storing in an airtight container for up to 3 days.

NUTRITION FACTS (SERVING SIZE: 1 COOKIE): CALORIES 101; FAT 7 G (SAT 2.5 G); PROTEIN 2 G; CARB 8 G; FIBER 2 G; SUGARS 6 G (ADDED SUGARS 6 G); SODIUM 107 MG

DAIRY-FREE OPTION Substitute ¼ cup (60 ml) of avocado oil for the butter and lightly spray the baking sheet with cooking spray to prevent sticking.

4 tablespoons butter, melted and cooled

¼ cup (55 g) brown sugar

2 tablespoons molasses

1 egg, room temperature

2 teaspoons lemon zest

1 teaspoon vanilla extract

1 cup (96 g) almond flour

¼ cup (28 g) coconut flour

½ teaspoon baking soda

¾ teaspoon ground ginger

½ teaspoon ground cinnamon

½ teaspoon allspice

½ teaspoon ground nutmeg

¼ teaspoon salt

Turbinado sugar (optional)

Gf *gluten-free*

Ve *vegetarian*

Df *dairy-free**

Sp *sheet pan*

Pa *prep ahead*

chocolate chip almond butter cookies

HANDS-ON: 12 MINUTES :: TOTAL: 21 MINUTES :: SERVES 20

I'm always skeptical about messing with a classic, but this flourless chocolate chip cookie might be better than the original. Almond butter, which takes the place of butter, is the secret ingredient that adds protein and keeps saturated fat levels down.

1 cup (240 ml) almond butter

½ cup plus 1 tablespoon (124 g) brown sugar

2 large eggs

1 tablespoon vanilla extract

1 cup (80 g) gluten-free old fashioned rolled oats

1 teaspoon baking soda

½ teaspoon salt

⅔ cup (112 g) semisweet chocolate chips

1 Preheat the oven to 350°F (180°C).

2 Combine the almond butter, sugar, eggs, and vanilla in a large bowl and beat with a hand mixer until smooth.

3 In a small bowl, combine the oats, baking soda, and salt. Add the oat mixture to the almond butter mixture, stirring to combine. Gently fold in the chocolate chips.

4 Scoop the dough by 1½ tablespoons, evenly placing the dough across two baking sheets. Bake for 9 minutes, until set in the middle. Let cool on the baking sheet for 10 minutes. Transfer to a wire rack to cool completely.

NUTRITION FACTS (SERVING SIZE: 1 COOKIE): CALORIES 150; FAT 10 G (SAT 2 G); PROTEIN 4 G; CARB 15 G; FIBER 2 G; SUGARS 10 G (ADDED SUGARS 9 G); SODIUM 150 MG

DAIRY-FREE OPTION Use ⅔ cup (149 g) vegan dark chocolate baking morsels in place of the chocolate chips.

TIP The taste testers in my house were partial to the almond butter, but peanut butter can be used instead, if desired.

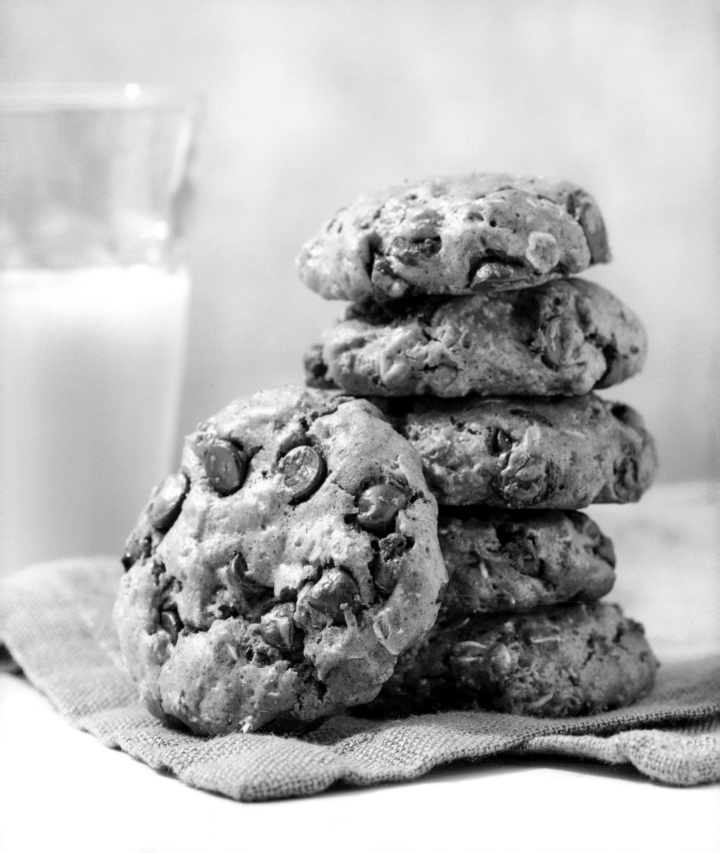

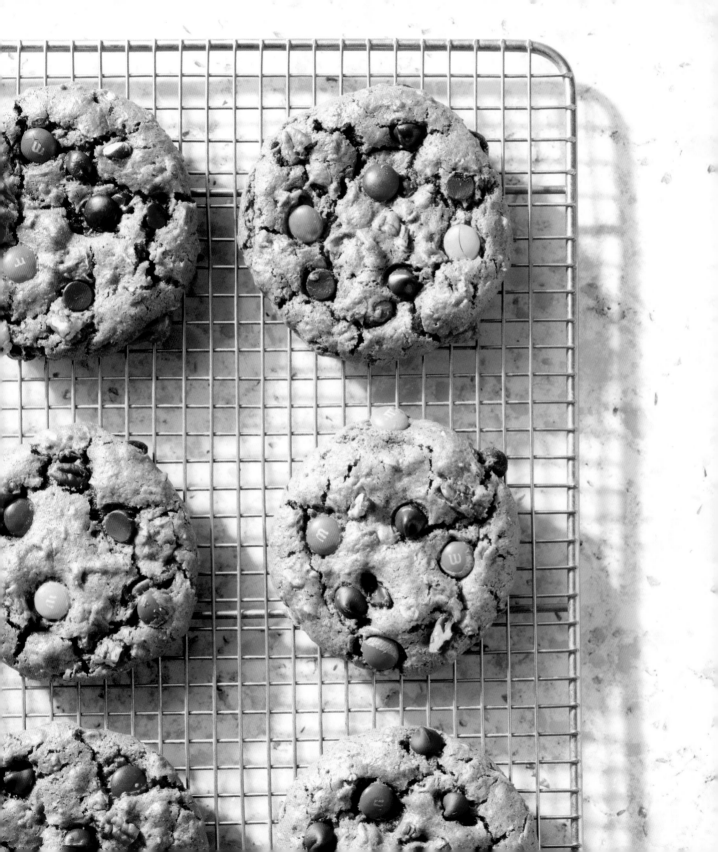

flourless monster cookies

HANDS-ON: 10 MINUTES :: TOTAL: 25 MINUTES :: MAKES 14 COOKIES

More than your average cookie in both size and flavor, these Monster Cookies use chocolate chips and chocolate candies, which adds sweetness and texture. They're crisp on the edges and chewy on the inside.

1 Preheat the oven to 350°F (180°C). Line a large baking sheet with parchment paper.

2 Stir together the almond butter, sugar, eggs, vanilla, baking soda, cinnamon, nutmeg, and salt in a large bowl. Add the oats, stirring until well combined. Fold in the chocolate chips, candies, and pecans.

3 Use a cookie scoop or measuring spoon to scoop 2½ tablespoons of dough into rounded balls and place on the baking sheet, leaving a 1-inch (2.5 cm) space in between for the cookies to spread.

4 Bake for 8 to 11 minutes, until the edges are starting to turn golden brown. Let cool on the baking sheet for 10 minutes, then transfer to a wire rack to cool completely. Store in an airtight container for up to 3 days.

NUTRITION FACTS (SERVING SIZE: 1 COOKIE): CALORIES 204; FAT 13 G (SAT 2.5 G); PROTEIN 5 G; CARB 20 G; FIBER 3 G; SUGARS 14 G (ADDED SUGARS 11 G); SODIUM 83 MG

DAIRY-FREE OPTION Use ¼ cup (52 g) vegan, milklike chocolate candies in place of the chocolate candies and ¼ cup (56 g) vegan dark chocolate baking morsels in place of the chocolate chips.

1 cup (240 ml) natural almond butter

⅔ cup (147 g) packed brown sugar

2 eggs

1 teaspoon vanilla extract

½ teaspoon baking soda

¼ teaspoon ground cinnamon

¼ teaspoon ground nutmeg

¼ teaspoon salt

1 cup (80 g) gluten-free old fashioned rolled oats

¼ cup (60 g) dark chocolate chips

¼ cup (52 g) chocolate candies (such as M&Ms)

¼ cup (27 g) chopped pecans

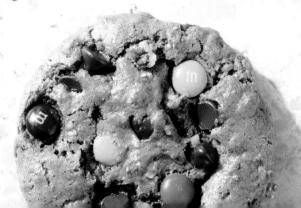

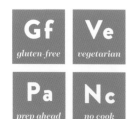

Gf
gluten-free

Ve
vegetarian

Pa
prep ahead

Nc
no cook

Mp
muffin pan

1½ cups (360 g) dark chocolate chips

½ cup (128 g) creamy peanut butter

½ teaspoon flaky sea salt

dark chocolate peanut butter cups

HANDS-ON: 15 MINUTES :: TOTAL: 1 HOUR 15 MINUTES :: MAKES 12 CUPS

One of my all-time favorite combos is the salty-sweet mix of chocolate and peanut butter found in peanut butter cups. But I wanted one made with high-quality chocolate and fewer added sugars, so I created this quick homemade version. Now, I prefer these over store-bought versions. For the most anti-inflammatory-friendly version, look for a creamy peanut butter without any added sugars or salt.

1 Line a muffin pan with 12 liners.

2 Place the chocolate chips in a microwave-safe bowl. Microwave for 1 minute, stopping to stir every 15 seconds, until melted and smooth.

3 Spoon 1 tablespoon of the melted chocolate into the bottom of each muffin liner. Place the pan in the freezer for 5 minutes, or until the chocolate is slightly hardened.

4 Place the peanut butter in a small microwave-safe bowl. Microwave for 15 to 20 seconds until the texture has loosened and is easier to stir. Spoon 2 teaspoons of peanut butter on top of the chocolate in each cup.

5 Reheat the remaining chocolate for 15 seconds if needed. Spoon over the peanut butter, dividing the chocolate evenly among the 12 cups. Smooth the tops with the back of a spoon and sprinkle with flaky sea salt. Refrigerate for at least 1 hour, or until the chocolate has hardened and is firm enough to remove from the liner.

NUTRITION FACTS (SERVING SIZE: 1 CUP): CALORIES 200; FAT 17 G (SAT 8 G); PROTEIN 4 G; CARB 18 G; FIBER 5 G; SUGARS 11 G (ADDED SUGARS 10 G); SODIUM 95 MG

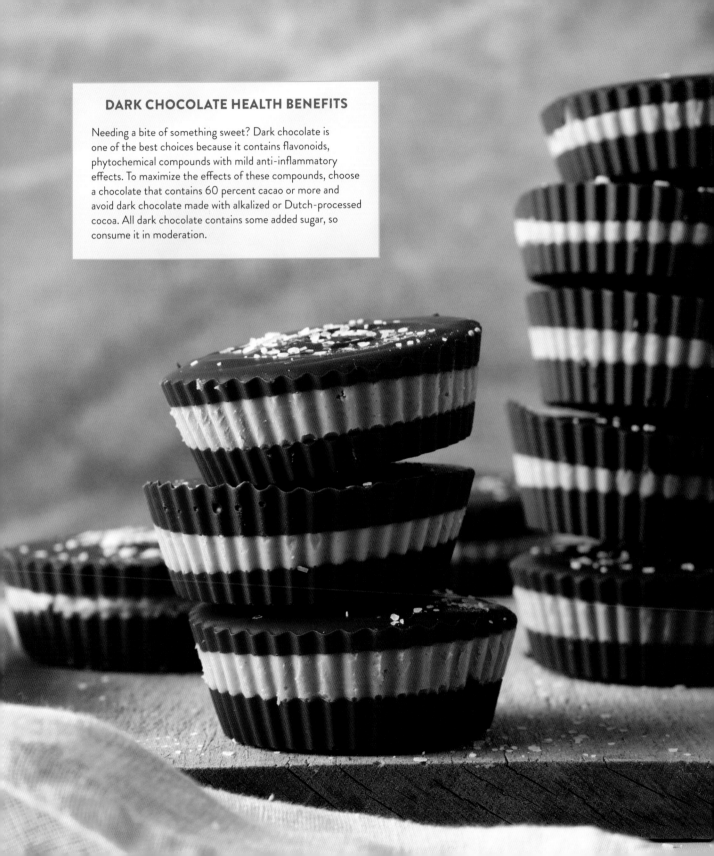

DARK CHOCOLATE HEALTH BENEFITS

Needing a bite of something sweet? Dark chocolate is one of the best choices because it contains flavonoids, phytochemical compounds with mild anti-inflammatory effects. To maximize the effects of these compounds, choose a chocolate that contains 60 percent cacao or more and avoid dark chocolate made with alkalized or Dutch-processed cocoa. All dark chocolate contains some added sugar, so consume it in moderation.

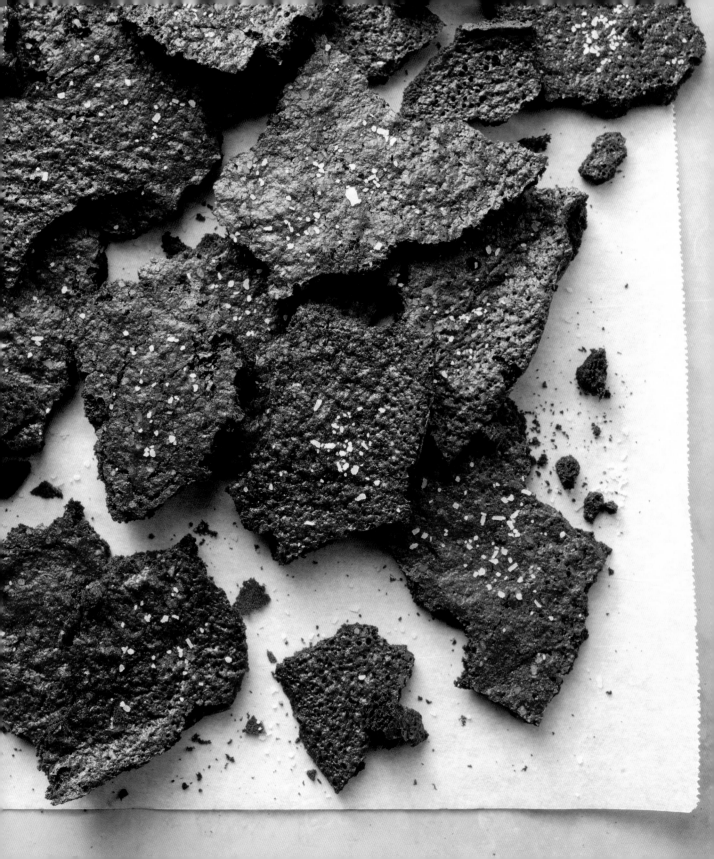

gluten-free brownie brittle

HANDS-ON: 10 MINUTES :: TOTAL: 40 MINUTES :: SERVES 24

These thin brownie pieces are crispy but still have a little chewiness. They're a perfect way to get a quick chocolatey brownie fix.

1 Preheat the oven to 300°F (150°C). Line two 9 x 13-inch (23 x 33 cm) sheet pans with parchment paper.

2 Combine the brownie mix, butter, egg whites, and ½ cup (120 ml) water in a large bowl. Beat with a hand mixer until well combined. Spoon or pour the batter into the center of the baking sheets, evenly dividing the batter between the two. Use a spatula to spread the batter to the edges. Sprinkle with sea salt.

3 Bake for 35 minutes, until the edges are beginning to crisp and the center appears set. Let cool completely before breaking into pieces. Store in an airtight container for up to 1 week.

NUTRITION FACTS (SERVING SIZE: 1/24 OF BRITTLE/29 G): CALORIES 120; FAT 4 G (SAT 2 G); PROTEIN 1 G; CARB 20 G; FIBER 1 G; SUGARS 13 G (ADDED SUGARS 12 G); SODIUM 149 MG

DAIRY-FREE OPTION Use a brownie mix that is gluten-free and dairy-free or provides directions for making a dairy-free version. Use ¼ cup (60 ml) avocado oil in place of the melted butter.

One 20-ounce (566 g) box gluten-free double chocolate brownie mix

4 tablespoons butter, melted and cooled

2 egg whites, room temperature

¾ teaspoon flaky sea salt

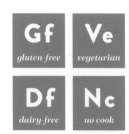

Gf
gluten-free

Ve
vegetarian

Df
dairy-free

Nc
no cook

Pa
prep ahead

no-churn strawberry-lemon sorbet

HANDS-ON: 15 MINUTES :: TOTAL: 6 HOURS 15 MINUTES :: SERVES 7

Ripe, sweet strawberries and fresh lemon juice create the perfect balance of sweet and tart. The addition of vodka may seem odd, but just a tablespoon prevents big ice crystals from forming, giving this sorbet a slightly softer texture that's easier to scoop.

4 cups (576 g) hulled strawberries

⅓ cup (80 ml) honey

¼ cup (60 ml) lemon juice

1 tablespoon vodka

2 teaspoons lemon zest

1 Combine the strawberries, honey, lemon juice, vodka, and lemon zest in the bowl of a food processor or heavy-duty blender. Puree until smooth, 1 minute.

2 Pour the strawberry puree into a large storage container. Add a layer of plastic wrap flush against the surface of the puree, then secure the lid. Freeze until firm, 6 hours.

NUTRITION FACTS (SERVING SIZE: ½ CUP/110 G): CALORIES 82; FAT 0 G (SAT 0 G); PROTEIN 1 G; CARB 20 G; FIBER 2 G; SUGARS 17 G (ADDED SUGARS 13 G); SODIUM 3 MG

TIP Frozen strawberries can be used instead of fresh. Thaw for 30 minutes at room temperature to soften before pureeing. Taste the mixture at the end of step 1 and adjust the sweetness with an additional tablespoon or two of honey as needed.

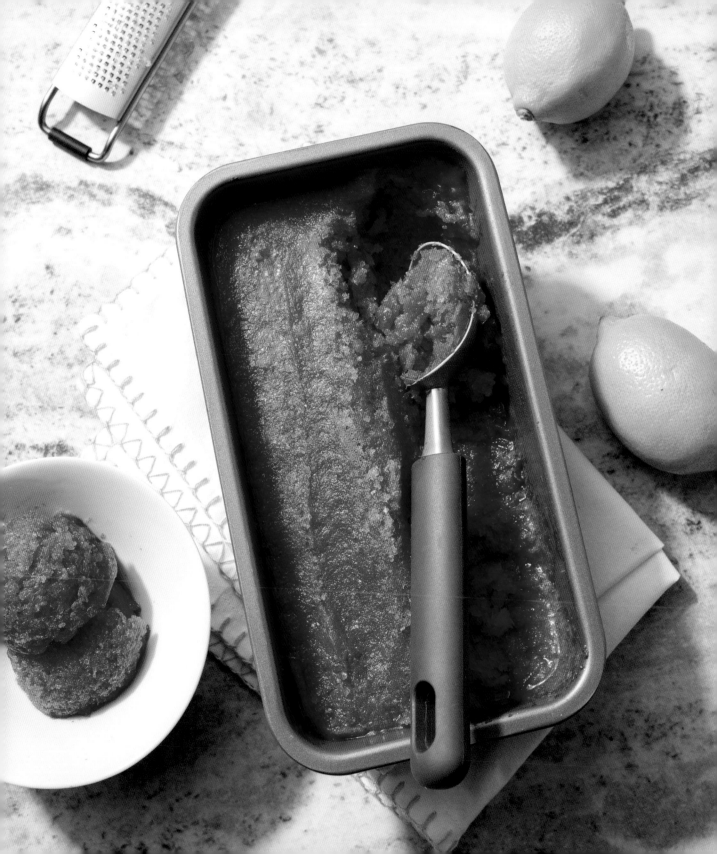

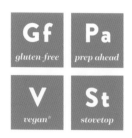

Gf gluten-free

Pa prep ahead

V vegan*

St stovetop

1¾ cups (420 ml) extra-creamy plain oat milk

½ cup (120 ml) maple syrup

2 tablespoons cocoa powder

2 tablespoons cornstarch

1 teaspoon vanilla extract

⅛ teaspoon salt

¼ cup (60 g) dark chocolate chips (optional)

1 tablespoon coconut oil (optional)

dairy-free fudgesicles

HANDS-ON: 15 MINUTES :: TOTAL: 24 HOURS AND 15 MINUTES :: MAKES 6 POPSICLES

Fair warning that if you make these fudgesicles you will get asked, "Are you sure these are really dairy-free?" because of their creamy decadence. The key is purchasing a creamy oat milk. I recommend comparing brands and choosing the one with the highest fat per serving. For an even creamier pop, use canned coconut milk instead. The chocolate drizzle makes the popsicles a showstopper, but they taste just as good without it.

1 Combine the milk, maple syrup, cocoa powder, and cornstarch in a small saucepan over medium heat, whisking constantly. Cook until the mixture is the consistency of very thin pudding, stirring frequently, 10 minutes.

2 Remove from the heat and stir in the vanilla and salt. Set the mixture in the fridge until cooled completely, about 1 hour. Pour into popsicle molds. Freeze overnight until solid.

3 To add the optional drizzle, place the chocolate chips and coconut oil in a small microwave-safe bowl. Cook on high in 15-second increments, stirring between each, until melted and smooth.

4 Line a large baking pan or small baking sheet with parchment or wax paper. Remove one popsicle from the mold and drizzle the melted chocolate over one side. Lay the popsicle on the pan, drizzle-side up, and place in the freezer. Repeat with the remaining popsicles.

NUTRITION FACTS (SERVING SIZE: 1 POPSICLE): CALORIES 155; FAT 5.5 G (SAT 0.5 G); PROTEIN 2 G; CARB 28 G; FIBER 1 G; SUGARS 20 G (ADDED SUGARS 16 G); SODIUM 62 MG

DAIRY-FREE/VEGAN OPTION Use vegan dark chocolate chips for the drizzle and decrease the coconut oil to 2 teaspoons. Then, follow the directions as written in step 3.

TIP Popsicle molds vary in their size and fluid ounce capacity. This recipe is designed for molds that hold approximately 3 fluid ounces (90 ml), but any size mold will work. This fudgesicle mixture makes approximately 2¼ cups (540 ml), so first find the capacity for each mold on the packaging. Then, divide among your molds. Liquids expand when freezing, so don't fill the molds completely to the top. I recommend filling ⅛ to ¼ inch (3.25 to 6.5 mm) below the rim.

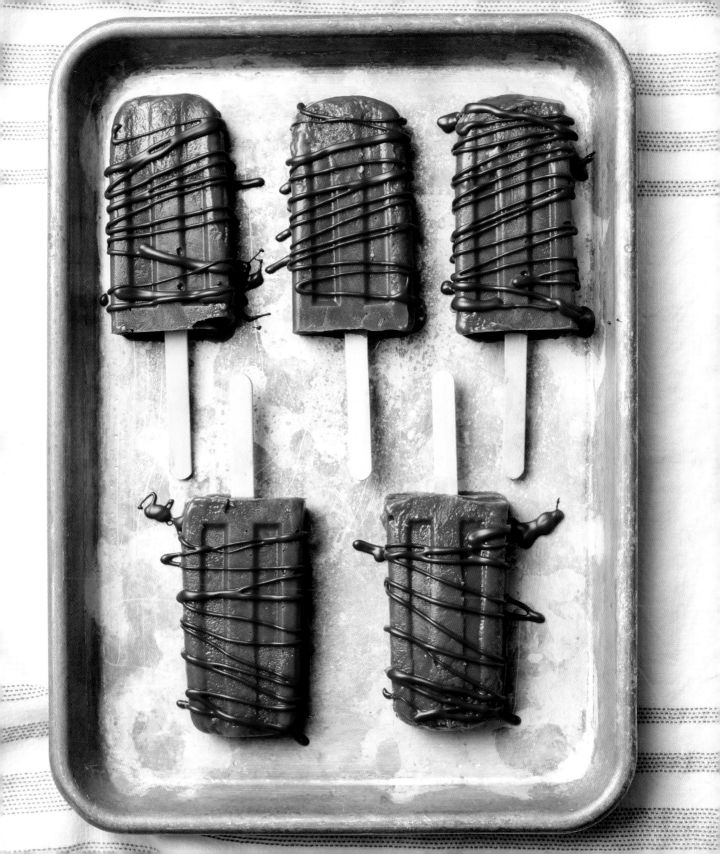

Gf *gluten-free*

Lc *low carb*

V *vegan*

Nc *no cook*

Df *dairy-free*

pomegranate-lime mocktail

HANDS-ON: 2 MINUTES :: TOTAL: 2 MINUTES :: SERVES 1

Periodically, I take breaks from consuming alcohol (for example, dry January). Every time I do, I realize that I don't miss the alcohol, but rather the ritual of having a glass of wine or cocktail to mark the end of the day and a time to decompress. I created this quick mocktail to sip on so I could keep my end-of-day routine without the alcohol.

3 tablespoons pomegranate juice

1 tablespoon sweetened lime juice

½ cup (120 ml) flavored fizzy water or light tonic water

Lime wedge (optional)

Pour the pomegranate and lime juices over ice in a glass. Top with fizzy water; stir well to combine. Serve with a lime wedge, if desired.

NUTRITION FACTS (SERVING SIZE: 1 DRINK): CALORIES 38; FAT 0 G (SAT 0 G); PROTEIN 0 G; CARB 10 G; FIBER 0 G; SUGARS 6 G (ADDED SUGARS 2 G); SODIUM 0 MG

ALCOHOL VARIATION Pour the juices and vodka over ice in a glass. Top with ⅓ cup (80 ml) light tonic-soda mixer; stir well.

NUTRITION FACTS (SERVING SIZE 1 DRINK): CALORIES 145; FAT 0 G (SAT 0 G); PROTEIN 0 G; CARB 13 G; FIBER 0 G; SUGARS 11 G (ADDED SUGARS 5 G); SODIUM 20 MG

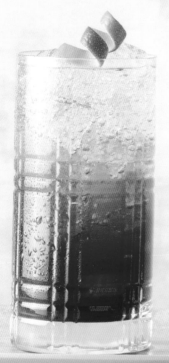 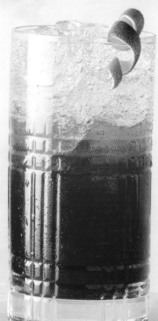

elderflower margarita

HANDS-ON: 2 MINUTES :: TOTAL: 2 MINUTES :: SERVES 1

St. Germain is a sweet French liqueur made from the small white blossoms of the elderberry bush. The liqueur's sweetness balances the tequila and lime juice just enough so that another sweetener (or sugar-laden mixer) isn't needed. It also lends a fresh floral edge to this classic drink.

Combine the lime juice, tequila, and St. Germain in a cocktail shaker. Shake well. Pour over ice in a salt-rimmed glass, and top with fizzy water, if desired. Serve with a lime wedge.

NUTRITION FACTS (SERVING SIZE: 1 DRINK): CALORIES 173; FAT 0 G (SAT 0 G); PROTEIN 0 G; CARB 9 G; FIBER 0 G; SUGARS 6 G (ADDED SUGARS 4 G); SODIUM 1 MG

TIP This cocktail can be made with or without fizzy sparkling water, but I prefer to add it because I sometimes find myself sipping quickly while socializing. Adding a little extra water creates a larger drink that slows your overall alcohol consumption.

3 tablespoons fresh lime juice

1½ ounces (45 ml) tequila

½ ounce (15 ml) St. Germain or other elderflower liqueur

Fizzy sparkling water (optional)

Lime wedge

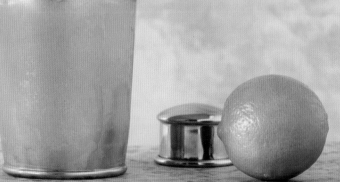

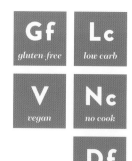

Gf *gluten-free* Lc *low carb*

V *vegan* Nc *no cook*

Df *dairy-free*

greyhound spritzer

HANDS-ON: 2 MINUTES :: TOTAL: 2 MINUTES :: SERVES 1

Using freshly squeezed grapefruit juice is a simple way to elevate this cocktail from run-of-the-mill to refreshingly delicious. It also means you don't have to use canned or bottled juices, which can be a sneaky source of added sugars. Seeking out a light tonic-soda mixer is another way I keep this cocktail low in sugar.

¼ cup (60 ml) freshly squeezed pink grapefruit juice

1½ ounces (45 ml) vodka

½ cup (120 ml) light tonic-soda mixer

Grapefruit or lime wedge (optional)

Pour the grapefruit juice and vodka over ice in a glass. Top with the mixer; stir well to combine. Serve with grapefruit or lime wedge, if desired.

NUTRITION FACTS (SERVING SIZE: 1 DRINK): CALORIES 136; FAT 0 G (SAT 0 G); PROTEIN 0 G; CARB 10 G; FIBER 0 G; SUGARS 8 G (ADDED SUGARS 4 G); SODIUM 21 MG

TIP I've kept the juice to ¼ cup (60 ml) and added a low-sugar soda-tonic mixer to keep calories and carbs low. Feel free to adjust these amounts if you want more grapefruit flavor or sweetness.

ANTI-INFLAMMATORY BENEFITS AND RISKS OF ALCOHOL

An anti-inflammatory lifestyle doesn't mean you need to give up an occasional cocktail or glass of wine. In fact, research suggests that consuming moderate alcohol amounts elicits a slight anti-inflammatory effect that may potentially reduce heart disease risk and ease inflammatory joint issues. But there's a catch: Alcoholic drinks need to be kept to around one to two a day. Exceeding this negates the beneficial effects because the alcohol also starts to turn inflammatory.

Here are the key things to know if you choose to incorporate alcohol into your anti-inflammatory lifestyle. These recommendations are for those who already choose to consume alcohol; potential health benefits are not great enough to suggest that anyone should start consuming alcohol if they currently choose not to drink.

- Consume alcohol in moderation: no more than 1 drink per day for women and no more than 2 drinks per day for men.
- Choose an alcoholic beverage that doesn't contain excessive calories. If you choose liquor, minimize added sugars (and calories) by combining with a low- or no-calorie mixer.
- Choose wine, liquor, or beer, as no one type appears to offer significantly greater benefits over another.
- Gluten-free individuals should avoid beer since most all types are brewed using gluten-containing grains like wheat, rye, or barley.

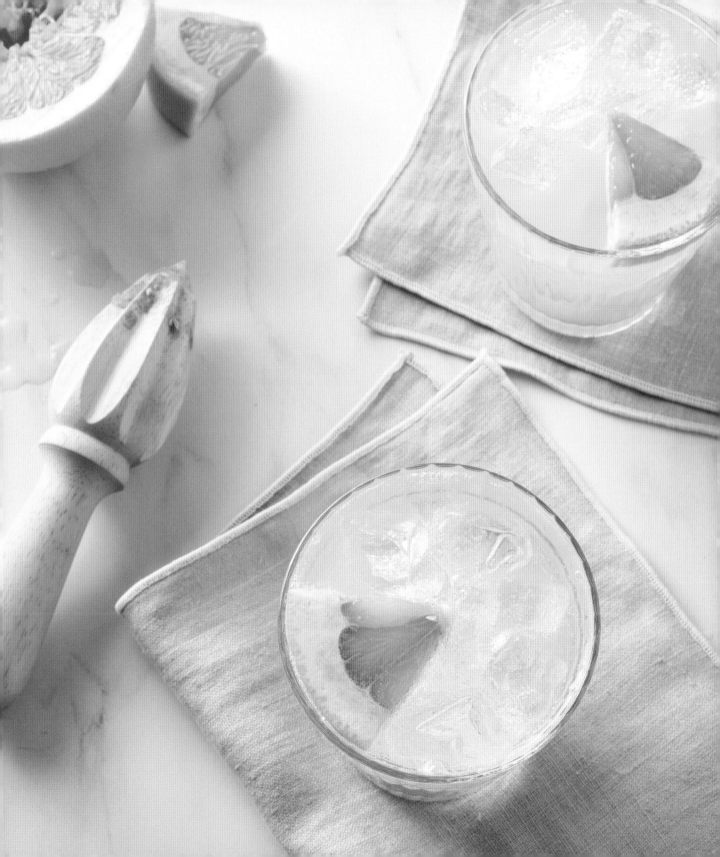

references

Adan, R. H., et al., "Nutritional Psychiatry: Towards Improving Mental Health by What You Eat," *European Neuropsychopharmacology: The Journal of the European College of Neuropsychopharmacology* 29, no. 12 (2019): 1321–32.

Arnett, D., et al., "2019 ACC/AHA Guideline on the Primary Prevention of Cardiovascular Disease: A Report of the American College of Cardiology/American Heart Association Task Force on Clinical Practice Guidelines," *Circulation* 140, no. 11 (2019): e596–646.

Atkinson, F., et al., "International Tables of Glycemic Index and Glycemic Load Values 2021: A Systematic Review," *The American Journal of Clinical Nutrition* (2021).

Babizhayev, M. A., et al., "Management of the Virulent Influenza Virus Infection by Oral Formulation of Nonhydrolized Carnosine and Isopeptide of Carnosine Attenuating Proinflammatory Cytokine-Induced Nitric Oxide Production," *American Journal of Therapeutics* 19, no. 1 (2012).

Bazzano, L., et al., "Effects of Low-Carbohydrate and Low-Fat Diets: A Randomized Trial," *Annals of Internal Medicine* 161, no. 5 (2014): 309–18.

Beavers, K., et al., "Effect of Exercise Training on Chronic Inflammation," *Clinica Chimica Acta* 411, no. 11–12 (2010): 785–93.

Bennett, J., et al., "Inflammation-Nature's Way to Efficiently Respond to All Types of Challenges: Implications for Understanding and Managing 'the Epidemic' of Chronic Diseases," *Frontiers in Medicine* 5 (2018).

Bordoni, A., et al., "Dairy Products and Inflammation: A Review of the Clinical Evidence," *Critical Reviews in Food Science and Nutrition* 57, no. 12 (2017).

Changwei, C., et al., "Diet and Skin Aging—From the Perspective of Food Nutrition," *Nutrients* 12, no. 3 (2020): 870.

Charlot, A., et al., "Beneficial Effects of Early Time-Restricted Feeding on Metabolic Diseases: Importance of Aligning Food Habits with the Circadian Clock," *Nutrients* 13, no. 5 (2021): 1405.

Charoenngam, N., et al., "Immunologic Effects of Vitamin D on Human Health and Disease," *Nutrients* 12, no. 7 (2020): 1–28.

Chen, G., et al., "Sterile Inflammation: Sensing and Reacting to Damage," *Nature Reviews Immunology* 10, no. 12 (2010): 826–37.

Cline, J., "Nutritional Aspects of Detoxification in Clinical Practice," *Alternative Therapies* 21, no. 3 (2015): 54–62.

Cole, W., and E. Adamson, *The Inflammation Spectrum: Find Your Food Triggers and Reset Your System* (New York: Avery, 2019).

Cooper, S., "Promoting Physical Activity for Mental Well-Being," *ACSM's Health and Fitness Journal* 24, no. 3 (2020): 12–16.

Drake, V., "Cognitive Function In Depth," Linus Pauling Institute, Oregon State University, lpi.oregonstate.edu/mic/health-disease/cognitive-function. Accessed September 20, 2021.

Drake, V., "Immunity In Depth," Linus Pauling Institute, Oregon State University, lpi.oregonstate.edu/mic/health-disease/immunity. Accessed September 20, 2021.

Drake, V., "Inflammation," Linus Pauling Institute, Oregon State University, lpi.oregonstate.edu/mic/health-disease/inflammation. Accessed September 20, 2021.

Franceschi, C., et al., "Chronic Inflammation (Inflammaging) and Its Potential Contribution to Age-Associated Diseases," *The Journals of Gerontology. Series A, Biological Sciences and Medical Sciences* 69, no. 1 (2014): S4–9.

Franceschi, C., et al., "Inflammaging: A New Immune–Metabolic Viewpoint for Age-Related Diseases," *Nature Reviews Endocrinology* 14, no. 10 (2018): 576–90.

Fung, J., *The Obesity Code* (Vancouver: Greystone Books, 2016).

Furman, D., et al., "Chronic Inflammation in the Etiology of Disease across the Life Span," *Nature Medicine* 25, no. 12 (2019): 1822–32.

Gammoh, N., et al., "Zinc in Infection and Inflammation," *Nutrients* 9, no. 6 (2017): 624.

Glaser, R., et al., "Stress Damages Immune System and Health," *Discovery Medicine* 5, no. 26 (2009): 165–69.

Golbidi, S., et al., "Health Benefits of Fasting and Caloric Restriction," *Current Diabetes Reports* 17, no. 12 (2017).

Gómez-Pinilla, F., "Brain Foods: The Effects of Nutrients on Brain Function," *Nature Reviews Neuroscience* 9, no. 7 (2008): 568–78.

Gregor, M., et al., "Inflammatory Mechanisms in Obesity," *Annual Review of Immunology* 29 (2011): 415–45.

Greten, F., et al., "Inflammation and Cancer: Triggers, Mechanisms, and Consequences," *Immunity* 51, no. 1 (2019): 27–41.

Grivennikov, S., et al., "Immunity, Inflammation, and Cancer," *Cell* 140, no. 6 (2010): 883–99.

Grundy, S., et al., "Diagnosis and Management of the Metabolic Syndrome," *Circulation* 112, no. 17 (2005).

Gupta, R., et al., "Prevalence and Severity of Food Allergies Among US Adults," *JAMA Network Open* 2, no. 1 (2019): e185630.

Higdon, J., "Cruciferous Vegetables," Linus Pauling Institute, Oregon State University, lpi.oregonstate.edu/mic/food-beverages/cruciferous-vegetables. Accessed September 20, 2021.

Higdon, J., "Glycemic Index and Glycemic Load," Linus Pauling Institute, Oregon State University. Accessed September 20, 2021.

Higdon, J., "Magnesium," Linus Pauling Institute, Oregon State University, lpi.oregonstate.edu/mic/minerals/magnesium. Accessed September 20, 2021.

Higdon, J., "Vitamin C," Linus Pauling Institute, Oregon State University, lpi.oregonstate.edu/mic/vitamins/vitamin-C. Accessed September 20, 2021.

Higdon, J., et al., *An Evidence-Based Approach to Phytochemicals and Other Dietary Factors*, 2nd edition (New York: Theme Medical Publishers, Inc., 2013).

Hollander, J., et al., "Beyond the Looking Glass: Recent Advances in Understanding the Impact of Environmental Exposures on Neuropsychiatric Disease," *Neuropsychopharmacology* 45 (2020): 1086–96.

Huang, Q., "Linking What We Eat to Our Mood: A Review of Diet, Dietary Antioxidants, and Depression," *Antioxidants* 8, no. 9 (2019).

Hurst, R., et al., "Establishing Optimal Selenium Status: Results of a Randomized, Double-Blind, Placebo-Controlled Trial," *The American Journal of Clinical Nutrition* 91, no. 4 (2010): 923–31.

Iddir, M., "Strengthening the Immune System and Reducing Inflammation and Oxidative Stress through Diet and Nutrition: Considerations during the COVID-19 Crisis," *Nutrients* 12, no. 6 (2020): 1592.

"Dietary Reference Intakes," *Nutrition Reviews* 55, no. 9 (1997): 319–26.

Irwin, M., et al., "Sleep Disturbance, Sleep Duration, and Inflammation: A Systematic Review and Meta-Analysis of Cohort Studies and Experimental Sleep Deprivation," *Biological Psychiatry* 80, no. 1 (2016): 40–52.

Jacobson, T., et al., "National Lipid Association Recommendations for Patient-Centered Management of Dyslipidemia: Part 1 - Full Report," *Journal of Clinical Lipidology* 9, no. 2 (2015): 129–69.

Jensen, M., et al., "2013 AHA/ACC/TOS Guideline for the Management of Overweight and Obesity in Adults: A Report of the American College of Cardiology/American Heart Association Task Force on Practice Guidelines and the Obesity Society," *Circulation* 129, no. 25, suppl. 1 (2014).

Kelley, D., et al., "A Review of the Health Benefits of Cherries," *Nutrients* 10, no. 3 (2018): 368.

Kern, H., et al., "Role of Nutrients in Metabolic Syndrome: A 2017 Update," *Nutrition and Dietary Supplements* 10 (2018): 13–26.

Korn, L., *Nutrition Essentials for Mental Health: A Complete Guide to the Food-Mood Connection* (New York: W. W. Norton & Company, 2016).

Kumar, M., et al., "Environmental Endocrine-Disrupting Chemical Exposure: Role in Non-Communicable Diseases," *Frontiers in Public Health* (2020).

Jonasson, L., et al., "Advice to Follow a Low-Carbohydrate Diet Has a Favourable Impact on Low-Grade Inflammation in Type 2 Diabetes Compared with Advice to Follow a Low-Fat Diet," *Annals of Medicine* 46, no. 3 (2014): 182–87.

Merrill, M., et al., "Consensus on the Key Characteristics of Endocrine-Disrupting Chemicals as a Basis for Hazard Identification," *Nature Reviews Endocrinology* 16, no. 1 (2020): 45–57.

Litao, M., et al., "Erythrocyte Sedimentation Rate and C-Reactive Protein: How Best to Use Them in Clinical Practice," *Pediatric Annals* 43, no. 10 (2014): 417–20.

Liu, Y-Z., et al., "Inflammation: The Common Pathway of Stress-Related Diseases," *Frontiers in Human Neuroscience* 11 (2017): 316.

Lomer, M. C. E., "Review Article: The Aetiology, Diagnosis, Mechanisms and Clinical Evidence for Food Intolerance," *Alimentary Pharmacology and Therapeutics* 41, no. 3 (2015): 262–75.

Margină, D., et al., "Chronic Inflammation in the Context of Everyday Life: Dietary Changes as Mitigating Factors," *International Journal of Environmental Research and Public Health* 17, no. 11 (2020): 4135.

McEwen, B. S., "Neurobiological and Systemic Effects of Chronic Stress," *Chronic Stress* (2017).

Medzhitov, R., "Origin and Physiological Roles of Inflammation," *Nature* 454 (2008): 428–35.

Miller, A. H., et al., "Therapeutic Implications of Brain-Immune Interactions: Treatment in Translation," *Neuropsychopharmacology* 42, no. 1 (2017): 334–59.

Minihane, A. M., et al., "Low-Grade Inflammation, Diet Composition and Health: Current Research Evidence and Its Translation," *British Journal of Nutrition* 114, no. 7 (2015): 999–1012.

Morey, J. N., et al., "Current Directions in Stress and Human Immune Function," *Current Opinion in Psychology* 5 (2015): 13–17.

Morris, M. C., et al., "Nutrients and Bioactives in Green Leafy Vegetables and Cognitive Decline: Prospective Study," *Neurology* 90, no. 3 (2018): E214–22.

Neto, H., et al., "Effects of Food Additives on Immune Cells As Contributors to Body Weight Gain and Immune-Mediated Metabolic Dysregulation," *Frontiers in Immunology* 8 (2017): 1478.

Nile, S. H., et al., "Edible Berries: Bioactive Components and Their Effect on Human Health," *Nutrition* 30, no. 2 (2014): 134–44.

Olden, K., et al., "Discovering How Environmental Exposures Alter Genes and Could Lead to New Treatments for Chronic Illnesses," *Health Aff (Millwood)* 30, no. 5 (2011).

Pae, M., et al., "The Role of Nutrition in Enhancing Immunity in Aging," *Aging and Disease* 3, no. 1 (2012): 91–129.

Pahwa, R. et al., "Chronic Inflammation," *Pathobiology of Human Disease: A Dynamic Encyclopedia of Disease Mechanisms* (2021): 300–14.

Paul, E., et al., "Loneliness and Risk for Cardiovascular Disease: Mechanisms and Future Directions," *Current Cardiology Reports 2021* 23, no. 6 (2021): 1–7.

Portier, C., et al., "A Human Health Perspective on Climate Change: A Report Outlining Research Needs on the Human Health Effects of Climate Change," *Environmental Health Perspectives* (2010).

Rakel, D., *Integrative Medicine*, 4th edition (Philadelphia: Elsevier, 2018).

Rathnavelu, V., et al., "Potential Role of Bromelain in Clinical and Therapeutic Applications," *Biomedical Reports* 5, no. 3 (2016): 283.

Rennard, B. O., et al., "Chicken Soup Inhibits Neutrophil Chemotaxis In Vitro," *Chest* 118, no. 4 (2000): 1150–57.

Rosenblum, M. D., et al., "Mechanisms of Human Autoimmunity," *Journal of Clinical Investigation* 125, no. 6 (2015): 2228–33.

Scrambler, T., "Autoinflammation," British Society for Immunology, immunology.org/public-information/bite-sized-immunology/immune-dysfunction/autoinflammation. Accessed September 19, 2021.

Seiler, A., et al., "The Impact of Everyday Stressors on the Immune System and Health," *Stress Challenges and Immunity in Space: From Mechanisms to Monitoring and Preventive Strategies* (2020): 71–92.

Sharma, D. K., "Physiology of Stress and Its Management," *Journal of Medicine: Study & Research* 1, no. 1 (2018): 1–5.

Slavich, G. M., "Understanding Inflammation, Its Regulation, and Relevance for Health: A Top Scientific and Public Priority," *Brain, Behavior, and Immunity* 45 (2015): 13.

Stevens, J. F., et al., "Acrolein: Sources, Metabolism, and Biomolecular Interactions Relevant to Human Health and Disease," *Molecular Nutrition & Food Research* 52, no. 1 (2008): 7.

Straub, R. H., "The Complex Role of Estrogens in Inflammation," *Endocrine Reviews* 28, no. 5 (2007): 521–74.

Strowig, T., et al., "Inflammasomes in Health and Disease," *Nature* 481 (2012): 278–86.

Thieme-Burdette, M., "7 Risk Factors for Autoimmune Disease," Global Autoimmune Institute, last modified June 10, 2019, autoimmuneinstitute.org/articles/7-risk-factors-for-autoimmune-disease.

Todoric, J., et al., "Targeting Inflammation in Cancer Prevention and Therapy," *Cancer Prevention Research* (2016).

Trasande, L., et al., "Food Additives and Child Health," *Pediatrics* 142, no. 2 (2018).

Trepanowski, J. F., et al., "Effect of Alternate-Day Fasting on Weight Loss, Weight Maintenance, and Cardioprotection Among Metabolically Healthy Obese Adults: A Randomized Clinical Trial," *JAMA Internal Medicine* 177, no. 7 (2017): 930–38.

Vojdani, A., "A Potential Link between Environmental Triggers and Autoimmunity," *Autoimmune Diseases* (Hindawi Publishing Corporation, 2014).

Wastyk, H. C., et al., "Gut-Microbiota-Targeted Diets Modulate Human Immune Status," *Cell* 184, no. 16 (2021): 4137–53.

Watson, J., et al., "Raised Inflammatory Markers," *BMJ* 344 (2012): 7843.

Weil, A., "Anti-Inflammatory Diet & Pyramid," WEIL, Andrew Weil, M.D., drweil.com/diet-nutrition/anti-inflammatory-diet-pyramid. Accessed September 20, 2021.

Wysoczański, T., et al., "Omega-3 Fatty Acids and Their Role in Central Nervous System—A Review," *Current Medicinal Chemistry* 23, no. 8 (2016): 816–31.

Yin, K., et al., "Vitamin D and Inflammatory Diseases," *Journal of Inflammation Research* (Dove Medical Press Ltd., 2014).

Yu, Z., et al., "Associations between Nut Consumption and Inflammatory Biomarkers," *The American Journal of Clinical Nutrition* 104, no. 3 (2016): 722.

Zeisel, S. H., et al., "Choline: An Essential Nutrient for Public Health," *Nutrition Reviews* 67, no. 11 (2009): 615.

Zheng, G., et al., "Effect of Aerobic Exercise on Inflammatory Markers in Healthy Middle-Aged and Older Adults: A Systematic Review and Meta-Analysis of Randomized Controlled Trials," *Frontiers in Aging Neuroscience* (2019): 98.

Zhuang, Y., et al., "Inflammaging in Skin and Other Tissues—the Roles of Complement System and Macrophage," *Inflammation & Allergy Drug Targets* 13, no. 3 (2014): 153–61.

"10 Chemicals of Public Health Concern," World Health Organization, last modified June 1, 2020, who.int/news-room/photo-story/photo-story-detail/10-chemicals-of-public-health-concern.

"About Genomics," National Human Genome Research Institute, genome.gov/about-genomics. Accessed June 20, 2021.

"Anti-Inflammatory Lifestyle, The," University of Wisconsin Integrative Health, https://www.fammed.wisc.edu/files/webfm-uploads/documents/outreach/im/handout_ai_diet_patient.pdf. Accessed September 20, 2021.

Autoimmune Association, aarda.org. Accessed September 19, 2021.

"Autoimmune Disease List," Global Autoimmune Institute, autoimmuneinstitute.org/resources/autoimmune-disease-list. Accessed June 8, 2021.

"Autoimmune Diseases: Clarity & Facts for Patients," Johns Hopkins Medicine, Department of Pathology, pathology.jhu.edu/autoimmune. Accessed June 8, 2021.

"Autoimmune Disease List," Global Autoimmune Institute, autoimmuneinstitute.org/resources/autoimmune-disease-list. Accessed June 8, 2021.

"Cancer: Carcinogenicity of the Consumption of Red Meat and Processed Meat," World Health Organization, last modified October 26, 2015, who.int/news-room/q-a-detail/cancer-carcinogenicity-of-the-consumption-of-red-meat-and-processed-meat.

"Cancer Causes and Prevention," National Cancer Institute, National Institutes of Health, cancer.gov/about-cancer/causes-prevention. Accessed June 8, 2021.

"Celiac Disease Foundation," celiac.org. Accessed May 1, 2021.

"Cooking with Fats and Oils: Can They Withstand the Heat?," Colorado State University, Kendall Reagan Nutrition Center, www.chhs.colostate.edu/krnc/monthly-blog/cooking-with-fats-and-oils. Accessed September 19, 2021.

"Dietary Supplement Fact Sheets," National Institutes of Health, Office of Dietary Supplements, ods.od.nih.gov/factsheets/list-all. Accessed September 20, 2021.

"Dietary Supplement Guides," University of Wisconsin Integrative Health, fammed.wisc.edu/integrative/resources/supplement-samplers. Accessed September 20, 2021.

"Elimination Diet, The," University of Wisconsin Integrative Health, fammed.wisc.edu/files/webfm-uploads/documents/outreach/im/handout_elimination_diet_patient.pdf.

"Endocrine Disrupters and Child Health: Possible Developmental Early Effects of Endocrine Disrupters on Child Health," World Health Organization, 2012.

"Endocrine Disruptors," National Institute of Environmental Health Sciences, last modified July 12, 2021, niehs.nih.gov/health/topics/agents/endocrine/index.cfm.

"EWG's 2021 Shopper's Guide to Pesticides in Produce," Environmental Working Group, ewg.org/foodnews/full-list.php. Accessed July 21, 2021.

"Glycemic Index," Glycemic Index Research and GI News, University of Sydney, glycemicindex.com. Accessed May 25, 2021.

"How Much Arsenic Is in Your Rice?," Consumer Reports, last modified November 2014, consumerreports.org/cro/magazine/2015/01/how-much-arsenic-is-in-your-rice/index.htm.

"Immune System Research," National Institute of Allergy and Infectious Diseases, last modified July 11, 2016, niaid.nih.gov/research/immune-system-research.

"Managing Dietary Carbohydrates for Better Health," University of Wisconsin Integrative Health, fammed.wisc.edu/files/webfm-uploads/documents/outreach/im/handout_glycemic_index_patient.pdf. Accessed September 20, 2021.

"Office on Women's Health," U.S. Department of Health & Human Services, womenshealth.gov. Accessed September 20, 2021.

"Omega-3 Fatty Acids," National Institutes of Health, Office of Dietary Supplements, last modified August 4, 2021, ods.od.nih.gov/factsheets/Omega3FattyAcids-HealthProfessional.

"Pediatric Environmental Health Toolkit," University of California San Francisco, peht.ucsf.edu/index.php. Accessed June 20, 2021.

"Persistent Organic Pollutants: A Global Issue, A Global Response," United States Environmental Protection Agency, epa.gov/international-cooperation/persistent-organic-pollutants-global-issue-global-response. Accessed July 19, 2021.

"POPs, The," UN Environment Programme, Stockholm Convention, chm.pops.int/theconvention/thepops/tabid/673/default.aspx. Accessed July 19, 2021.

"Test Catalog," Mayo Clinic Laboratories, mayocliniclabs.com/test-catalog/index.html. Accessed September 20, 2021.

"Your Genome: Discover More about DNA, Genes and Genomes, and the Implications for Our Health and Society," yourgenome.org. Accessed September 20, 2021.

acknowledgments

This book would not be possible without both my personal and professional support team and cheerleaders.

First and foremost, I want to thank my children, Madeline and Griffin, for their support and patience last year while I immersed myself in recipe testing, research, and editing, as well as enduring "the most boring summer ever." Your willingness to continuously taste new dishes has not gone unnoticed, and your feedback and opinions are reflected throughout.

To my parents, thank you for always listening, believing in my work, and enabling me to follow this serendipitous path that continues to unfold. Thank you also for being my sounding board for work and life; it's what enables me to keep going, follow my heart, and be brave enough to trust my gut.

Thank you to my colleague, dear friend, and podcast partner, Brierley Horton, MS, RD. I am beyond grateful for your friendship over the past two years, as we've navigated the ups and downs in both podcasting and life. And, of course, thank you for introducing me to our amazing Happy Eating producer, Les Nuby. Our weekly recording/therapy sessions are the highlight of my week!

Thank you to my amazing assistant and recipe tester, Jordan Mitchell, MS, RD. I could not have produced this book without your help in brainstorming, testing, and retesting recipes. Having Alex as a taste tester was a bonus!

To my agent, Eryn Kalavsky, thank you for believing in my work and helping me bring this book to fruition. This book wouldn't have happened without your support and willingness to hop on the phone. Thank you also to my attorney, Jesseca Salky, for your expertise and always being available to have my back.

Thank you to the entire team at The Experiment for your hard work and support, especially my editor Olivia Peluso who believed in this project and enabled me to bring it to life. Your insight throughout the process was invaluable, pushed me to go further, and challenged me to look at things differently. Your passion and love for this book is as strong as mine, and that means the world to me!

Last, but not least, thank you to all of my amazing friends and followers. A special shout-out goes to Chaney (the best next-door neighbor a girl could ever have) and our supper club: Jen, Wes, Chase, and Jon. Thank you for your ongoing support for my work . . . and life in general!

index

Page numbers in *italics* refer to photos.

chickpeas (*continued*)

    Skillet Shakshuka, *190*, 191

    Tomato, Cucumber, and
        Chickpea Salad, *224*, 225

Chile-Garlic Pork Chops and
    Broccoli, 160, *161*

Chile-Lime Crab Cakes, *180*, 181

chiles

    Chile Verde with Shredded Pork,
        128–29, *129*

    Chipotle-Lime Lentil Chili, *118*,
        119

    Creamy Southwestern Beef
        Soup, 130, *131*

    Southwestern Caesar Salad, *96*,
        97

chili-garlic sauce

    Chile-Garlic Pork Chops and
        Broccoli, 160, *161*

    Chile-Lime Crab Cakes, *180*, 181

chipotles

    Chipotle-Lime Lentil Chili, *118*,
        119

    Southwestern Caesar Salad, *96*,
        97

chocolate

    Chocolate Chip Almond Butter
        Cookies, 262, *263*

    Dairy-Free Fudgesicles, 272, *273*

    Dark Chocolate Peanut Butter
        Cups, 266, *267*

    Flourless Monster Cookies,
        264–65, 265

    health benefits, 267

    Pumpkin Chocolate Chip Mini-
        Muffins, 258, *259*

chronic ("bad") inflammation, 7–11

cocoa powder, 272, *273*

coconut milk, *138*, 139

coconut oil, 57

coffee, 256, *257*

cognitive/psychological stressors, 35

Cold Brew Breakfast Smoothie, 256,
    257

complex carbs, 52–55, 80, 81

cookies

    Chocolate Chip Almond Butter
        Cookies, 262, *263*

    Flourless Monster Cookies,
        264–65, 265

    Lemony Ginger Cookies, *260*, 261

    See also snacks and treats

corn

    Seared Scallops over Summer
        Corn Salad, 172, *173*

    Skillet Mexican Rice Casserole,
        204, 205

    Southwestern Caesar Salad, *96*,
        97

    Southwestern Flank Steak Salad,
        150, *151*

    Street Corn Salad, 226, *227*

    Tex-Mex Tuna Salad, *100*, 101

crab, *180*, 181

Creamy Buffalo Chicken Soup,
    122–23, *123*

Creamy Southwestern Beef Soup,
    130, *131*

Creamy Spinach-Artichoke Chicken,
    140, 141

Creamy Wild Rice and Chicken
    Soup, *126*, 127

Crispy Ranch Chickpeas, 250, *250–51*

cruciferous vegetables, 15, 44, 45–46

cucumbers

    Marinated Feta-Veggie Skewers,
        252, *253*

    Mediterranean Quinoa Salad,
        94, *95*

    Quick Poke Bowls, 182, *183*

    Thai-Inspired Beef Salad, 110,
        110–11

    Tomato, Cucumber, and
        Chickpea Salad, *224*, 225

    Tzatziki "Rice" Bowls with Gyro
        Meatballs, 154, *155*

Curried Butternut Soup with
    Spinach, 116, *117*

cytokines, 5, 6

D

Dairy-Free Fudgesicles, 272, *273*

dairy products, 60

Dark Chocolate Peanut Butter Cups,
    266, *267*

dietary inflamers

    food allergies and food
        reactions, 20–23

    toxins, chemicals, and
        compounds, 24–25

    universal, 18–20

Dijon mustard, *168*, 169

drinks

    Elderflower Margarita, 275, *275*

    Greyhound Spritzer, 276, *277*

    Pomegranate-Lime Mocktail,
        274, *274*

    See also smoothies

E

Easy Greek Frittata with Balsamic
    Tomatoes, 102, *102–3*

edamame

    about, 167

    Hoisin Salmon with Warm
        Broccoli-Edmame Slaw, 166,
        167

    Tuna, Edamame, and Rice Bowl,
        106, *106–7*

eggs

    about, 103

    Easy Greek Frittata with
        Balsamic Tomatoes, 102,
        102–3

    Roasted Vegetable Frittata, 188,
        189

    Skillet Shakshuka, *190*, 191

Elderflower Margarita, 275, *275*

elimination diet, 22–23

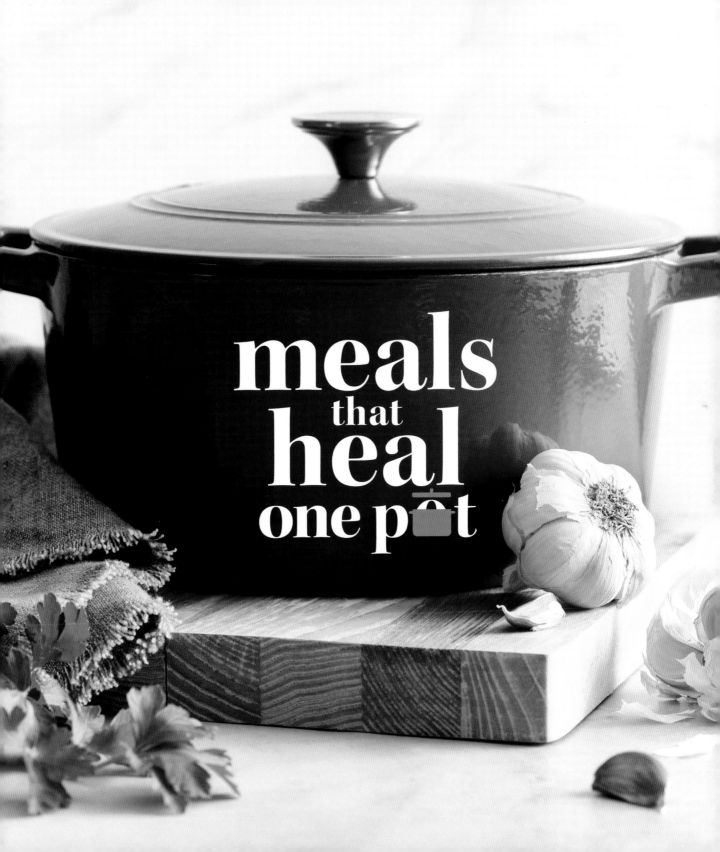

meals
that
heal
one p🍲t

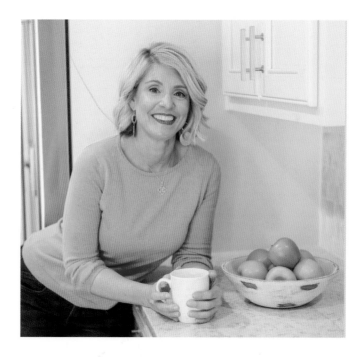

about the author

CAROLYN WILLIAMS, PhD, RD, is a leading culinary nutrition expert who creates quick, healthy recipes that you can't wait to eat. She is a 2017 James Beard Award winner with a knack for breaking down complex science. She serves as a contributing editor for *CookingLight* and *EatingWell* and writes for a variety of media outlets and lifestyle brands on nutrition topics ranging from inflammation to fasting to mental health. In 2021, Carolyn launched the *Happy Eating* podcast alongside her cohost and cocreator, Brierley Horton, MS, RD. The podcast explores the impact that diet and lifestyle have on brain health and mental wellness through interviews and candid but light-hearted conversations.

Carolyn's realistic approach to anti-inflammatory cooking, eating, and living helped make her first anti-inflammatory cookbook, *Meals That Heal: 100+ Everyday Anti-Inflammatory Recipes in 30 Minutes or Less* (Tiller Press, 2019), an instant hit! The cookbook's success also helped cement Carolyn's position as a leading expert on anti-inflammatory eating and managing chronic inflammation through lifestyle, and she regularly speaks at conferences and events.

Carolyn resides in Alabama with her two children, Madeline (15 years) and Griffin (12 years), and is a tenured college professor at a local community college teaching culinary arts and nutrition courses.

carolynwilliamsrd.com | ⧉ realfoodreallife_rd